THE ULTIMATE WOMEN'S GUIDE TO BEATING DISEASE

...and living a happy, active life

2020

FROM THE EDITORS OF BOTTOM LINE HEALTH

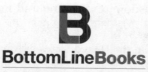

BottomLineBooks

BottomLineInc.com

CONTENTS

Contents

Contents

Contents

PREFACE

We are proud to bring to you *The Ultimate Women's Guide to Beating Disease and Living a Happy, Active Life 2020*. This essential volume features trustworthy and actionable life-saving information from the best health experts in the world—information that will help women beat the conditions that are most deadly to them.* In the following chapters, you'll find the latest discoveries, best treatments and scientifically proven remedies to keep you living a long, happy and active life.

Whether it's heart care, the latest on stroke, breast cancer prevention and treatment, breakthrough treatments for hot flashes or cutting-edge nutritional advice, the editors of *Bottom Line Health* talk to the experts—from top women's health doctors to research scientists to leading alternative care practitioners—who are creating the true innovations in health care.

Over the past four decades, we have built a network of literally thousands of leading physicians in both alternative and conventional medicine. They are affiliated with the premier medical and research institutions throughout the world. We read the important medical journals and follow the latest research that is reported at medical conferences. And we regularly talk to our advisors in major teaching hospitals, private practices and government health agencies for their insider perspective.

*"Leading Causes of Death in Females," Centers for Disease Control and Prevention (*http://www.cdc.gov/women/lcod/2014/index.htm*).

In this 2020 edition, we've gone beyond diseases and have included several chapters of life-enhancing health information on pregnancy, pain, depression, fitness, diet, quality medical care, sexuality and aging…all of which are essential to living a happy, active life. And it's all backed by breaking studies and top health experts. Also note that respiratory diseases, according to the Centers for Disease Control and Prevention, are now considered one of the top three causes of death in women of all ages (same percentage as stroke).

The Ultimate Women's Guide to Beating Disease and Living a Happy, Active Life 2020 is a result of our ongoing research and connection with these experts, and is a distillation of their latest findings and advice. We trust that you will glean new, helpful and affordable information about the health topics that concern you most…and find vital topics of interest to family and friends as well.

As a reader of a Bottom Line book, be assured that you are receiving well-researched information from a trusted source. But, please use prudence in health matters. Always speak to your physician before taking vitamins, supplements or over-the-counter medication…stopping a medication…changing your diet…or beginning an exercise program. If you experience side effects from any regimen, contact your doctor immediately.

Be well,
The Editors, *Bottom Line Health*
Stamford, Connecticut

Chapter 1

AGING GRACEFULLY

The Secret Anti-Aging Agent You Should Be Eating

Move over, vitamin C. Step aside, collagen. There's a new micronutrient stealing center stage. It's the flavonoid fisetin, and it's starting to get its share of attention as a promising way to slow down aging.

Yes, that's what we said. Previously, lab studies on animals and on human cells had found that fisetin can reduce diabetes complications, protect against stroke and enhance memory. Fisetin also has been shown to relieve allergic reactions by inhibiting cytokine production.

But now we can add one more benefit: Slowing down the aging process and increasing the prime-of-life years. When researchers from University of Minnesota and Mayo Clinic gave fisetin to older mice, the animals experienced a rejuvenation and longer-than-average span of time during which they were healthy (before any chronic diseases set in)—what researchers call their healthspan. The study looked at 10 flavonoids in all, each with the potential to stop the aging process,

but it was fisetin that stood out as the most potent.

Fisetin: Fighting Cell Damage

In our bodies, cells go through an aging process known as cellular senescence, in which the cell stops dividing. These types of cells have been linked to many age-related diseases. Certain flavonoids have been shown to help the body remove these cells, with fisetin being the most effective.

So where can you get it and how much do you need? Clinical trials are under way to help find the best human dosages for fisetin's different benefits—it's likely that a higher amount is needed for antiaging than for enhancing memory, for instance. It's found naturally in (in order of richness) strawberries, apples, persimmons, lotus root, onions, grapes, kiwis, peaches and cucumbers, but current thinking is that it will take more food than you can comfortably eat every day to get enough fisetin to fully reap its antiaging benefits. You can already buy concentrated fisetin supplements, generally in 100 mg tablets,

Paul Robbins, PhD, associate director of the Institute on the Biology of Aging and Metabolism at University of Minnesota, Minneapolis, and co-senior author of "Fisetin Is a Senotherapeutic That Extends Health and Lifespan," published in *EBioMedicine*.

but there are no guidelines stating whether that's the ideal amount. To give an idea of what that amount translates to in food, you'd need to eat a pound of strawberries to get 100 mg of fisetin—but at just 150 calories, that could be a wise choice.

In fact, despite the open questions on dosing, there's no reason not to choose fisetin-rich foods to get your recommended five to seven servings of fruits and vegetables each day…you'll also get the benefits of the many other nutrients in these foods.

How to Feel Younger Than Your Age

Study titled, "Feeling Young and in Control: Daily Control Beliefs Are Associated with Younger Subjective Ages," by researchers at North Carolina State University in Raleigh and Friedrich Schiller University in Jena, Germany, published in *The Journals of Gerontology: Series B*, reported by Bob Barnett, former editor, *Bottom Line Personal*.

Feel younger, live longer. It's a simple prescription for longevity, and one that is backed up by research. For older people, feeling younger than your chronological age is strongly linked with better memory, better health and improved longevity, studies show.

But what is the secret to feeling younger?

After all, there are many reasons why people feel older than their actual age—including health issues. But now new research has found a powerful factor in how young we feel—and it's one you can do something about. For older adults, the study finds, how young you feel has a lot to do with your sense of control.

How Old Do You Feel Day to Day?

Previous research has found that how old we feel (our subjective age), as well as how in control, both fluctuate from day to day as events and encounters with others influence our perceptions and mood. This new study was designed to investigate how those fluctuations might be linked in both older and younger adults.

Researchers at at North Carolina State University in Raleigh and at Friedrich Schiller University in Jena, Germany, recruited 116 men and women ages 60 to 90 and another 106 men and women ages 18 to 36. In the older group, 55% were still working and 45% were retired.

In daily surveys over nine days, participants were asked eight questions that tapped into their sense of control—to what extent they felt they could influence the events in their lives—and were also asked how old they felt that day. In addition, both groups submitted information about daily stressors they encountered such as disagreements or potential disagreements as well as stressful events at work, home or among friends. They also logged daily physical symptoms they experienced from a checklist of 28 (such as allergies, fatigue, joint pain, cough).

What Matters Over Age 60

For both the younger and older groups, subjective age varied day to day. But among the older participants, these variations were keenly tied to their sense of control.

Key finding: On the days when they felt more in control, they tended to feel younger. (For the younger participants, the number of stressors and physical symptoms made a difference, but their sense of control didn't.)

Given the challenges of growing older, it's easy to feel out of control some days. But the more you feel in control on a daily basis, the less likely you are to overreact to stress. In addition to physical health benefits of reduced stress, your cognitive abilities—how well your brain performs—benefit, too.

The findings have implications for elderly caregiving, the researchers note. In nursing homes, for example, letting residents have more choices in their daily lives—choices as simple as how the furniture is arranged, how they spend time with friends, even who takes care of the houseplants—have been shown to improve well-being.

For the rest of us who are in our 50s, 60s and older, there's no one-size-fits-all solution to feeling more in control. Setting priorities, finding time to disconnect from devices and spending time with friends are common advice. But one activity may be particularly effective—exercise.

Everyone knows that exercise is key to lifelong health. But one of the ways that it benefits us is by giving us a sense that we have a little more control over how the day goes. A regular exercise habit—something as simple as a daily walk—has been shown to improve mood, reduce anxiety, boost self-esteem…and increase a sense of control. In a separate pilot study from the group at the University of North Carolina, previously sedentary men and women aged 35 to 69 who started exercising regularly reported that they felt—you guessed it—younger.

Look Younger in Under an Hour for Less Than $100...Top 12 Ways

Adriane Berg, Esq., is the founder of Adriane Berg & Associates, a firm that helps companies market to the boomer and mature generations. Ms. Berg is the host of *Generation Bold: The Fountain of Truth*, syndicated on BIZTALK Radio. She is a well-known advocate for successful aging with multiple appearances on the *Oprah Winfrey Show, Good Morning America* and other national shows. She is author of 14 books including *How Not to Go Broke at 102: Finding Everlasting Wealth* and *The Totally Awesome Money Book for Kids*. She is also an attorney and helped found the National Academy of Elder Law Attorneys.

I brand myself as the pro-aging advocate, ready to stamp out ageism as a destructive force. So it might seem hypocritical for me to focus on helping readers look younger. Here is my reasoning.

In the battle against ageism, we are searching for new and exciting images of aging.

We want others to see the vitality, adventure, charm and surprise we experience as we grow older. Of course, there is a definite connection between how we feel and how we look, including whether we have a youthful view of life or a view that has dimmed with age. Vibrant older people need to be more visible and relevant if we hope to change the cultural image of aging.

Similarly, we need a vocabulary for external beauty that goes beyond, "You look young for your age."

But for now, this is what we have—by looking younger, you get seen for the dynamo you are…you contribute to the revolution.

So, what can you do to preserve your youthful appearance? *Here are my top 12…*

#1. Sugar. It's the enemy to good skin when ingested, but it makes a great scrub, as does salt. Mix it with facial oils, especially rose oil. It exfoliates the top layer of skin (epidermis) to allow for regeneration. I've been exfoliating with sugar every month for many years. It makes my skin feel smoother and look brighter.

#2. Posture. Your overall posture is what people see first. Sit and stand up straight. Do what the news anchors do. Before you sit down, grab the bottom of your jacket, shirt, sweater or blouse and pull it down with both hands. Sit down still holding the garment. Remove your hands and the tightened material will cause you to sit up straight.

Alternatively, if your shirt doesn't reach, watch where you gaze. Joel Harper, personal trainer to the stars, offered a great posture tip in his book *Mind Your Body*. Simply look straight ahead. In our heads-down world, we tend to cast our eyes downward, pulling our head and shoulders down. By simply keeping your gaze up, your seated posture straightens. Voilà!

If you spend a lot of time sitting, consider buying a balance ball chair that will get your core stronger and your back aligned. I bought the Gaiam Classic for my daughter, $69.99.

#3. Gait. Walk tall and balanced. Stride out PROUD. Even folks who use walkers can do this—the new ones are now higher, so there's no more "walker slouch." Try balance, yoga and Tai Chi exercises for gentle ways to improve your posture and gait.

#4. Dress with flair. As Albie, the protagonist in the film *The Birdcage*, said so pointedly, "One wants a bit of color." If you're in a fashion rut, check out the website, Advanced Style (Advanced.Style), which features stylish seniors. Or choose your favorite store, whether Chanel or H&M, Men's Wearhouse or John Varvatos. Look at their windows and mannequins. Copy what you see…it's all in your closet already.

#5. Remove your hair. No, I don't mean on your head. I mean on your chin! Nothing signals that you gave up on your looks more than inappropriate facial hair—women's top lip and cheeks…men's eyebrows, ears and nose hairs.

#6. Condition your hair. Follicles get ultra-dry as you age. Good news, white and grey are "in" for hair color. Even young fashionistas are stripping their hair to make it look white—but you still need luxurious strands.

#7. Grey hair is in…grey teeth are out. Try nonperoxide whitening toothpaste and/or whitening strips, or get professional whitening from your dentist. I tried Zoom, Supersmile and whitening mouth wash. They all help, but I can't get my teeth Chicklet white. My default? Bright red lipstick. Take care of your gums. Do you remember what Julia Roberts got caught doing in *Pretty Woman*? She was flossing. Good job!

#8. Wear glasses, contacts and hearing aids if you need them. They don't make you seem as old as you do when you can't see or hear.

#9. Lift away flabby upper arms. They are caused by sarcopenia, loss of fat and elasticity. Before you put on that sleeveless blouse or tee shirt, do 25 or more upright rows and triceps curls. No weights? Use soup cans. Or do push-ups. You can do them on your knees if the full push-up is painful.

#10. Don't sag. Here's where the plastic surgery and filler industry racks up trillions. I have no objection to any of these, though as many celebrities have learned, there are good and bad plastic surgeons. For an immediate fix under $20, try a Frownie. These are sticky patches invented in 1889 that pull back the skin. So help me, they work. If you don't have the patience to use them each day, just wear a headband, like the girls in Grease. It will pull back the facial skin and bring back memories.

#11. Wear a hat. The screen stars of the 1940s understood the importance of being seen in the right light. Since you can't travel with a lighting director…women, wear a broad-brimmed hat, and men, a fedora for just the right amount of light and shadow. Wow. You look marvelous.

#12. Cream yourself and use sunscreen. Skin gets dry, itchy, acidic and inflamed, starting around age 50…not attractive. My mother, who had great skin into her 90s, gave me sage advice—"Moisturize." She sought eternal beauty…so she used Revlon's Eterna 27.

But there may be more to moistening the skin than just good looks. A pilot study published in *Journal of the European Academy of Dermatology and Venereology* showed that skin inflammation lets cytokine molecules loose in the bloodstream. Cytokines make us more prone to heart disease, cancer and Alzheimer's. Subjects between the ages of 58 and 95 creamed their body twice a day for 30 days with a cream containing lipids, like cholesterol, free fatty acids and ceramides. The result was the reduction of three cytokines—interleukin-1 beta, interleukin-6 and tumor necrosis factor (TNF) alpha—to the levels of people in their 30s.

Full disclosure: The research for this study was supported by the National Institute on Aging, the National Institute of Arthritis and Musculoskeletal and Skin Diseases, the National Natural Science Foundation of China and NeoPharm, the company that makes the over-the-counter cream.

This study reinforces the importance of my mother's sage advice—use sun protection and moisturize.

Bottom Line: glow from the inside and you will look better on the outside. Good nutrition, exercise and joyful living all contribute to good looks.

---

7 Mindless Ways We Undermine Our Skin Health

Ginger Hodulik Downey, CNS, co-owner and vice president of R&D for DermaMed Solutions. In addition to her work at DermaMed, Ginger devotes time to working with patients in private clinical practice. As a contributor, Ginger hopes to continue to share her passion for holistic health and wellness. She writes the blog "Beyond Beauty" at BottomLineInc.com/blogs.

O ne of the questions I hear often is, What am I doing wrong? I'm using my high-quality skincare products every day, but my skin still does not have the healthy glow I'm looking for.

While quality "product" is an important part of good skincare, there are lots of ways people undermine their skin without even realizing it. *Here are seven big skincare mistakes that might be keeping you from looking your best, and how to do better…*

• **Not nourishing from the inside out.** Our skin is a reflection of our internal health, and the food and nutrients we put into our bodies are reflected in our skin. Good food in means good skin on the outside. Collagen is the material that gives our skin structure. In order to make collagen, we need to eat foods rich in vitamins A, C and E, trace minerals like iron, zinc and copper and, of course, plenty of protein from clean sources. You can reach this goal very easily by eating five to seven servings of colorful plant food every day along with a handful of nuts and seeds. Great protein sources include eggs, chicken and fish.

• **Skipping the bedtime routine.** We collect all sorts of dirt, germs and pollutants on our skin throughout the day, in addition to the makeup and skincare products we put on ourselves. Cleansing the skin before bed is critical! It's also a great time to use a vitamin A-containing serum to encourage healthy skin cell turnover, followed by a moisturizer to retain precious water that would be lost during sleep. This can all be done in under 2 minutes and will make a tremendous difference in the quality of your skin.

• **Ignoring daily sun protection.** UVA and UVB radiation from the sun is the number-one cause of premature wrinkling, sagging skin and age spots. Not only must you apply sunscreen to your face every day—rain or shine, winter and summer—but you must reapply it if you will be outdoors for extended periods of time. Always choose a mineral sunscreen with at least SPF 30. I also suggest you skip the chemical sunscreens, which have been shown to inflame the skin.

• **Stripping away the good stuff.** It is very important to cleanse the skin daily, and I'm an advocate of using some alpha hydroxy acids (like glycolic) to refresh and renew the skin. But be careful not to overcleanse or strip the skin. When you take too much oil from the skin it reacts by producing more. There is a fine line to walk here, and each person needs to take care to observe the best balance for her skin. I suggest using a gentle cleanser in the morning and at night…a weekly exfoliating scrub or enzyme mask…and to limit use of professional acid peels to once per quarter. Oily or aging skin types may tolerate a daily glycolic lotion as well but, again, it's very personal. We want the skin to look refreshed and clean, not stripped and feeling tight and dry. I also recommend using a product with probiotics to replace the protective bacteria stripped away by the acids to restore immune function and the natural barrier.

• **Thinking you don't need to moisturize.** Our skin loses water every single day, which can leave it looking dry and flaccid. The amount of moisture loss varies based on the weather, our personal hydration status and environmental inputs like airplane travel. Even oily, acneic skin needs to be moisturized! The key is to use the right product for the current conditions surrounding the skin. For oily skin, perhaps all that is needed is a water-based product containing some aloe vera, sodium hyaluronate and honey. Mature or dry skin calls for more emollient ingredients like shea butter, allantoin and jojoba. Find the right product for your skin and re-evaluate your choice as your skin changes throughout the year, but do not skip the moisturizer!

• **Following your teenage regimen.** The way we treat our skin during our teen years is very different from the way we should treat our skin at age 50. There are a few common themes—sun and anti-oxidant protection, good cleansing habits and daily moisturizer—but as we age our skin needs change. In general, the skin gets thinner and drier as we age. Skin cell regeneration slows, and we need to encourage the process by daily use of vitamin A—an interesting skincare ingredient. Our skin gets used to the type and strength of the vitamin A (sometimes called retinol) we use, and we typically need to use stronger products to get the desired benefits after a period of time. We may also find that we need to exfoliate two times per week instead of one time to keep the skin glowing, and that a heavier nighttime face cream is needed. Work with your professional aesthetician to develop a skincare regimen that is appropriate for you and your time of life. I highly recommend a quarterly facial. Taking care of your skin should be viewed as a priority, not a luxury.

• **Skimping on your beauty rest.** Cell turnover and regeneration—including for the cells that support our skin—occur during sleep. When we skimp on sleep we do not allow for our skin to be renewed and refreshed, leading to dull, damaged skin cells (and maybe a short fuse and grumpy disposition too). In addition, when we do not get enough sleep, our cortisol production increases. Cortisol is a hormone released in response to stress. We need cortisol to deal with the ups and downs of daily living—it gives us the energy we need to react to stressors. However, when we overproduce cortisol, collagen is depleted, leading to sagging, wrinkled skin. Additionally, the hormone melatonin is released during sleep and counteracts the effects of too much cortisol production. That's why getting your seven to eight hours of rest each night supports your skin. Do your best to make good sleep a staple in your beauty routine.

Does Getting Shorter Make You Fatter?

Louis J. Aronne, MD, director, Comprehensive Weight Control Center, Weill Cornell Medicine and New York-Presbyterian, New York City.

Even if you haven't gained weight since college, you've probably lost some height as you've aged. Since BMI is calculated based on height vs. weight, does that mean you're now fatter?

The answer to that is a little complicated. Losing height as we age is inevitable, but even health professionals don't agree whether body mass index (BMI) for older people should be calculated using current height... or height before inches were lost.

BMI is one way to estimate body fat and provide a clue to overall health and risk for chronic health problems such as heart disease and diabetes. However, BMI is not the only way to do that—or even necessarily the best way.

For one thing, BMI doesn't take into account muscle mass. Muscle weighs more than fat by volume, which means that a fit, muscular athlete can have a BMI score within the "overweight" zone while actually having low body fat and low risk for fat-related health conditions.

Losing muscle mass occurs naturally with aging and needs to be taken into account when deciding whether you are too heavy. And even if you are overweight, losing weight that is mostly muscle is not good for you. If you had to choose between the two—losing muscle to lose weight or staying a bit overweight to retain muscle—keeping the muscle (and the weight) through exercise and good nutrition would be the healthier choice. You need the strength that muscles provide!

BMI also doesn't take into account different body builds. Take two hypothetical people with the same BMI, for example. If one of them has a slight build (less muscular) and the other a heavy build (more muscular), the slight one will have more body fat—and yet the same BMI.

We also lose bone mass as we age, so our bones weigh less, and whatever we weigh is proportionately more fat (because of less bone and muscle) than when we were younger.

There are two other measurements that can help give you an idea whether your weight is just right or needs paring down—one is your waist circumference and the other is your waist-to-hip ratio.

A waist of more than 40 inches for men and more than 35 inches for women is considered a general marker of being overweight—but depending on your height and build, your healthful waist circumference might be far less. For example, it's recently been shown that a waist measurement more than 50% of your height is an indicator of health risks from being overweight. To get your waist-to-hip ratio, divide your waist measurement by your hip measurement. For men, a healthy ratio is 0.95 or less, and for women it's 0.85 or less.

As for how to measure BMI when you've lost height, as a practical matter, we use patients' current, lower heights. You may end up with an uptick in your BMI, but take that with a grain of salt. Consider the rest of your overall health—and concentrate more on maintaining muscle than on losing weight.

Give Yourself a "Butt Facial" at Home

Ginger Hodulik Downey, CNS, co-owner and vice president of R&D for DermaMed Solutions. In addition to her work at DermaMed, Ginger devotes time to working with patients in private clinical practice. As a contributor, Ginger hopes to continue to share her passion for holistic health and wellness. She writes the blog "Beyond Beauty" at BottomLineInc.com/blogs.

Believe it or not, many spas are now offering Fanny Facials—a treatment focused solely on clearing and firming the skin on your butt. The reviews sound great, but not everyone has the budget or comfort level to engage in this type of luxury, so I'd like to talk about how you can keep your backside looking great with some good at-home care.

We need to begin by understanding that the skin on your buttocks differs from the skin on your face. It is thicker and has smaller pores. Therefore, when you get an inflamed hair follicle or pimple it does not form a white head, but rather a condition called folliculitis—an infection of the hair follicle. Folliculitis is usually caused by *Staphylococcus aureus*, a type of staph bacterium that is always present on the skin. The infection happens when it manages to break through the skin and travel down the hair follicle. This is very common and treatable through some good home care. In some cases, the infection grows and forms a very painful boil. Boils should not be squeezed or popped. This will not clear them, but rather will spread the infection and make things worse. Boils should be treated by your dermatologist or general doctor.

Keeping Your Rear Clear

Keeping your fanny smooth does not require too much time and effort. Your daily care routine and personal habits will go a long way to creating a healthy environment for your behind.

• **Cleanse daily with soap and water.** Yes, you need to use soap, not just water. If you are prone to bumps, you can choose a body wash that contains salicylic or lactic acid.

• **Exfoliate gently with a loofah or clean washcloth.** Do not use harsh scrubs as they will cause more inflammation, not less. I personally like to use Alba Organics Acnedote Face & Body Scrub once per week. It is a very gentle exfoliator with salicylic acid.

• **When you are experiencing a breakout, you can try using a tea tree oil spray once per day.** It is anti-bacterial and will help clear the folliculitis. Zinc ointments are also very effective if you can get past the memory of putting it on your baby's bottom and think of the good it will do for you.

• **Change out of wet clothes immediately after a workout** and choose loose fitting pants and underwear made from breathable fabrics like cotton to encourage airflow. Workouts and any activity that cause you to sweat can cause breakouts. Bacteria and yeast love moist environments.

• **For those who wax the hair back there,** do so with care! Excessive waxing can cause folliculitis as well.

Preventing and treating those annoying bumps on your butt is a good practice for general self-care and hygiene even if your fanny will never see the light of day this summer (or any other day of the year). We all like to look and feel our best!

Weight Issues Run in the Family? Here's How Women Can Beat Their "Fat" Genes

Study titled, "Physical Activity Modifies Genetic Susceptibility to Obesity in Postmenopausal Women," by researchers at University of Buffalo, Buffalo, New York, and elsewhere, published in *Menopause*.

Is weight gain as you pass through middle age and later inevitable? After all, hormonal changes from menopause land a one-two punch—boosting fat accumulation while simultaneously making it harder to hang on to calorie-burning muscle. The result is often increased weight, especially belly fat—aka, the "menopot." It's even worse if weight issues run in your family genes.

But you can triumph over your genes when it comes to this weight gain and without eating so little that you feel you're starving, according to new research published in *Menopause*. The secret might not sound surprising at first—it's exercise—but not just any kind of exercise. And you don't have to exercise every day. It turns out that getting enough exercise each week...of the right kind...is so powerful that it can override a genetic predisposition to putting on pounds.

It may even get easier as you get older.

This Exercise Knocks Out Genetics

The researchers developed a genetic risk score based on 95 variants in the building blocks of DNA and used it on data from 8,206 women, ages 50 to 81, from the Women's Health Initiative, an ongoing study of postmenopausal women. The goal was to examine the effect of obesity genes on body mass index (BMI)—a measure of body fat based on weight in relation to height—later in women's lives and to see to what extent lifestyle behaviors, including exercise, might mitigate that effect. Past studies have suggested that genetics play a role in ratcheting up BMI, but not much was known about the interplay of genetics and weight as people age—or how lifestyle might influence that interplay.

Many of the findings weren't surprising. After controlling for various lifestyle factors, the researchers found, as they expected, that women who exercised the most had the lowest BMIs, regardless of their age. Women who got a "moderate" amount of exercise—basically, met the minimum recommendation of getting 150 minutes per week of moderate-intensity aerobic activity (such as walking at three miles per hour) or 75 minutes of vigorous-intensity exercise (running, doing activities that make you break a sweat)—weighed less compared with those who got little or no exercise.

Women who exceeded those minimum recommendations—getting about 20% more exercise weekly than the minimum—did even better. These "high" exercisers weighed, on average, about nine pounds less than their sedentary peers. Exercise partly overcame genetic risk. When the researchers looked more closely at the genetic markers for obesity, they found that physical activity reduced the impact of a woman's genetic predisposition to obesity.

But the real surprise was that the genetic risk dropped the most in the oldest age group—women 70-plus. Exercise habits were more strongly linked with lower BMI in women in their 70s than those in their 60s or 50s. Chalk it up as an unexpected benefit of aging—and of the importance of physical activity at any age.

If you, your mom or your grandmother is postmenopausal, keep in mind that staying active will improve your health in myriad ways such as preventing muscle loss…improving bone strength…balance…mood…concentration…keeping your brain healthy—and now, curbing any genetic tendency you might have toward being overweight.

Why Do the Veins in My Hands Bulge So Much?

Susan B. Fox, DO, an expert in vein and vascular diagnosis and treatment with a private practice in Hollywood and Pembroke Pines, Florida. She is board certified in internal medicine, vascular medicine and phlebology (the treatment of veins). FoxVein Experts.com

---

The older we are, the more likely hand veins are to bulge from time to time. That's because our skin gets thinner and we lose collagen and fat under the skin, which can make the veins much more noticeable. *The following also can contribute to bulging hand veins…*

Forehead Wrinkles Warning

People with the most and deepest horizontal forehead wrinkles had nearly 10 times the risk of dying from heart disease as those with no wrinkles, according to a 20-year study of 3,200 adults ages 32 to 62.

Theory: Some of the factors that lead to premature skin aging and wrinkles also are linked to aging of the arteries and atherosclerosis.

Yolande Esquirol, MD, PhD, associate professor of occupational health, Centre Hospitalier Universitaire de Toulouse, France.

• **Hydration.** The more hydrated a person is, the more visible veins are.

• **Body temperature.** Hot weather and vigorous exercise also can cause your hand veins to bulge. Feeling cold will make them less noticeable.

• **Hand position.** Veins protrude more when hands are below your heart—for example when hanging down by your sides. That's because gravity allows fluids to accumulate in the hands, making the veins more noticeable.

Bulging hand veins are most likely due to a combination of factors, and in some cases can be treated. If their appearance bothers you, veins will look less prominent with the injection of fillers in the hands. The veins also can be treated with a solution that closes them off by scarring them. But I generally do not advise this—these veins may be needed at some point for IV medication or fluids.

Important: If your hand veins start to ache or are prominent all the time, consult a vein specialist (also known as a phlebologist). In some cases, bulging hand veins can be due to phlebitis, a condition that causes a vein to become inflamed, or deep vein thrombosis, resulting from a blood clot deep in an arm vein.

Varicose veins also can occur in the hands. These can be treated with the scarring solution (described above) or laser therapy.

To find a vein specialist, consult the American Vein and Lymphatic Society, Healthy Veins.org.

Wear Sunglasses to Protect Your Eyes

Ginger Hodulik Downey, CNS, co-owner and vice president of R&D for DermaMed Solutions. In addition to her work at DermaMed, Ginger devotes time to working with patients in private clinical practice. As a contributor, Ginger hopes to continue to share her passion for holistic health and wellness. She writes the blog "Beyond Beauty" at BottomLineInc.com/blogs.

In addition to wearing SPF on your face every day, I recommend wearing sunglasses to protect the very delicate skin around the eyes from those harmful rays. *There's a lot more to the story though…*

Let's begin with a little primer on how our bodies make melanin, the compound that adds color to our skin. In the dermal layer of our skin, the one just beneath the thin, top layer (the epidermis), there's a powerhouse of activity going on. It's in the dermis that sweat and hair are produced through a network of nerves and blood vessels. In ad-

dition, this is where our melanin-producing cells (melanocytes) spring forth. These cells are stimulated by sunlight, in particular UV radiation. The origination of this process is an internal protection mechanism created by our bodies—adding pigment to the skin protects the skin from burning; the melanin is there to absorb light. This is why people native to places with more sun and warm temperatures have darker skin. Melanin is also the stuff that brown spots, freckles and patches are made of. Many of us, me included, fight these spots very hard and we do not want to encourage melanin production.

The plot thickens from there! The pituitary gland, a very small gland located behind your eyes and in front of your brain, is connected to the optic nerve. This tiny gland has a diverse and large purpose in our bodies, acting as the mastermind behind all of our hormones, including melanocyte-stimulating hormone. Aha!

Here's the connection: the pituitary is very sensitive to sunlight that comes in through the optic nerve, i.e., our eyes. When we do not wear sunglasses, our skin produces more melanin.

My takeaway here is that wearing SPF may not be enough protection for those of us looking to reduce the production of unwanted pigment in our skin. Always wear your SPF, preferably in the form of UVA/UVB/IR mineral sunscreen, but also wear your sunglasses at all times when in the sun.

When choosing sunglasses, be sure to get those with 100% UV protection. Larger frames are better—and stylish right now too! For extra glare protection you can choose polarized lenses. The color of your lenses and frames does not make a difference, so you can let your personal style be the guide here. Slip on those sunglasses and save your skin from unwanted pigment!

Fiber Fix Extends Life

New finding: Healthy adults who ate the most fiber (25 g to 29 g per day) had a 15% to 30% lower risk for heart disease, colorectal cancer, type 2 diabetes—and even death from any cause—compared with those who ate the least fiber, according to a review of 240 studies over 40 years. Americans eat, on average, only 15 g of fiber daily.

Good options: Whole grains (such as oatmeal and brown rice), lentils, beans, artichokes, raspberries and pears.

Jim Mann, PhD, professor in human nutrition and medicine, University of Otago, Dunedin, New Zealand.

Little-Known Causes of Wrinkles

Roundup of experts on skin care, reported in *Reader's Digest*. RD.com

Inserting contact lenses: Raising eyebrows to put contact lenses in can cause forehead skin to wrinkle.

Sleeping on your stomach: The pillow can cause wrinkles. And stomach sleeping prevents fluid from draining away from your face, increasing eye puffiness.

Air pollution: Use a gentle cleanser every night to wash away residue, and consider using skin-care products that are high in antioxidants.

Smartphones and other electronics: The blue light they emit penetrates deeper skin layers and can cause premature skin aging and wrinkling.

Your "Memory Problems" May Actually Be Due to Hearing Loss

The study "Considering Age-Related Hearing Loss in Neuropsychological Practice: Findings from a Feasibility Study" was conducted by a neuropsychology and cognitive health research team at Baycrest, a geriatric care program affiliated with University of Toronto, and published in *Canadian Journal on Aging*.

Forgetfulness can be frustrating…and frightening, causing you to worry that you have early symptoms of Alzheimer's disease if you can't remember what your spouse told you to pick up at the grocery store, for example, or the name of the restaurant where your friend said to meet.

But don't be too quick to panic.

A Canadian team of researchers recently took a closer look at 20 older adults who were undergoing cognitive evaluations and discovered that "forgetfulness" may have more to do with a person's hearing than an actual memory problem.

When clinical neuropsychologists analyzed the cognitive evaluations of the study participants, along with assessments of their hearing, 56% of those being tested because they were concerned about memory/thinking problems and possible brain disorders had some degree of hearing loss, ranging from mild to severe, with only about 20% of them wearing hearing aids. Interestingly, 25% of the individuals who were worried about potential memory problems had no signs that a brain disorder was causing their forgetfulness.

Because none of us can remember what we never heard, this research suggests that hearing difficulties can masquerade as forgetfulness. Even when a person's brain is otherwise healthy, hearing loss can cause communication problems, social isolation and loneliness—all of which are associated with an increased risk for dementia. Getting treatment for hearing loss can help preserve your physical and mental well-being.

Takeaway: If you're concerned about your memory, ask your primary care doctor to perform a hearing examination in addition to cognitive testing. On the basis of your results, your doctor may give you tips on how to communicate better…suggest an over-the-counter sound amplifier…or recommend that you see an audiologist for a full workup. These hearing professionals can determine the best way to improve your hearing…and if that includes the use of a hearing aid, they can explain how to correctly operate and maintain it. To find an audiologist near you, visit the American Academy of Audiology's website for a searchable list.

Important: Today's hearing aids are not the big, ugly, screechy appliances that your grandparents used. They are much more sophisticated now, and some are barely noticeable. They can be expensive, though—typical costs, which aren't covered by insurance, range from $800 to $4,000 per ear—so be sure to work with a professional who can help you find what's right for you.

How to Make Hearing Aids Work for the Ones You Love

Marcy Cottrell Houle, MS, professional biologist and award-winning author of four books and numerous articles. Her most recent book, *The Gift of Caring: Saving Our Parents—and Ourselves—from the Perils of Modern Healthcare*, coauthored with geriatrician Elizabeth Eckstrom, MD, MPH, MACP, shares the latest medical knowledge and best ways we can advocate for our loved one's health care as well as our own. MarcyCottrellHoule.com

When one is a caregiver to a senior, a difficulty often becomes apparent over time. We see our loved one begin to lose the crispness of their senses as well as their mobility. Older people can lose their hearing and their eyesight. Their gait can become increasingly impaired, a result of severe arthritis, a stroke, lessening vision, or loss of sensation in feet from diabetes. All of this is distressing not only to them, but to those of us who are caring for them.

As a caregiver to both of my parents for 14 years, I found there is something we can do to help them soldier through such declines: We need to encourage the use of aids. Aids should not be thought of as a sign of defeat. Rather, they are just the opposite. As Dr. Eckstrom, coauthor of our book *The Gift of Caring,* says, we all need to embrace the use of aids because they give us independence.

My mother was, I think, like many seniors. She was reluctant at first to use aids. "I will never use a walker in public," she professed. To her, using a walker to make her way down the sidewalk meant a loss of dignity and freedom. After some coaching by her doctor and those who cared for her, she came to see aids differently. Aids provided her liberation. They meant all the difference between being stuck at home and having the ability to take safe and enjoyable outings.

There are four major categories of aids, all of which I found very useful in caring for my mother. I will discuss each one separately in my upcoming posts. Today, I'll start with one that made a huge difference to my mother's quality of life as she aged: hearing aids.

Dr. Eckstrom stresses that the importance of good hearing to health cannot be overemphasized. Numerous studies show that decreased hearing is associated with an increased risk of mortality. Also, impaired hearing is associated with an accelerated risk of memory decline. Therefore, investing in hearing aids is essential for our loved ones who suffer from hearing loss.

There is a problem however, and I experienced it with my mother. It's not always easy to find ones that work. People can spend a lot of money to acquire hearing aids only to be disappointed with the results. They find the aids may work well in a quiet room but in a noisy situation like a restaurant, they amplify all the background noise, which can be exceedingly frustrating. This makes many people, like my mom, just want to give up.

But don't give up and, more importantly, don't let them give up. Hearing is too critical to life satisfaction. As I had to do with my mother, explain to your loved one that it will take time and several appointments to get the right adjustment. Find an audiologist and ear, nose and throat doctor who will work with you in these cases.

As I discovered, if your loved one knows they must have patience at the outset of the process, it makes the initial discouragement slightly easier to bear.

What about people who can't afford hearing aids? Or what about seniors who have memory problems that make this option not workable? Dr. Eckstrom suggests another venue, one that I personally saw work very successfully with my son-in-law's grandmother: pocket amplifiers. At 97 years old, after suffering from hearing loss for many years, it changed her life.

Pocket amplifiers are low in cost and can provide terrific results. They are packaged in a small box and easy to use. There is a microphone, attached by a wire to the box, that one person speaks into. The hearing impaired, wearing headphones or earbuds attached to the same box, can hear the spoken words. Fancier versions employ wireless sound systems. Sometimes, this is the first time they have clearly heard a loved one's voice in years. And while pocket amplifiers only work between two people, that can still vastly improve a person's quality of life!

Pocket amplifiers are great tools to have when trying to communicate in a noisy restaurant. They remove all the disturbing background interference. In addition, wireless models mean you don't have to raise your voice to be heard from different parts of the house. They are also very helpful at doctor appointments. A patient with hearing difficulties can actually hear what the doctor is saying! This is so important that Dr. Eckstrom encourages all doctors' offices to have pocket amplifiers available for their patients who are hard of hearing. As caregivers, we can advocate that our providers' offices have them if they don't already.

Like many caregivers, I often had to remind my mother that the aids she used should never be thought of as a form of embarrassment or a symbol signifying loss. In time, she realized this truth. Instead of considering them as a defeat, we all came to see that these tools promoted better ways to relate, encouraged greater independence, and made for better caring and for more meaningful living.

Good for the Heart, Good for the Ears

Diets good for the heart also are good for ears. People who ate a Mediterranean-style diet or the antihypertension DASH diet were about 30% less likely to develop moderate or severe hearing loss over a 22-year period than people whose eating habits were less healthful.

Analysis of 71,000 women in the Nurses' Health Study II by researchers at Brigham and Women's Hospital, Boston, published in *Journal of Nutrition*.

"Yo-Yo" Cardio Danger

When blood sugar, blood pressure, cholesterol and weight fluctuate—go up and down—by more than 5%, it can shorten a person's life span, according to a new Korean study that followed 6.7 million people for five-and-a-half years. Those who had the highest fluctuations were 41% more likely to have a stroke...and 43% more likely to have a heart attack than those whose numbers did not fluctuate by more than 5%.

Seung-Hwan Lee, MD, PhD, associate professor of internal medicine, College of Medicine, The Catholic University of Korea, Seoul.

Do You Really Need a Blood Test to Tell You You're in Menopause?

Tarun Jain, MD, board-certified reproductive endocrinology and infertility specialist, Northwestern Medicine, and associate professor of obstetrics and gynecology, Northwestern University Feinberg School of Medicine, Chicago.

Night sweats, hot flashes, irregular periods. If you're a woman of a certain age, you know that these are the hallmarks of menopause. So you might be skeptical about a blood test designed to confirm something your body will tell you naturally. But there are good reasons to consider having it.

The Change in Determining "The Change"

Before this blood test, called **MenoCheck**, became available, doctors would confirm menopause only after the fact—once a woman hadn't had a period for 12 straight months. Some doctors might check blood levels of follicle-stimulating hormone (FSH), which increases as women approach menopause. However, FSH ebbs and flows during the time leading up to menopause, so it's not a reliable indicator.

MenoCheck is more reliable and more specific than FSH tests because it measures levels of AMH (anti-Müllerian hormone), a marker of your ovaries' reserve. As the ovaries' pool of follicles (which contain eggs) further diminishes when you start the transition to menopause, levels of AMH hormone also continue to decline.

While AMH could be measured in blood tests before—often to help gauge fertility for family planning, MenoCheck is better able to measure declining concentrations and pinpoint where a woman is on the menopause path.

So do you really need a menopause test? Having a more accurate picture of how close you are to menopause can help guide your overall health care, including prevention steps. The loss of estrogen during menopause increases the risk of certain health conditions, including heart disease, osteoporosis and diabetes. So knowing definitively that the transition has started could prompt you to redouble your efforts to get enough calcium and vitamin D and engage in regular bone-building exercise to protect bones…and make sure that your blood pressure, cholesterol, blood sugar and weight are under control.

Knowing your menopause status is especially important for women having menopausal symptoms before the average age of 51—such as in your early to mid-40s. Early menopause makes women even more vulnerable to the health conditions listed above.

If the test confirms that bothersome symptoms are indeed due to menopause rather than another health issue, you can begin to explore treatments to relieve them. If you opt for hormone replacement therapy, your MenoCheck results may help determine the lowest possible effective dose.

MenoCheck may also help answer another big question—can you still get pregnant? Because of how accurately the blood test measures AMH, it can let you know whether you should still use birth control to avoid an unwanted pregnancy.

For women who are already in perimenopause (and who feel like it's dragging on!), the test can help evaluate how much longer the transition will take.

MenoCheck can be done in your doctor's office, and results are typically available within five to 10 days. The test costs roughly $100 and, as of this writing, is not yet covered by insurance. Keep in mind that the test is simply a measure of a particular hormone, so the results need to be interpreted in the context of other health factors.

Relief at Last for Severely Itchy Skin

Laurie Steelsmith, ND, LAc, naturopathic physician, acupuncturist and coauthor of three books—*Natural Choices for Women's Health*, *Great Sex, Naturally* and *Growing Younger Every Day*. A leading advocate for natural medicine, Dr. Steelsmith is the medical director of Steelsmith Natural Health Center in Honolulu. DrSteelsmith.com

The patient: "Laurel," a 48-year-old librarian.

Why she came to see me: Laurel arrived with a complaint that at first seemed better-suited for a dermatologist. Lifting the sleeves of her shirt, she pointed to the red, bumpy, dry skin on her forearms before showing me a similar patch on the T-zone of her face. Both places were consistently, if not relentlessly, itchy. The irritation had turned from mild to severe in the past three months and while she'd tried a number of treatments—from CBD oil to a consult with one of the city's top dermatologists—she hadn't been able to find any relief. She was intent on determining the root cause of this flare…and she was equally keen on treating it naturally.

How I evaluated her: We began with a thorough exploration of Laurel's medical history and lifestyle. Three years sober, Laurel prioritized health. She followed a low-fat diet, practiced Pilates five times a week and meditated daily. She'd also quit smoking eight years earlier—a gift to herself on her 40th birthday. She was in a steady, happy relationship, loved her job at the library downtown and felt pleased with her overall progress and place in life, which, she said, made her recent health concerns all the more vexing.

The itchiness had started out of the blue and was at first only felt on her forearms and above her elbows before traveling upwards to her face. She'd switched to a mild, natural laundry detergent and made a point to use only using chemical-free soaps, sunscreens and lotions. But the itchiness and redness grew from mild to severe and oftentimes delayed her ability to fall asleep, frequently woke her up in the middle of the night and served as something of a social embarrassment.

Probing deeper, I found that a number of other symptoms had also started to emerge in Laurel's life, including insomnia, mood swings and difficulty maintaining her weight, particularly around her midsection. Her once-predictable periods had become irregular as well, arriving every other month or so. When they did show up, they were heavier and carried with them more intense and aggravating PMS symptoms.

While I assumed that these skin problems and other symptoms were associated with her age, I ordered a PAP smear, a blood test, a kidney exam and a thyroid test to rule out any underlining medical issues. In addition, I ordered a hormone test that would allow me to assess where she stood in terms of hormone production.

What my evaluation revealed: While Laurel's PAP and other exams were clear, her hormone test revealed precisely what I expected: She was in perimenopause and, as such, demonstrated lowered hormone levels, particularly estrogen.

As I explained to Laurel, this was not necessarily cause for concern—it is completely normal for hormones to decline in the years leading up to a woman's final period. (Men see a fall in hormones with age as well, FYI.) As the ovaries mature, they release fewer hormones, which leads to decreased amounts of estrogen as well as progesterone and testosterone. In turn, a woman may experience any one of the symptoms Laurel was enduring, as well as hot flashes, vaginal dryness, memory loss, incontinence and more.

The hormonal decline that accompanies the onset of menopause can also impact the skin. As estrogen drops, so does the skin's capacity for holding water and keeping it elastic. Estrogen also plays a key role in shielding skin against oxidative stress and in stimulating collagen—an essential protein that profoundly influences skin health. This waning of estrogen can manifest as wrinkling, dry skin, pigmentary changes, photo-aging—and the very itchiness Laurel was lamenting. This itchiness, technically known as pruritus, may be irritating but, as I assured her, it's neither grave nor a life sentence.

How I addressed her problem: I wanted to treat not only Laurel's itchy skin but also the discomfiting symptoms that were taking a toll on her otherwise-ideal life.

Before she considered estrogen replacement therapy—which, as the National Institutes of Health (NIH) reports, has been implicated as "a risk factor in breast and uterine cancer"—I urged Laurel to alter her diet to include more phytoestrogens. These plant-based compounds, first discovered in the early 1920s by Bernhard Zondek (who also, incidentally, developed the first pregnancy test), can mimic estrogen in the body and thus help moderate hormones. To this end, I encouraged her to add the following foods to her diet: soy, hummus, tempeh, rye bread, flax and sesame seeds, dried fruit (such as prunes and apricots), alfalfa sprouts, yams and apples.

I also suggested she add cruciferous vegetables such as Brussels sprouts, broccoli and cauliflower to her grocery list as they organically bolster estrogen metabolism through their inclusion of indole-3-carbinol. Furthermore, I recommended adding healthy fats—salmon, avocado and walnuts, to name just a few—to her diet. Rich in Omega-3 fatty acids, these foods naturally strengthen the skin's oil barrier, which is a crucial component to keeping skin hydrated (and itch-less). They also enhance the body's production of anti-inflammatory compounds, further protecting the skin from aging and the itchiness that can arrive with it. Additionally, I persuaded Laurel to eat more grapes, which contain a particular phytoestrogen that brims with resveratrol and has powerful antioxidant (read: skin-boosting) properties.

I recommended cutting sugar from her diet entirely. Sugar causes insulin to spike, which may prompt inflammation and the itchiness and signs of aging that can come with it.

I then urged Laurel to start using sea buckthorn oil. Obtained from the sea buckthorn plant, this oil nurtures the health and beauty of skin through its balanced combination of fatty acids and vitamins and has the potential to treat dry, flaky or rapidly aging skin. (According to the NIH, sea buckthorn oil also "improves blood circulation, facilitates oxygenation of the skin, removes excess toxins from the body and easily penetrates through the epidermis.") It can be taken as a supplement or applied topically in a face oil (one to try: Kora Organics Noni Glow Face Oil, a terrific product that also includes skin-soothing rosehip oil).

To achieve fast relief during a bout of itchiness, I advised her to take an oatmeal bath by adding a cup of colloidal oats to a warm, not hot, bath (heat can further dry out the skin), soaking for at least 10 minutes and locking in moisture with a thick, quality cream.

Finally, I encouraged Laurel to supplement with 1,000 mg per day of Vitamin C, which has been shown to help prevent dry, itchy skin, and with 500 mg twice a day of dong quai. Known to some as the "female ginseng," dong quai is a revitalizing tonic that operates as a phytoestrogen and can support skin and hormone health.

The patient's progress: Within a month, the patches of irritation on Laurel's forearms and T-zone had diminished to little more than a few bumps. As a result, she was sleeping better and feeling more apt to socialize. What's more, she reported less fatigue and fewer mood swings and, thanks to her diet, she'd shed the last five pounds she'd aimed to lose when she got sober.

Above all, she claimed to feel far less anxious—not only about her skin and its itchiness, but also about getting older. She felt emboldened and powerful, which, I explained to her, are the two best- and least-known "side effects" of aging.

How Drinking Can Weaken Your Muscles

Study titled "Associations between High-Risk Alcohol Consumption and Sarcopenia among Postmenopausal Women," by Hee-Taik Kang, MD, Chungbuk National University College of Medicine, Republic of Korea, and colleagues, published in *Menopause: The Journal of the North American Menopause Society.*

There's a very common habit you may have that is silently robbing your body of the muscle mass and strength you'll need as you get older. The habit is drinking alcohol.

Surprised? You knew that alcohol could hurt your liver—but shrink your muscles?

It's true. A new study finds, in fact, that drinking is strongly linked to worsening sarcopenia, the age-related loss of muscle mass and strength. Sarcopenia is increasingly recognized as an important contributor to falls and fractures as well as many chronic diseases.

How much you drink is the key. A little bit—not to worry. If you're still drinking like you did when you were younger, however, it's time to ask yourself, Is my drinking setting me up for a fall?

Background: The US Centers for Disease Control and Prevention recently recognized sarcopenia, a combination of low muscle mass and weakness in older adults, as a diagnosable medical condition. It can affect balance and walking and interfere with the ability to take care of the activities of daily living that allow for independence. Muscle mass is also key to metabolic and cognitive health—sarcopenia is linked with increased risk for heart disease, diabetes and cognitive impairment. In short, minimizing or preventing sarcopenia can help you remain healthy, functional and independent at older ages.

We naturally start losing muscle mass in our 40s. By the 50s, the average man or woman loses 1.5% a year. After age 60, that goes up to 3% a year. Sarcopenia, as opposed to just normal age-related muscle loss, is defined as a substantial loss of both muscle mass and strength—so much so that walking is affected. While statistics vary, it is estimated that as many as 15% of Americans age 60 and older and 50% of those age 80 and older have sarcopenia.

A healthy lifestyle that includes regular exercise and a good diet helps prevent sarcopenia. But too little has been known about the role of alcohol, which is what researchers set out to address in the latest study.

Study: Using data from a large national patient registry, South Korean researchers pulled medical records on about 2,400 postmenopausal women. (The issue affects men, too.) The records included measurements of lean body mass (aka, muscle). The women filled out questionnaires about their frequency and quantity of alcohol use, whether they drank alcohol in the morning (a sign of problem drinking), guilt or concern about drinking and known alcohol-related injuries. Based on their responses, they were classified as either at low, medium or high risk for alcohol problems. On average, the women were 62 years old. About 8% had sarcopenia.

Results: Women who were at risk for alcohol problems were at substantially increased risk for sarcopenia. *Here are the percentages of women who had sarcopenia associated with their drinking habits…*

Low risk—7.6% had sarcopenia.
Medium risk—11%.
High risk—22.7%.

Heavy drinkers, of course, also tend to have otherwise less healthy lifestyles than light drinkers or teetotalers. But even after adjusting for age, weight, blood pressure, cholesterol levels, blood sugar, smoking and exercise habits, high-risk drinkers in this study were more than four times more likely than those in the low-risk group to have sarcopenia.

Bottom line: It's not exactly shocking to learn that something that we already knew was bad for us—drinking too much—causes additional harms. (According to Dietary Guidelines for Americans, moderate drinking for women is an average of no more than seven drinks a week and for men, no more than 14. According to the National Institute on Alcohol Abuse and Alcoholism, over age 65, "low-risk drinking" for men and women is the same—no more than seven drinks a week and no more than three drinks in a single day.) But this new research might be a wake-up call to look at your own habits. Unfortunately, drinking problems are increasing faster among people over 65 than in any other age group. Plus, over the age of about 45, alcohol can be harder on your body than when you were younger—even if you're still just drinking like you used to. And there's new evidence that even moderate drinking may not be so great for your brain.

Surefire Ways to Prevent Muscle Loss

Stuart M. Phillips, PhD, professor, department of kinesiology and Michael G. DeGroote School of Medicine, McMaster University, Ontario, Canada. He is director of the McMaster Centre for Nutrition, Exercise and Health Research and a fellow of the American College of Sports Medicine and the American College of Nutrition.

Starting in your 30s, your muscles began shrinking, making you imperceptibly but steadily weaker. And now, as each year ticks by, you keep weakening—losing muscle mass at a rate of 0.5% to 1% a year—so that the loss of strength is more obvious. At some point, if it hasn't happened already, you'll be in your kitchen wrestling with a jar of spaghetti sauce and thinking, Why do they make these lids so much tighter than they used to?

Loss of muscle mass and strength isn't just an inconvenience. It's one of the most accurate indicators—for seniors and the middle-aged and the young—that disease and death may be in your near future.

Scary findings: Study after study shows that people with less strength are more likely to be hospitalized or to die of any cause, including heart disease, stroke, cancer and pneumonia, within a given period. Scientists haven't figured out all the reasons that strength predicts health and well-being, but it's not only because unhealthy people get weaker—in fact, a reduction in strength is a better predictor of dying from cardiovascular disease than is high blood pressure.

If you've told your doctor that you're a bit weaker these days, and he/she said it's a "normal part of aging"—ignore him. You can and should preserve and build muscle mass and strength at any age—it's as important to health and longevity as keeping your arteries free of plaque and your cells free of cancer. And you can do it with a surprisingly simple three-pronged strategy—a routine of three simple strengthening exercises (no gym required)…the right diet…and three particular nutritional supplements that are proven muscle protectors. *Here's how to do it…*

Best Exercises

Preserve and build the muscles in your arms, legs, hips and back that you need for everyday strength and activity by doing these three exercises two or three times a week at home or anywhere else…

• **Body-weight squat.** Stand directly in front of a stable, not-too-high chair with no armrest and with your back toward the chair seat and your feet shoulder-width apart. Slowly bend your legs, keeping your back straight and arms at your sides and knees over your toes, and lower yourself onto the chair. Then stand up slowly by reversing the motion. Do this 30 times. If you can't do 30 repetitions

at first (and many people can't), start with what you can do, and over a period of days or weeks, work up to 30. (The same goes for the next two exercises.) If you can do even more, all the better—but 30 should be your minimum target.

• **Lunge.** While standing, keep your upper body straight and your shoulders back, and step forward with one leg, lowering your hips until both knees are bent at a 90-degree angle. Return to the standing position. Do 15 times on each side for a total of 30.

• **Push-up or modified push-up.** This oldie but goodie develops the upper back, shoulders, arms, chest and wrists. If you can't yet do "full" push-ups (with only your hands and toes on the ground), start with modified push-ups in which your toes and knees are on the ground…or even with easier "wall push-ups" where you stand facing a wall and place your hands on the wall at shoulder height. Your ultimate goal is at least 30 full push-ups.

Also important: Aerobic exercise to maintain fitness. You don't have to run miles and miles. A 25-minute jog or vigorous cycling just three times a week…or a 30-minute brisk walk five times a week will do the trick.

Best Foods

The ideal strategy for staying strong is like a three-level pyramid. The base of the pyramid—the essential factor—is exercise as described above, and the most important dietary component for your muscles is protein, the material out of which muscles are made. And believe it or not, despite the prevalence of meat in the typical Western diet, many Americans don't get enough protein for the best possible muscle strength.

The government's Recommended Dietary Allowance (RDA) for protein is 0.36 grams (g) of protein per pound of body weight per day. But that level is the minimum, not the optimum. For preserving and building muscle, we need at least 50% more—0.54 g of protein per pound of body weight per day. And some studies indicate that 0.73 g per pound of body weight is even better. (More than that doesn't build more muscle or strength.)

Problem: Most seniors get only two-thirds of the RDA, or about 0.24 g of protein per pound of body weight per day.

How much protein should you eat? Don't go by the government's RDA. Instead multiply your body weight in pounds by 0.54 to get the minimum number of grams per day…and multiply your body weight by 0.73 to get the maximum daily grams of protein likely to help your muscles. Then each day, aim to eat an amount in between those two results.

Example: A person who weighs 150 pounds would multiply 150 by 0.54 to get a minimum daily protein goal of 81 g…and multiply 150 by 0.73 to get a maximum useful daily protein amount of 109 g.

Equally important: Not only do you need enough protein—you need the kind that your muscles can easily use. The best muscle-building protein has two features. It is digestible— the amino acids that are the building blocks of protein are easily absorbed. Protein from meat, poultry, fish and other seafood, eggs and dairy is far more digestible than protein from plants. And the best protein for muscles has a high level of the amino acid leucine, which kick-starts muscle-building. The digestible sources of protein mentioned above also have the most leucine.

To optimize muscle-building, you also need to get protein at every meal, because unlike unused carbohydrates and unused fat, unused protein is not stored by the body for later use.

Best strategy: Eat a highly digestible form of leucine-rich protein, chosen from the above sources, at every meal.

Examples: For breakfast, eat two eggs (12 g protein) and one-half cup of yogurt (6 g). For lunch, cut up four ounces of chicken breast (35 g protein) into a salad. For dinner, eat a six-ounce serving of high-quality (preferably organic) meat or fish (around 40 g protein) along with vegetables and whole grains. For a bedtime snack, have one-half cup of cottage cheese (12 g protein).

Grand total: 105 g of protein, or just about the perfect amount to help preserve strength for our 150-pounder.

Note: Some medical conditions, for example kidney disease, can make it dangerous to consume even moderate amounts of protein—check first with your physician.

Best Supplements

In a recent study by my colleagues and me at McMaster University, we added three nutritional supplements to the diets of older men who also were engaged in an exercise program—and the supplements increased strength and muscle mass more than exercise alone (of course, check with your physician to make sure that any new supplement is safe for you)…

•**Whey protein.** Milk has two main proteins—casein and whey. Whey is separated from casein during cheese-making, and whey protein powder is a supplement containing that by-product. It is unusually rich in leucine.

Suggested amount: If you are meeting your target range of daily protein from food as described above, you don't need a protein supplement. If you fall a bit short, mix enough protein powder into the drink of your choice (many people use milk) to reach the total daily range of protein for your body weight as described above. (Check the label of your whey product to determine how much powder provides that much protein.) Don't get more than 50 g of daily protein from whey powder—it is not a total substitute for protein-rich food. When buying whey powder, look for "NSF" on the label—NSF is a third-party organization that certifies products that have met rigorous manufacturing standards.

Best timing: Take whey protein soon after exercise, which maximizes muscle-building. If you can't consume whey because of an allergy or some other reason, consider a soy protein supplement instead.

•**Creatine.** This amino acid boosts the body's ability to produce energy and helps build muscle.

Your Diet Can Affect Menopause Onset

A healthy diet can delay menopause by nearly three years, while a refined-food diet can start it a year and half sooner. Later menopause—associated with a diet high in oily fish, beans, greens, etc.—may reduce risk for osteoporosis and heart disease.

University of Leeds

Recent finding: In a study published in *Nutrients*, just six days of creatine supplementation improved upper-body strength by nearly 3%.

Suggested amount: Two capsules per day, in divided doses, that together total 4 g to 5 g.

• **Fish oil.** The omega-3 fatty acids in fish oil (EPA and DHA) make your muscles more sensitive to protein, encouraging muscle-building.

Suggested amount: 750 milligrams (mg) of EPA and 500 mg of DHA per day.

If Your Voice Is Getting Deeper...

Gina R. Vess, MA, CCC-SLP, director of clinical voice programs, Duke Voice Care Center, Duke University Medical Center, Durham, North Carolina.

One of the most common causes of a deeper, lower pitch (the rate of vibration of the vocal cords) in a person's voice is fluid buildup in the vocal cords due to chronic smoking. This change is permanent and will not resolve even after the smoker gives up cigarettes.

Of course, a deeper voice could also be due to something as common as viral laryngitis (inflammation of the larynx, or "voice box"), in which case you should be sounding like yourself in a few weeks. Other potential causes of a lower and/or raspier voice include hormonal changes (menopause, for example, which can also cause fluid build-up) or conditions such as hypothyroidism, in which the thyroid gland doesn't produce enough of certain hormones. (In this case, your voice should return to normal with thyroid medication.)

Noncancerous vocal cord lesions (polyps and cysts) are another possible cause of voice changes and hoarseness. These lesions are caused by repetitive use and are usually found in people who use their voices extensively, such as singers or rabid sports fans who scream a lot at games.

If voice issues last for more than a few weeks, see an ear, nose and throat doctor (otolaryngologist), who can determine the cause. In many cases, conservative treatment such as voice therapy (which might include vocal and/or respiratory exercises) performed by a qualified speech pathologist will be recommended, but surgery may be advised if the cause turns out to be a polyp or cyst.

See Better Than Ever!

Robert Abel, Jr., MD, an ophthalmologist at Delaware Ophthalmology Consultants in Wilmington and founder/medical director of Medical Eye Bank of Delaware. Dr. Abel is author of *The Eye Care Revolution: Prevent and Reverse Common Vision Problems.*

When you're nearly blinded by oncoming headlights or can't read the menu in a candlelit restaurant, you've officially entered the world of "age-related vision loss."

For many people, such vision loss starts in their 40s or 50s. By age 65, about one-third of Americans will have vision loss due to common conditions such as presbyopia (trouble focusing close up)...or more serious eye problems such as cataracts or glaucoma.

Latest development: New advances are rapidly improving treatments for cataracts and glaucoma—especially when the problem is caught early.

Here are the breakthroughs to consider—and what to watch out for...*

Cataracts

Cataracts are caused by a clouding of the lens that results in such symptoms as blurry vision, cloudy vision, poor night vision and even double vision. The preferred treatment is cataract surgery—a procedure that's become increasingly effective in recent years. *Latest advances...*

•**Extended depth of focus lens.** With cataract surgery, a surgeon can remove the cloudy, vision-impairing lens of the eye in a matter of minutes and replace it with a clear corrective lens. But until recently, the replacement lens would only enhance either near or far vision in each eye.

This meant that doctors might treat one eye for near vision and the other eye for seeing at a distance...or they might use a "multifocal" implant that offered some improvement in both near and far vision. Most people simply choose to correct for far vision and use reading glasses the rest of the time.

The new extended depth of focus (EDOF) lens is an important advance because it can correct distance vision while also improving your ability to see up close. For eye surgeons, it's one step closer to the holy grail—the ability to completely reverse age-related vision loss without the need for glasses. With EDOF, you might actually see better than you ever did.

Drawbacks: The new lenses are expensive. If your insurance doesn't pick up the tab, you can expect to pay $1,500 to $2,500 more per eye than you would for traditional replacement lenses.

Even though the new lenses are better for brightness, contrast and seeing colors—and they do improve vision at in-between distances—you still might need reading glasses in some cases.

Best for: Active middle-aged and older adults who want to avoid wearing glasses.

*The treatments included in this article may not be covered by insurance. Check with your insurer for details.

•**RxSight Light Adjustable Lens.** The FDA approved an artificial lens in 2017 that can be adjusted repeatedly after cataract surgery—important because slight errors in lens manufacturing (or eye changes that occur during healing) can skew the vision-correcting effects.

This adjustable lens contains a unique material that shifts in response to UV light. If your vision isn't optimal after the surgery, your doctor can fine-tune it with three or four laser treatments that modify the curvature of the lens, delivered about three weeks after the procedure.

The lens can provide vision improvements that are comparable to vision-correcting procedures such as LASIK. But for now (despite the FDA's approval), the lens has not yet become widely adopted and is mainly available for patients who are participating in ongoing studies.

Best for: Any cataract surgery patient who is looking for precise vision correction that is permanent.

Glaucoma

Glaucoma results from fluid buildup that damages the eye's optic nerve, potentially causing vision loss and even blindness. Depending on the extent of the disease, treatment has traditionally included medication (such as eyedrops or pills)...laser surgery (to help make sure that fluid drains out of the eye)...or conventional surgery (to create an opening for fluid to leave the eye). *Latest advances...*

•**iStent.** Because most types of glaucoma are accompanied by excessive fluid buildup (often leading to high pressure within the eye), one of the main treatments is to surgically install a stent (or a related device called a shunt) to improve drainage and keep eye pressure low.

The iStent is a game-changer. It's the first FDA-approved device that can be implanted during cataract surgery for patients who have mild-to-moderate open-angle glaucoma, which accounts for at least 90% of all glaucoma cases. The device, which is about one-third the size of a grain of rice, creates a permanent opening to improve fluid drainage.

Previous devices worked similarly, but they required the surgeon to open a flap of skin from outside the eye, install the stent, then close things up. The iStent doesn't require a separate procedure when performed with cataract surgery.

Bonus: Patients who have the stent often can reduce their dependence on pressure-reducing medications, which tend to be less reliable and may cause side effects, including extremely low pressure. It's a phenomenal development!

Best for: Any glaucoma patient who is undergoing cataract surgery.

• **Pressure-reducing eyedrops.** More than 95% of adults with glaucoma use eyedrops (at least initially) to reduce glaucoma-causing fluid buildups.

About half of patients require two or more eye medications—and patients using multiple drugs are less likely to follow dosing instructions. The most commonly used medications are prostaglandin analogs (PGAs), which improve the functioning of the drainage pathway known as the uveoscleral outflow.

What's new: Latanoprostene bunod ophthalmic solution (Vyzulta), approved by the FDA in 2017. Unlike other PGAs, it increases the outflow of fluid through both the uveoscleral pathway and the trabecular meshwork (an area of tissue near the base of the cornea). In studies, it lowered intraocular pressure more than the older drugs...and the dual action means that some glaucoma patients can use only one eyedrop.

My take: All of the PGAs, including Vyzulta, can cause inflammation and red or puffy eyes. For this reason, I believe that glaucoma patients will often do better with other (non-PGA) eyedrops or laser treatments.

Best for: Vyzulta can be a reasonable choice for advanced glaucoma patients who must use eyedrops but are resistant to other products and are not significantly troubled by mild eye inflammation.

Guard Against Dry Eye

The condition is more common in winter because humidity outside is low and people keep homes and offices heated as well as dry—so eye moisture evaporates both outdoors and indoors. It helps to use a humidifier in heated environments and avoid directing heat right at your face—for example, direct car vents downward toward your lower body.

Also: Drink lots of fluids so that your whole body stays hydrated...wear eye protection outdoors or use a hat with a visor. If you wear contact lenses, keep them very clean to reduce the risk of itching and infection. See your doctor if dry eye persists.

Marissa K. Locy, OD, instructor, department of ophthalmology, University of Alabama at Birmingham.

Great New Devices That Make Life Easier

Chris Cusack, partnership manager of *Disability Horizons* magazine, a UK-based online lifestyle publication for the disabled. He was a judge for the Accessible Tech in Employment Hackathon event held on Google's London campus in 2017. DisabilityHorizons.com

Clever new "assistive technologies" now reaching the market can help you or a loved one better use a computer if it is difficult...enjoy the outdoors if you need extra support to walk...navigate better if you have low vision or blindness...and much more. Also, some of these devices are useful for people who are not disabled but would just like to make things easier.

Mobility

Wheelchairs and conventional walkers are not the only devices that can help you get around...

• **More comfortable crutch.** Ergobaum distributes users' body weight over the length of their forearms instead of in the armpits. Many people find this less stressful for the arms, particularly when crutches are needed for more than a few days. ($189 for a pair,* ErgoActives.com)

• **"Walker" you can use for jogging.** Afari Mobility Aid has three large wheels plus bicycle-like steering controls and brakes. It lets people who need extra stability when walking move at faster speeds than with a traditional walker. It also works on unpaved surfaces. It is currently being produced in small quantities, so availability is limited. ($1,875, Mobility-Tech.com)

Alternative: Trionic Veloped is another walker capable of traveling off-road. There are versions for golfing...hiking...and hunting—the golfing model can carry golf clubs, for example. ($1,089, Trionic.us/en)

• **Strong, portable lift.** Molift Smart 150 is a hoist capable of picking up a person who weighs as much as 330 pounds to transfer him/her from a bed to a wheelchair or vice versa. Yet this hoist folds down into two sections weighing less than 30 pounds apiece (including rechargeable battery) that can easily fit into the trunk of a car. It gives you the freedom to travel even if you can't get yourself up out of bed and your partner can't lift you. ($3,955.50, Etac.com/en-us/products)

• **Clothing tailored for wheelchair users.** Chairmelotte designs mostly women's garments specifically for wheelchair users. (The company also has a small selection for men.) The clothing is cut to be comfortable, stylish and flattering while seated, not while standing...there are extra zippers where people who use wheelchairs are likely to need them, such as up the side seam of skirts and pants...and the sleeves are cut to allow the full arm motions needed to propel a hand-operated wheelchair. (Chairmelotte.com)

Hand Use

Many conditions can lead to hand tremors or hand-strength problems. *Among the tech that can help...*

*Prices are from online retailers and may be below the manufacturers' retail prices. Prices and availability subject to change.

• **Gadget that controls tech with head movements.** GlassOuse lets you control the cursor on a PC or Mac computer screen using small movements of your head rather than with a traditional computer mouse. It can control Bluetooth-enabled Android phones, tablets and smart TVs, too. GlassOuse is worn on the face like eyeglasses, only with no lenses. (If you wear actual eyeglasses, it can sit just above them.) Users can operate its "mouse button" by tapping a finger pad...biting a specially designed switch...or blowing a puff of air—these button units are sold separately. ($499 for GlassOuse plus $29 to $129 for the attachments, GlassOuse.com)

• **Software that takes dictation.** Dragon NaturallySpeaking is not the only software program that converts spoken words into typed text on a screen, but it is the most accurate. While most apps and programs that attempt this are prone to misunderstandings, NaturallySpeaking learns your accent and speech patterns so that the more you use it, the more accurate it becomes. The company that makes this software has been improving its speech-recognition software for decades, so its products are some of the most sophisticated. (Nuance.com/dragon, purchase at Amazon.com)

• **Spill-avoiding spoon.** S'up Spoon has an easy-to-grip handle and a very deep head (almost like a pipe) to cut down on spills. ($24.34, with shipping from the UK, Sup-Products.com)

Alternative: Liftware Steady is a high-tech spoon that has sensors and motors hidden in its handle to counteract hand tremors. The head of the spoon remains largely steady even if your hand does not. Fork and spork attachments also are available. ($195, Liftware.com/steady)

• **Pour hot liquids without spills.** "Kettle tippers" such as Maxi Aids' The Tipper are not new or high-tech, but they are quite useful. They support the weight of a kettle as you pour, reducing the odds of spills and burns. ($37.95, MaxiAids.com/the-tipper)

Limited Eyesight or Blindness

Useful items for people who have vision problems…

• **Glasses that use sound to paint a picture of your surroundings.** Eyesynth smartglasses scan the area in front of the wearer and convert the visual environment into a tonal soundscape. With practice, users can learn to interpret its sounds so that they can navigate indoor and outdoor areas—it's a little like having sonar. Eyesynth creates its soundscape using only tones, not words, and it does so through small vibrations in the user's facial bones rather than with an earpiece, so it is not overly distracting. The company is getting ready to release the product, but you can reserve one for a deposit of about $600. (Final price expected to be about $2,800. Eyesynth.com/?lang=en)

• **Cane that warns of obstacles.** UltraCane uses ultrasonic waves (people can't hear them) to identify upcoming obstacles. It then silently warns its user about these obstacles via vibrations in its handle. Unlike conventional canes, it identifies obstacles at head or chest height, such as low tree branches, in addition to those at or near ground level. ($1,295, UltraCane.com, shipped from the UK)

• **Easy way to access the Internet via voice.** Amazon Echo speakers weren't designed for the blind, but devices such as this that offer access to a "virtual assistant" can be tremendously useful for people who cannot see (and for people who have limited use of their hands, too). You can ask Echo's virtual assistant, Alexa, to check your messages, place a phone call, look up information online, play music and more—all with your voice. ($99.99, Amazon.com)

Alternative: The Amazon Echo Plus does everything the Echo does and serves as a smarthome hub. Together with compatible smarthome devices, you could tell Alexa to lock or unlock your doors…adjust your thermostat…or turn on or off any device that plugs into a power outlet. ($149.99 plus chosen smarthome devices)

Hearing/Speaking

A pair of products for people who suffer from hearing loss or who communicate via sign language…

• **Headphones that let you hear even if your eardrums cannot.** AfterShokz headphones convey sound through small vibrations in the cheekbones, bypassing the eardrums.

They're a way for people who have eardrum damage or certain other ear problems to hear again. These headphones can be used to listen to music or podcasts, but if you combine AfterShokz with a smartphone and the Petralex sound-amplification app (Petralex.pro, free for iOS or Android), it could improve your ability to hear ambient sounds around you, too. Note that although AfterShokz headphones bypass the eardrums, a functioning inner ear still is needed for them to successfully convey sound. ($49.95 to $179.95 depending on model selected—higher-end models are lighter and offer wireless Bluetooth connectivity, among other advantages, AfterShokz.com)

Chapter 2

BRAIN HEALTH

For Most Older Women with Breast Cancer, Brain Function Stays Intact After Chemo

If you're an older woman with breast cancer, we have some good news...and some not-so-good news. The largest US study looking at the question of brain function following treatment for breast cancer contains a bit of both.

Background: Because aging adults often worry about their memory and cognitive abilities, researchers from Georgetown University Medical Center wanted to investigate how breast cancer and its treatment may affect brain function in older patients.

Study details: To analyze this question, researchers compared 344 women who had been newly diagnosed with nonmetastatic breast cancer (cancer that has not spread beyond the breast) with 347 women without cancer. The women in both groups were age 60 and older and similar in their education levels, lifestyles and other factors.

When the research began—and before the women with breast cancer started their treatment—both groups of women took a series of 13 neuropsychological tests that assessed their attention, thinking, learning and memory skills. At that time, none of the study participants had cognitive problems or dementia. The women with cancer then received treatment with chemotherapy with or without hormonal therapy. All the women then took the same series of tests one year and two years later.

Good news: The study found that most older women treated for breast cancer do not experience any cancer-related cognitive difficulties, including having trouble remembering or taking longer to complete everyday tasks, within the first two years of diagnosis and treatment.

However: For a small subset of women—those who have one or two copies of the APOE4 gene, which has been found to significantly increase risk of developing Alzheimer's disease—a steady decline in cognitive function occurred after chemotherapy compared with patients without the APOE4 gene and noncancer study participants.

"It is not that the chemotherapy causes Alzheimer's disease, but that these patients

The study "Cancer-Related Cognitive Outcomes Among Older Breast Cancer Survivors in the Thinking and Living with Cancer Study," conducted by researchers at Georgetown University Medical Center and published in *Journal of Clinical Oncology.*

may be at risk for both cancer-related cognitive problems and Alzheimer's—perhaps through a process of accelerated aging or other shared disease processes," explained Jeanne Mandelblatt, MD, MPH, lead author of the study and professor of oncology at Georgetown Lombardi Comprehensive Cancer Center.

Bottom line: Most older women with breast cancer do not have to worry about the cognitive effects of treatment. But women who are APOE4-positive do appear to be more vulnerable to such adverse effects. If these preliminary results are replicated and confirmed by other trials, testing for the APOE4 gene may become part of breast cancer care to ensure that each woman receives the safest and most effective treatment.

Breakthrough Way to Prevent Mild Cognitive Impairment and Early Dementia

Jeff D. Williamson, MD, MHS, professor of gerontology and geriatric medicine, department of internal medicine, Sticht Center for Healthy Aging and Alzheimer's Prevention, Wake Forest School of Medicine, Winston-Salem, North Carolina. Study titled, "Effect of Intensive vs Standard Blood Pressure Control on Probable Dementia," by researchers at the SPRINT Research Group, National Institutes of Health, published in *JAMA*.

Mild cognitive impairment (MCI) isn't dementia…but for approximately one out of five people who has it, dementia is the inevitable result. Exciting new research now finds that a treatment that protects your brain from stroke may also help avert MCI…and perhaps dementia down the road.

MCI is age-related cognitive decline in memory, language, thinking and judgment that is more than normal aging but not as serious as actual dementia. It has long been known that high blood pressure, a prime

risk factor for stroke, is linked to memory loss. It is thought that high blood pressure may damage tiny blood vessels in the brain, which leads to inflammation, a prime factor in both MCI and dementia.

Researchers from the National Institutes of Health SPRINT Research Group looked at whether intensively treating high blood pressure would reduce the risk for both MCI and dementia. They conducted a randomized, controlled trial of more than 9,000 adults age 50 or older who had no history of stroke or diabetes and had high blood pressure (systolic: 130 to 180…140 average).

Half the participants received drugs to lower their blood pressure with a target of systolic below 140 (standard treatment). The other half were treated to lower their blood pressure to a target systolic below 120 (intensive treatment). Both groups were treated for three and a half years and followed for about five years…and were tested for evidence of MCI and probable dementia before, during and at the end of the study.

Results: Participants in the standard group maintained an average systolic blood pressure of about 135…while the intensive group maintained an average systolic pressure of about 122. Compared with the standard treatment group, participants who got intensive treatment had a statistically significant 19% lower risk for MCI. The intensive group also had a 17% lower risk for dementia—a result that is not considered statistically significant and could still be from chance.

According to the researchers, as well as other experts in the field, these results are impressive! In fact, the Alzheimer's Association has sponsored a continuation of the study for another round of cognitive testing at eight years, since it can take additional years for dementia to develop.

While more research is needed to determine the best practical application of these results, if you're older than age 50 and are being treated for high blood pressure it makes sense to discuss with your doctor whether your blood pressure is controlled enough. And if you and your doctor agree that it is not and more treatment might be a good idea, be sure to discuss both the benefits and the risks.

New Ways to Make Your Brain Act 20 Years Younger

Sandra Bond Chapman, PhD, founder and chief director of the Center for BrainHealth at The University of Texas at Dallas, Dee Wyly Distinguished University Professor at its School of Behavioral and Brain Sciences, lead researcher of the study "Enhancing Innovation and Underlying Neural Mechanisms Via Cognitive Training in Healthy Older Adults," published in *Frontiers in Aging Neuroscience*, and author of *Make Your Brain Smarter: Increase Your Brain's Creativity, Energy, and Focus*, which includes all nine of the strategies used in the study.

I f it seems like you've heard conflicting advice in the media about brain games and other ways to make your brain "younger," you're right. A few years ago, pricey brain-game software (and hours at the computer) were thought to accomplish this…and then, soon after, almost completely discredited. In fact, physical exercise, like Ping-Pong and dancing, have held the brain-preservation spotlight recently.

Well, our knowledge about what can really keep your brain humming keeps getting better, and now, according to a new study from the Center for BrainHealth at The University of Texas at Dallas, simple yet direct brain-training exercises—not games—should be part of any plan to keep your brain young because they can make your brain act 20 years younger. Will this be the last word on brain preservation? Of course not. But when it comes to these latest exercises, they are proved scientifically…they don't take up a lot of time…and it won't cost you anything to try them.

For the 12-week study, 58 cognitively normal people ranging in age from 56 to 75 were randomly divided into three groups—a cognitive-training group, a physical exercise group and a control group.

Members of the cognitive-training group attended weekly 60-minute sessions where they participated in cognitive exercises designed by the researchers that were intended to strengthen "innovative cognition," which is needed for adaptive and flexible thinking—the ability to react to challenging and changing life demands. They also spent two hours a week on homework assignments involving these exercises (we'll share three of them below).

Members of the exercise group did three 60-minute physical workouts per week, alternating between a treadmill and stationary bike. The control group just went on with their lives as usual.

Using MRI scanners, researchers measured how well participants' neurons were working (their "connectivity"), blood flow in the brain and the amount of glucose (energy) their brains used at the beginning, middle and end of the study. Only members of the cognitive-training group showed significant changes—a 30% increase in neuron connectivity on average, an 8% increase in blood flow, the brain's energy supply, and a 17% increase in regional white matter, the fiber bundles that connect different parts of the brain.

Translation? At the end of the study, the cognitive-training group had, on average, improved their brains' fitness so that they worked in many ways like the brains of people 20 years younger. The improved blood flow and regional connectivity were associated with an enhanced ability to think creatively and perform complex reasoning. Thus, greater brain fitness produced higher cognitive performance.

Important: Even though the physical exercise group did not show improved brain function, don't skip fitness workouts. Exercise still conveys benefits ranging from increased fitness and overall physical health to reduced inflammation—and inflammation can be harmful to the brain. So physical exercise does help your brain but in different ways.

Brain Exercises That Work

Here are three of the study's cognitive exercises that you can use to improve your brain function starting right now...

•**Strategic attention.** Every day, identify two daily tasks that require fairly deep thinking, such as tracking and analyzing your budget, following a complex new recipe, writing meaningful, personal thank-you notes—or pondering the actionable takeaways from an article about the benefits of cognitive exercises.

Then carve out two 30-minute uninterrupted sessions to focus on them. Choose the time of day you usually feel sharpest. But no matter when it is, make sure that the environment is quiet—no cell phones or any other devices to distract you. And don't get up for a snack or a drink or do anything that will take you off your task during these 30-minute blocks. Why? Because it can take up to 20 minutes to get back on track after an interruption.

Benefit: Over time, you'll find that you can accomplish tasks more quickly and with greater focus.

•**Five by five.** Five times a day, intentionally do nothing for five minutes. Stop whatever you're doing—step away from your desk or laptop, for instance—and let your brain rest, empty out and reset. Just as the muscles in your body need a rest after a long run or strenuous workout, your brain needs to rest after working hard. Do not use the time to plan your vacation or the rest of your day in your head or anything of the sort. You can take a walk or sit still, but don't read, play music or listen to an audiobook. Enjoy the silence and lack of stimulation.

Sometimes it will be obvious when you need these breaks, such as when pushing yourself to keep going on a task is netting little result.

Benefit: Taking brain breaks helps you find clarity, collect your thoughts and, often, see things in a new way.

•**Innovative thinking.** Become aware of and increase the moments when your brain innovates—in other words, create more "aha" moments. You say that it's not possible to purposely create innovative thoughts? Oh, yes, it is! The trick is to get yourself out of your familiar ruts—try a new experience, take on a new challenge, seek ways to improve an existing relationship or an ongoing logistical challenge. Brain "aha" moments usually come when you have brain downtime, when you are in the shower, driving without the radio on or in nature with no earbuds. The more you embrace the brain's capacity to improve even routine activities, tasks and conversations, the greater will be your innovative brainpower.

Start by trying to have at least one innovative thought each day, and work your way up from there as you get better at it. But don't just think these thoughts. As soon as you realize that you see a better way to do or say something, write it down and put some aspect of it into practice. Keep an innovation diary, and challenge yourself to see how many times you innovate each day or week. The strongest brain changes come with the implementation of innovative ideas—just thinking them is not enough.

Benefit: By challenging yourself to do and act on innovative thinking, you put your brain in unknown territory and activate the neurotransmitter norepinephrine, the brain's wonder drug that speeds learning and makes it longer lasting. Additionally, innovative problem-solving helps reduce your fear of failure and fear of the unknown—the awe of a new experience actually recharges the brain.

Carving out blocks of time and keeping a tally of your brain breaks and innovation attempts can seem daunting at first. It's OK to start slowly and gradually add to the time you spend on cognitive exercises. Once you start seeing the benefits in your daily life, you'll want to make more time for these exercises, and they will become a habit.

And that's key: For cognitive exercises to work, you need to do them regularly.

Beware of "Skinny Fat" —a New Dementia Risk

The study "Sarcopenic Obesity and Cognitive Performance" led by researchers at Florida Atlantic University Comprehensive Center for Brain Health in the Charles E. Schmidt College of Medicine in Boca Raton, Florida, and published in *Clinical Interventions in Aging*.

For most people, losing muscle mass as they get older is as natural as going gray. But unlike the silver streak in your hair, reduced strength and muscle mass may signal a dangerous risk—especially if you're carrying extra body fat.

Background: We've long known that loss of muscle mass (a condition known as sarcopenia) is bad for our health, increasing our risk for falls and a loss of physical independence. It's also widely known that being overweight or obese sets us up to develop heart disease, diabetes and other chronic ailments.

When it comes to brain health, research has also shown that sarcopenia and obesity are independently linked to cognitive impairment.

Exception: In people over age 70, extra body weight seems to protect against dementia, for reasons that aren't fully understood.

With this evidence in hand, researchers wanted to learn how the combination of sarcopenia and obesity affects one's risk for various forms of dementia, including Alzheimer's disease.

To study this question, researchers took precise body measurements and performed a thorough cognitive assessment on 353 adults, with an average age of 69. The researchers then determined which of the participants had sarcopenia and were also obese based on their percentage of body fat mass—a condition known as sarcopenic obesity or

"skinny fat." Interestingly, the "skinny" term comes into play because people with sarcopenic obesity tend to look less overweight than those who are simply obese.

In analyzing the data, researchers had to contend with some tricky definitions that are used for both sarcopenia and obesity. Traditionally, sarcopenia has been defined as low muscle mass. Now, some experts also include low muscle function in the definition—as determined, for example, by grip strength. Obesity, too, has been defined various ways. The conventional definition is tied to body mass index (BMI), which is the ratio of a person's weight-to-height…or it can be defined based on the percentage of body fat.

Study results: Adults who could be described as "skinny fat"—that is, they had sarcopenia, defined by the combination of low muscle mass and low muscle strength, along with a high percentage of body fat—were the most likely to have lower cognitive function. The combination of those features was more strongly linked to cognitive decline, followed by sarcopenia alone and then obesity alone.

Takeaway: Maintaining muscle strength while preventing excess body fat may help protect your cognitive ability as you get older.

Why Your Brain Needs a Glucose Fix

Lisa Mosconi, PhD, associate director of the Alzheimer's Prevention Clinic at Weill Cornell Medical College, NewYork-Presbyterian Hospital in New York City, where she is also associate professor of neuroscience in neurology…and adjunct faculty member in the department of psychiatry at New York University School of Medicine, also in New York City. She is author of *Brain Food: The Surprising Science of Eating for Cognitive Power*. LisaMosconi.com

For health-conscious people everywhere, "glucose"—a specific type of sugar—has become the enemy. After all, a high-sugar diet has been linked to obesity, diabetes and many more health problems. *But…*

Did you know that while the organs and tissues in your body are mainly fueled by carbohydrates and fats, 99% of the fuel the brain uses comes from glucose? In fact, glucose is essential to keep your brain in top form. *In the brain, glucose…*

• **Turns into ATP,** the fuel that powers all cellular activity, including the activity of billions of brain cells (neurons).

• **Helps produce neurotransmitters,** the chemical messengers that send signals across synapses from neuron to neuron. Without neurotransmitters, you couldn't think, feel or move. For example, the brain's most abundant neurotransmitter—glutamate, an "excitatory" (or energizing) neurotransmitter active in 90% of synapses—can't be manufactured without glucose. Similarly, GABA, an "inhibitory" (or calming) neurotransmitter, depends entirely on glucose for its production.

• **Stimulates the plasticity of neurons so that they don't shrivel and die off.**

When your brain doesn't get the glucose it needs, memory, focus and reasoning decline. In a worst-case scenario, without sufficient glucose, you could end up with Alzheimer's disease.

New study: In a scientific paper published in *Frontiers in Aging and Neuroscience,* Lisa Mosconi, PhD, associate director of the Alzheimer's Prevention Clinic at Weill Cornell Medical College/NewYork-Presbyterian Hospital and her colleagues stress that Alzheimer's disease develops over decades, and that preventing or delaying the disease requires addressing the factors that lead to it.

Perhaps the most notable factor identified in the development of Alzheimer's was a slowdown in glucose metabolism, or the rate at which the brain burns glucose. Getting sufficient glucose speeds glucose metabolism and is a must for mental performance—particularly as you age.

Here, Dr. Mosconi tells how to make sure your brain gets the glucose it needs…

The Best Way to Get Glucose

Getting enough glucose for your brain does not mean eating a diet rich in refined sugar and carbohydrates such as candy, bread, pasta and baked goods. These foods do contain a very small amount of glucose but also a massive amount of other sugars. These other sugars get converted to glucose but, in the process, are hard on the liver and pancreas, increasing insulin levels.

The best foods to provide immediate glucose to the brain are root and other vegetables, fruits and whole grains—key components of the Mediterranean diet.

These foods provide the glucose needed while minimizing the total amount of sugar ingested to avoid high blood sugar and other health problems.

New study: In a three-year study I coauthored and published in *Neurology,* individuals who closely followed a Mediterranean-style diet preserved glucose metabolism in their brains—while those who ate a typical Western diet had decreases in glucose metabolism. Additionally, declining rates of glucose metabolism were associated with increased Alzheimer's plaques.

Glucose-rich foods: 88% of the sugar in scallions is glucose…turnips (76%)…rutabagas (56%)…dried apricots (52%)…kiwifruit (48%)…grapes (40%)…onions (38%)…whole grains (36%)…red beets (31%)…and raw honey (30%).

To put this in perspective—two red beets contain 20% of your brain's daily glucose requirement, which is 62 g of glucose…and one cup of grapes will give your brain 17% of the glucose it needs for a day…but you would need to eat 16 pounds of chocolate chip cookies to achieve your daily goal!

In a study published in *Psychology and Aging,* older adults (ages 65 to 82) were among those given either a drink containing a small amount of glucose or a drink with an artificial sweetener. After consuming these drinks, they were asked to perform difficult mental tasks. The older adults who drank glucose had better memory, a more positive mood and were more engaged with the mental tasks, compared with those given the artificially sweetened drink.

For a quick mental boost: Add one teaspoon of glucose-rich raw honey to a cup of tea. Refined honey, like table sugar, is more likely to give you an energy crash later.

And for a brain-building breakfast or lunch: Try avocado toast with whole-grain bread. It delivers a hearty supply of glucose and brain-healthy monounsaturated fat.

The Vitamin That Can Boost Brain Health

George T. Grossberg, MD, Samuel W. Fordyce Professor of psychiatry and director of geriatric psychiatry at the Saint Louis University School of Medicine and coauthor of the study "The Role of Vitamin D in Cognitive Disorders in Older Adults," published in *Touch Neurology*.

The hardest vitamin to obtain through diet could be one of the most important ones for brain health. You already know vitamin D as a key building block for bones—but it also has a starring role in maintaining normal brain functions and protecting brain cells from damage, a role that grows as the brain ages.

With age, brain cells become more susceptible to damage from calcium-induced stress. Vitamin D may help prevent calcium from entering brain cells by blocking off key channels. It may also prevent brain-cell loss and increase the ability of nerve cells to communicate with one another, possibly by increasing activity of the neurotransmitter acetylcholine.

Vitamin D helps regulate the brain's immune system and inhibit the inflammatory mediators (cytokines) involved with immunity and inflammation. So when levels of vitamin D are low, the body has less ability to fight inflammation in the brain, inflammation that typically increases with age. This is important because inflammation that destroys brain cells may contribute to the cognitive decline seen in conditions such as Alzheimer's disease and Parkinson's disease. Low levels of vitamin D have also been linked to other forms of dementia, memory loss and depression. A research review in *Touch Neurology* pointed out that 70% to 90% of older adults with cognitive problems are deficient in the vitamin.

Making Up the "D"-ifference

The National Institutes of Health suggests that people age 50 to 70 get 600 IU of D a day, 800 IU per day for people age 71 or older. It's a challenge to get vitamin D naturally, especially as we age. Vitamin D is made by the skin, but only when the skin is exposed to enough sunlight. Seniors face two problems here. Many people spend more time indoors as they age. And even when you get enough sunlight, "older" skin—skin that has become thinner and more fragile—isn't as efficient at making vitamin D as it used to be. At age 70, your skin makes 50% less vitamin D than it did at age 20.

It also becomes progressively harder to get vitamin D through diet because problems such as gastritis and decreased liver metabolism, common in seniors, limit the body's ability to absorb vitamin D through the digestive system. Some people avoid dairy altogether because of lactose intolerance and/or GERD.

To treat or prevent vitamin-D deficiency, supplements are often the answer. But first it's important to find out your exact level of D with a blood test. In fact, if you're over age 60, you should get your vitamin-D level checked annually, or more often, if needed.

If you are low on D, talk to your doctor about a plan to get up to a brain-healthy level. Studies suggest a daily dose of 1,000 IU. (It's possible to overdose with vitamin-D supplements, but very unlikely as you would need to take the amount associated with toxicity of 10,000 to 40,000 IU per day.) Some people might need a high dose for a short period of time and then a lower maintenance dose. Your doctor can recheck your blood levels after a few months and adjust the dose as needed. The two forms available are D-2 and D-3. Most doctors agree that D-3 is more effective at raising levels of vitamin D.

Cell Phones Affect Your Memory

Cell phones may interfere with memory. After one year, nonverbal memory scores declined more for study subjects who spent more time talking on their cell phones. Nonverbal memory is processed in the right side of the brain, where most subjects held their phones. Texting and gaming did not affect memory. A high-quality connection and using wireless or wired headphones can drastically cut exposure to the brain.

Martin Röösli, PhD, is head of the environmental exposures and health unit, Swiss Tropical and Public Health Institute in Basel, Switzerland, and coauthor of a study of teenagers published in *Environmental Health Perspectives.*

Probiotics Can Cause Brain Fog

Satish S.C. Rao, MD, PhD, professor of medicine, director of neurogastroenterology, Medical College of Georgia, Augusta University, and coauthor of study titled "Brain Fogginess, Gas and Bloating: A Link between SIBO, Probiotics and Metabolic Acidosis," published in *Clinical and Translational Gastroenterology.*

Andrew Rubman, ND, naturopathic physician, medical director of the Southbury Clinic for Traditional Medicines in Southbury, Connecticut, and author of the Bottom Line blog "Nature Doc's Patient Diary."

Taking the healthful bacteria called probiotics can be great for gut health, but new research has uncovered a serious potential side effect—trouble thinking straight, aka brain fogginess.

Why would researchers even look for such a connection? It all started when Satish S.C. Rao, MD, director of neurogastroenterology at the Medical College of Georgia at Augusta University, noticed that a number of his pa-

tients with gastrointestinal symptoms had also been experiencing mental symptoms—confusion, impaired judgment, short-term memory problems and difficulty concentrating. The brain fogginess happened intermittently but usually after the patients ate—for four of them, the fogginess was so severe that it was interfering with their careers.

So he conducted a study of 38 patients who had GI complaints of bloating, stomach distention, pain and gas without any obvious cause. Thirty of these patients had not only the GI symptoms but also had complained of brain fogginess.

A variety of tests revealed that the patients with brain fogginess had up to three times the normal level of D-lactic acid, which is made in the gut. Under normal circumstances, D-lactic acid is produced in very small amounts, easily cleared by the kidneys. But when the body produces large amounts of D-lactic acid, the kidneys can't clear it all and it accumulates. The D-lactic acid is then able to enter the brain and cause brain fogginess. (*Note*: This is different from L-lactic acid, which can accumulate in muscle and cause muscle cramps during exercise.)

How did the patients get those high levels of D-lactic acid? The researchers were able to trace it back to their intake of probiotics. They found that in 68% of the patients on probiotics, the probiotics and other bacteria had colonized in the small bowel and produced a condition called SIBO, small intestinal bacterial overgrowth. Every time these bacteria came into contact with sugar—from the carbs in the patients' diets—D-lactic acid production went into overdrive. The result was the brain fogginess along with the GI symptoms. Once they stopped taking probiotics and were treated for bacterial overgrowth with antibiotics, both types of symptoms went away.

Probiotics, the Right Way

The problem isn't with probiotics themselves—Dr. Rao does prescribe them to some patients with GI issues. The problem is when people self-prescribe them (only four people in the group of 30 patients with brain fogginess were taking them after consulting with a health-care provider) and have other aggravating factors that can help set the stage for SIBO and high D-lactic acid levels.

Two known culprits are the heartburn drugs proton pump inhibitors, or PPIs, and opioid pain relievers, says Andrew Rubman, ND, medical director of Southbury Clinic for Traditional Medicines in Southbury, Connecticut.

PPIs make your stomach less acidic, but in doing so they change your gut microbiome and expose the small bowel to bacteria overgrowth. (To ease the occasional acid stomach, Dr. Rubman recommends skipping PPIs in favor of drinking a half-teaspoon of baking soda mixed into a half-cup of water between meals.)

Opioids slow your gut motility and can paralyze the small bowel, making it easier for bacteria to colonize there.

If you'd like to get only the benefits of probiotics, follow these guidelines…

• **Eat probiotic foods.** These include yogurt and kefir, pickled vegetables such as kimchi and sauerkraut, and tempeh and miso.

• **Eat prebiotic foods.** The fiber in these foods basically goes unchanged through the stomach and small bowel and acts as fuel for healthful bacteria in the colon. Prebiotic foods include onions, leeks, garlic, aspara-gus, Jerusalem artichoke, bananas, whole wheat, yams and sweet potatoes.

• **Get healthful guidance.** Have a medical evaluation to help you determine the right type and amount of supplemental probiotics for you. This is especially important if you have any health conditions, GI or otherwise, in order to avoid an adverse reaction. Don't take a probiotic supplement on your own.

Lithium: Not Just for Bipolar Disorder

James Greenblatt, MD, chief medical officer and vice president of medical services at Walden Behavioral Care in Waltham, Massachusetts. He has been studying the effects of low-dose lithium for 30 years and is author of *Nutritional Lithium: A Cinderella Story.* JamesGreenblattMD.com

Low-dose lithium may help prevent Alzheimer's…calm chronic irritability and anger…and ease depression.

Wait a second, you say to yourself—isn't lithium a serious drug for psychiatric conditions like bipolar disorder? Yes, in high doses of 150 mg to 1,800 mg. But in very low doses (say, 1 mg to 5 mg), lithium is a nutritional treatment, uniquely effective for a range of problems. *Here's what you need to know…*

Alzheimer's Disease

It's becoming widely accepted by scientists that the neurochemical changes that lead to Alzheimer's develop over a period of decades—and that prevention is the goal.

In my medical opinion, lithium may be the most effective preventive agent. *Research is ongoing, but here are some key studies that support that statement…*

• **Low-dose lithium helps lower the risk for Alzheimer's.** A Brazilian study published in *British Journal of Psychiatry* involved 41 seniors with mild cognitive impairment, the memory loss and mental decline that often precedes Alzheimer's. Half were given low-dose lithium and half, a placebo. After one

---

Taking a Photo Undermines Your Memory

Possible reasons: Using a camera causes the photographer to decrease engagement, relying instead on the camera. Or the effort of taking a photo may make photographers feel as if they are immersed in whatever they are photographing—even though, in reality, they are not absorbing it as they normally would.

Study by researchers at University of California, Santa Cruz, published in Journal of Applied Research in Memory and Cognition.

year, more of the people taking lithium had no mental decline, better memory, more focus and clearer thinking. Just 19% of those on lithium developed Alzheimer's compared with 35% in the placebo group.

● **Low-dose lithium helps treat Alzheimer's.** In another study, published in *Current Alzheimer Research*, 94 people with mild-to-moderate Alzheimer's were similarly divided into two groups. The lithium group had no cognitive decline during the 15 months of the study, while mental decline progressed by 20% in the placebo group.

● **Lithium improves sleep and eases agitation and psychosis.** In a case study report on three Alzheimer's patients with these symptoms, researchers from Columbia University Medical Center found that prescribing low-dose lithium led to dramatic changes in just two weeks—a normal sleep cycle and a marked decrease in symptoms.

How it helps: Lithium is a GSK-3 inhibitor—that means it blocks the enzyme GSK-3 to, in turn, stop the accumulation of plaques (beta-amyloid) and tangles, the changes that signal the development and advance of Alzheimer's. It improves the connections between neurons, triggers the growth of new neurons and boosts a protein that stops neurons from dying.

Lithium also protects against brain inflammation and oxidation and increases serotonin, which regulates mood and behavior.

Irritability and Anger

Because it improves problems with impulse control, nutritional lithium has a uniquely calming effect, demonstrated in research involving people with post-traumatic stress disorder (PTSD) and published in *Journal of Traumatic Stress*.

Depression and Suicide

Lithium may be an effective way to combat the rise in suicide. Research done around the world has found that the lower the levels of lithium in the water and soil (it's a naturally occurring trace element), the higher the rate of suicide.

A study published in *Journal of Psychiatric Research* compared the suicide rate in 226 Texas counties with 3,123 lithium samples from the public water supply.

Finding: Lower suicide rates were linked to higher lithium levels in the water.

Research done in Lithuania and published in *Journal of Trace Elements in Medicine and Biology* found the same was true for men, in particular, and suggested that lithium may decrease suicide risk, which is two to four times higher among men than women.

Bipolar Disorder

Pharmaceutical lithium is an effective treatment for bipolar disorder, but high doses can cause hand tremors, increased thirst, nausea, diarrhea, abdominal distress and even kidney disease. Low-dose lithium may produce positive results…without the health problems.

In fact, research published in *Experimental and Therapeutic Medicine* found that personalized dosing at lower levels than commonly prescribed can be helpful without causing the side effects of the typical prescription dose.

How to Use Lithium

Besides drinking water, naturally occurring lithium is in vegetables, grains, eggs and milk, but you can't reliably get enough lithium from your diet to make a symptom-controlling difference.

My advice: I recommend 2.5 mg of over-the-counter lithium (see next page) daily for prevention of cognitive decline or for chronic irritability…and 2.5 mg to 5 mg if you have symptoms of cognitive decline.

Also: If you have a personal or family history of bipolar disorder, substance abuse, suicide (or suicide attempts) or use prescription medication, see a physician before taking any lithium on your own.

Caution: Thyroid disorders and kidney disease can be caused by pharmaceutical lithium. If you have any health problem involving the thyroid or kidneys, talk to your doctor before using any lithium.

The Right Lithium...

For low-dose nutritional lithium, look for lithium orotate or lithium citrate, available over-the-counter. Avoid lithium aspartate, which can cause neurons to transmit impulses at a rapid rate and trigger headaches and brain inflammation in some people.

When to Start Levodopa for Parkinson's Disease

Study titled "Randomized Delayed-Start Trial of Levodopa in Parkinson's Disease," led by researchers at University of Amsterdam, the Netherlands, published in *The New England Journal of Medicine*.

L evodopa (Sinemet) is the most effective medicine used to treat Parkinson's disease. In fact, nearly everyone who has the disease will need it eventually. But there has long been a debate over whether it's better to start the drug as soon as symptoms start—or hold out as long as possible to put off dealing with the risks associated with taking levodopa. *New research now has the answer...*

But first, some background...Parkinson's disease (PD) is a progressive brain disease in which nerve cells in the brain that produce the chemical dopamine, a neurotransmitter needed to send signals between cells, gradually die. As the brain cells die, symptoms such as body tremors and slowed movement begin to interfere with daily activities. There is no cure for PD. Instead, symptoms are managed, typically with levodopa, a drug that converts to dopamine in the brain. Some research has found that starting levodopa soon after diagnosis—before symptoms curtail lifestyle—may slow progression of the disease. But other research has found that starting levodopa early actually may speed the loss of dopamine-producing brain cells... that the brain starts to depend more on drug-

dopamine than on naturally produced dopamine. The resulting irregular brain levels of dopamine increase risk for dyskinesia, uncontrolled, jerky or writhing movement.

To learn more, researchers from University of Amsterdam in the Netherlands compared early versus delayed start of levodopa in 445 recently diagnosed PD patients whose symptoms were not severe enough to need the drug and who had never received any other treatment for their PD.

Half the patients were randomly assigned to receive a standard dose of levodopa for 80 weeks. The other half received a placebo for 40 weeks...and then levodopa for 40 weeks. Neither patients nor researchers knew which patients were in which group. Patients had their PD rated according to a standard test that measures mental and physical symptoms of the disease, as well as how much activities of daily life are affected. The average score for both groups at the start of the study was between 28 and 29 (out of a possible score of 176, with a higher score meaning more severe disease).

Results: The researchers expected to find that the early starters would have about a four-point advantage in their PD score at the end of the study. But in fact, there was no significant difference between the groups—a one-point improvement for early starters compared with a two-point improvement for late starters.

While it's true that the study didn't find any benefit to starting the drug early, it didn't find any added risk in doing so either—88% of patients in the delayed group and 90% of patients in the early group had no evidence of dyskinesia. These results indicate that it's safe to start the drug whenever a patient (and his/her doctor) feels that it's the right time.

Yet even without dyskinesia, levodopa still has side effects (including drowsiness, nausea, dry mouth, diarrhea, constipation, insomnia among others) that you may want to put off dealing with until the PD symptoms become truly bothersome. But at least now you have more choice.

The Parkinson's Rx: A Strong Dose of Exercise

Marilyn Moffat, PT, DPT, PhD, professor of physical therapy at New York University in New York City, immediate past president of the World Confederation for Physical Therapy and past president of the American Physical Therapy Association. She is coauthor of *Age-Defying Fitness: Making the Most of Your Body for the Rest of Your Life.*

You might assume that anyone who moves slowly, isn't sure-footed and has hand or arm tremors should shy away from exercise. But when these symptoms are caused by Parkinson's disease (PD), nothing could be further from the truth.

What you need to know about exercise if you or a loved one has PD…

Rx for Heart and Brain

After Alzheimer's disease, PD is the most common neurodegenerative disease in the US. It causes serious motor changes—such as rigid muscles, tremors and balance problems—along with non-motor symptoms such as fatigue, depression and constipation…and it almost always worsens over time.

Drug treatments, such as *carbidopa-levodopa* (Sinemet) and *ropinirole* (Requip), can ease some of the symptoms, but the effectiveness of medications tends to wane over time. That's why researchers have looked for other treatments that can both improve symptoms and prevent the disease from worsening.

Aerobic workouts that tax the cardiovascular system appear to be the ticket. While weight training can improve balance and muscle strength (both important for PD), it doesn't seem to confer the wide-ranging benefits that accrue from fast biking, treadmill training, challenging dance sessions or other cardiovascular workouts.

Harder Is Better

Until recently, doctors routinely advised patients with PD, particularly those who weren't regular exercisers, to take it slow and easy. It seemed unrealistic—and possibly unsafe—to encourage physically impaired patients to go all-out.

New thinking: An increasing body of evidence now shows that intense workouts are more effective for patients with PD than slow walks, easy bike rides and other light physical activity.

Complex Beats Simple

Intense exercise is believed to offer such significant benefits because it increases blood flow to the brain. But additional research suggests that intensity is just part of the picture. Learning-based workouts—things that require close attention and involve frequent changes of direction, tempo, balance, etc.—are better than merely moving at a fast clip because they incorporate a cognitive component.

Physical therapists who specialize in PD also have developed workouts that draw from tai chi, kayaking, boxing, Pilates and other exercises that involve challenging combinations of movements. The workouts are more effective than repetitive types of exercise, such as straight-ahead walking or weight lifting.

A good example is a boxing-style workout known as Rock Steady Boxing. Designed for patients with PD, it emphasizes full-body movements that challenge gait, speed, hand-eye coordination and balance. During a session, participants (depending on their physical abilities/limitations) will do myriad boxing maneuvers, heel-walks, skipping, jumping rope, etc.

The workouts require participants to constantly monitor what their bodies are doing and to make adjustments—in balance, tempo, etc.—on the fly. A study in *Physical Therapy*, the journal of the American Physical Therapy Association, found that patients with PD who attended two to three boxing sessions a week for nine months had both short- and long-term improvements in balance and other physical parameters. They also reported having a better quality of life.

Exercise for Life

If you've been diagnosed with PD, your neurologist will probably refer you to a physical therapist. If he/she doesn't, insist on it. Insurance usually covers a certain number of visits.

Most large cities will have dozens of therapist-led exercise programs for PD. (Search online for "Parkinson's disease physical therapy centers" to find one near you. Or contact the American Parkinson Disease Association, 800-223-2732, APDAparkinson.org. Click on "APDA in your community" to locate your local chapter for resources, including exercise programs, in your area.) The key is to find something you like...that addresses all of the body's systems affected by the disease...and that you think you'll keep doing. *My advice...*

• **Start at your level.** Avoid overdoing it when you first start working out—but don't stay at a beginner level any longer than you have to. If you're new to exercise and/or have advanced symptoms, you might start out by, say, holding weighted poles while sitting and performing kayaking movements or doing slow Nordic walking (using walking poles). However, don't waste too much time on "baby steps." Push yourself to the next level as soon as you can.

• **Go for intensity.** As discussed earlier, intense workouts are more effective than easygoing exercises. An intense workout is one that increases your heart rate to 70% to 85% of your maximum capacity. If you don't use a heart-rate monitor, you can gauge intensity by how you feel—your breathing will be rapid...you'll be sweating within a few minutes...and you'll only be able to speak a few words.

• **Keep it interesting.** You want a program that not only challenges your body but also forces you to master (and memorize) complex routines and movements.

Examples: Forward and backward walking on a treadmill...tai chi...dance movements with frequent changes of tempo and direction...and boxing-style workouts.

• **Make a commitment.** While patients with PD can work out on their own, many enjoy the dynamics of a group exercise program, which also helps them to push themselves harder. The key is to find a high-intensity workout that fits one's lifestyle and allows for a long-term commitment to enhance well-being and functional ability.

PD Drugs That Work Against Each Other

People with Parkinson's disease (PD) may be taking "opposing" drugs. About 45% of PD patients taking an acetylcholinesterase inhibitor to treat cognitive impairment, which is common in PD, were also prescribed an anticholinergic medication.

Problem: Anticholinergic drugs, which treat overactive bladder, allergies and PD symptoms, decrease cognition.

Allison W. Willis, MD, MS, assistant professor of neurology and epidemiology, Perelman School of Medicine, University of Pennsylvania, Philadelphia.

What Is Charcot-Marie-Tooth Disease?

Janice F. Wiesman, MD, FAAN, clinical associate professor of neurology, New York University School of Medicine, New York City, and author of *Peripheral Neuropathy: What It Is and What You Can Do to Feel Better.*

Charcot-Marie-Tooth disease (or CMT) is one of the most common inherited neurological diseases, affecting about one in every 2,500 Americans. People with CMT have a genetic mutation that affects the way the peripheral nerves in the arms, hands, feet and legs function.

The first signs of CMT are often clumsiness, frequent tripping and/or a feeling of numbness and/or coldness in the hands and/or feet. Symptoms can appear in childhood, adolescence or middle age and progress slowly, but a patient may eventually have muscle wasting in the lower legs and feet and/or atrophy in the hands.

Anyone who has a family member with CMT or who experiences the symptoms above should get checked out by a neurologist with expertise in this field (find one at CMTAusa.org).

CMT is diagnosed with a neurological exam, including a check of reflexes, skin sensation and gait. But further testing may be needed. MRI scans may be used in diagnosis and to monitor progress of the disease.

It's treated with physical and occupational therapy. Some patients may need leg braces, custom footwear and/or hearing aids. There's no cure, but people can manage symptoms with treatment.

Seasonal Brain "Aging"

The ability to think, concentrate and remember was better in the late summer and early fall than in the winter and spring among more than 3,000 older adults in a recent Canadian study. Called seasonal plasticity of cognition, the difference in cognition was the equivalent of almost five years of brain age.

One theory: Seasonal changes in hormones affect cognition.

Marc E. Agronin, MD, senior vice president for behavioral health, Miami Jewish Health, Florida.

The Nose Knows

To test memory retrieval, researchers asked study participants to breathe through their noses or through their mouths for one hour after learning 12 different smells on two separate occasions. This is the period when memory is generally consolidated—between learning and memory retrieval.

Result: After breathing through their noses, participants remembered the smells about 8% better. Researchers theorize that nose breathing may aid communication between sensory and memory networks in the brain.

Artin Arshamian, PhD, assistant professor, department of clinical neuroscience, Karolinska Institutet, Stockholm, Sweden.

Bacteria on the Brain

Oral bacteria can travel to the brain and might trigger Alzheimer's disease. A laboratory study found that animals exposed to periodontal-disease bacteria had higher amounts of amyloid beta, the same plaque that occurs with Alzheimer's.

PLOS ONE.

Curcumin Fights Dementia

Bill Gottlieb, CHC, is a natural health coach in Middletown, California, certified by the American Association of Drugless Practitioners. He is author of 16 health books that have sold three million copies including *Speed Healing*. His Bottom Line videos can be found at Bottom LineInc.com/author/bill-gottlieb. BillGottliebHealth.com

Specially formulated supplements of curcumin—the active ingredient in the spice turmeric—improve memory and focus in people who don't have dementia. They also may reduce the risk of developing Alzheimer's disease.

Scientific evidence: Researchers at UCLA Longevity Center recruited 40 healthy middle-aged and elderly people. For 18 months, 21 of them took a curcumin supplement twice daily, while 19 took a placebo. At the beginning and again at the end of the study, their short-term verbal and visual memory abilities—such as recalling memorized words and images—were tested. And their brains were scanned for toxic amyloid plaques and tau tangles, two signs of Alzheimer's.

Key findings: After 18 months, participants taking curcumin had significantly improved results on the memory tests. (*Bonus:* They also had improved mood.) Participants taking the placebo had little or no improvement in memory. What's more, the follow-up brain scans showed that the curcumin group, compared with the placebo group, had lower levels of amyloid and tau deposits.

The Right Kind of Curcumin Supplement

While curcumin in its natural state—in the spice turmeric and in many supplements—is poorly absorbed by the body, there are five formulations that research has shown are well-absorbed. The UCLA researchers used one of them, Theracurmin, at a dose of 90 mg twice daily. (A one-month supply costs about $53.) The other four are Meriva, Curcumin C3 Complex, BCM-95 and CurcuWIN. All are available online.

More research is needed before we know whether curcumin supplements actually prevent Alzheimer's disease. Curcumin supplements have a strong safety record, but they can cause stomach upset in some people. And they act as blood thinners, so doctors generally say that curcumin should not be taken by people using blood-thinning drugs. To determine whether curcumin is safe for you—and what a proper dose might be—it's best to work with a doctor who has studied this supplement.

If you take curcumin, though, you may find that you experience more benefits. It's a powerful anti-inflammatory and antioxidant that has been found to help relieve arthritis pain, ease muscle soreness after exercise and relieve allergy symptoms.

Simple Memory Strategy

Want to remember something important? Read it out loud. That was the conclusion of researchers who asked 95 people to use four different strategies to remember material—reading silently…listening to someone else read it…listening to a recording of their own voice reading it…or reading it aloud. Why reading aloud works: The physical act of voicing the words and then hearing them spoken aloud makes the material more distinctive…and therefore more memorable.

Colin MacLeod, PhD, professor of psychology, and Noah Forrin, PhD, researcher, University of Waterloo, Ontario, Canada.

Gentle Exercise Can Reverse Cognitive Decline in Just Six Months

Gentle exercise may reverse cognitive decline in as little as six months. Among people with cardiovascular disease risks who never exercised and had verified cognitive concerns but not dementia, those who exercised three times a week for six months—while following the heart-healthy DASH diet—averaged 47 points on a scale testing executive-thinking skills at the end of the study. Those who exercised but did not follow the diet averaged 42 points…those who did not exercise or follow the diet averaged 38. Exercise included a 10-minute warm-up followed by 35 minutes of continuous walking or stationary cycling.

James Blumenthal, PhD, professor of psychiatry and behavioral sciences, Duke University School of Medicine, Durham, North Carolina, and leader of a study of 160 adults, published in *Neurology.*

To Improve Your Memory, Try Pink Noise

Michael Breus, PhD, clinical psychologist, Manhattan Beach, California, and a fellow of The American Academy of Sleep Medicine. He is author of *The Power of When: Discover Your Chronotype—and the Best Time to Eat Lunch, Ask for a Raise, Have Sex, Write a Novel, Take Your Meds, and More.* TheSleep Doctor.com

Lots of people use "white noise" machines while they sleep to drown out the sound of snoring bedmates, barking dogs or traffic. But research suggests that "pink noise" is more effective for falling and staying asleep…and sleeping with pink noise might make your memory stronger, too.

White noise sounds like radio static. Pink noise sounds similar, but because it emphasizes lower sound frequencies and deemphasizes the "sizzle" of high frequencies, most people find it calming and restful. Pink noise often is compared with the sound of a steady rainfall.

What about making your memory work better? A study at Northwestern University found that exposure to pink noise while sleeping significantly increased participants' ability to absorb and then recall information the next day. In the study, the noise wasn't constant all night but was synchronized with the sleepers' brain waves, an effect you can't reproduce at home. But sleeping with pink noise at home might help your memory if for no other reason than it encourages deeper, less interrupted sleep. Anything that does that has a positive effect on your mood and memory.

It's worth trying pink noise if you're struggling to fall asleep or remain asleep, even if there is no significant background noise to block out. Near total silence can keep people awake, too, because the brain becomes more alert to even slight or distant sounds. That's why people who live in cities sometimes have trouble sleeping when they visit the quiet countryside.

If you meditate, pink noise could be beneficial for this as well.

There are numerous free pink-noise apps available, including Sleepo and Pink Noise for Android devices and NoiseZ and White Noise Lite (which includes a pink-noise setting) for Apple devices. Or buy a sound machine capable of generating pink noise (and other sleeping sounds that some people prefer) such as the LectroFan Classic ($49.95, SoundOfSleep.com) or iHome Zenergy iZBT10 ($99.99, iHomeAudio.com), which adds an alarm feature including FM radio and music streaming.

CANCER BREAKTHROUGHS

What Matters Most When It Comes to Breast Cancer Risk

You probably know the odds—one in eight women will be diagnosed with breast cancer at some point in her life.

What you may not realize: In spite of all the focus on genetic testing and BRCA genes, most cases of breast cancer are not genetic. There's a lot of emphasis on family history when it comes to all forms of cancer, but 87% of women diagnosed with breast cancer do not have a single first-degree relative (mother, sister, daughter) with breast cancer. The older you are, the more likely it is that breast cancer is caused by things you eat or do, not your genes. This means there's a lot that's within your control! *An ever-growing body of research has shown what the myths are and what matters...*

The Myths

The following have zero to do with breast cancer...

Bras: Myths abound about underwires, cup size and how old you were when you started wearing a bra, but there is no research to support any increase in breast cancer risk due to bra usage.

Antiperspirant: Multiple studies have failed to find any conclusive links between the aluminum chlorohydrate in antiperspirants and breast cancer.

Hair relaxers: No association has been found between breast cancer and how often relaxers or straighteners are used, the number of burns experienced or the type of relaxer. Still it's always a good idea to choose products without parabens and phthalates, which have been linked to cancer.

Mobile phones and power lines: While much debate surrounds mobile phones and brain health, they do not emit the right type of energy—or a high enough amount—to damage breast cell DNA. The same goes for living near power lines. Multiple studies have debunked the idea that the electromagnetic fields (EMFs) generated by high-voltage power lines increase breast cancer risk.

Breast surgery: If you have had breast-reduction surgery, numerous studies support the finding that your risk for breast cancer

Kristi Funk, MD, board-certified breast surgeon and cofounder of Pink Lotus Breast Center in Los Angeles. She is author of *Breasts: The Owner's Manual.* PinkLotus.com actually decreases. On the flip side, research shows that most implants—no matter what type, the positioning or how long you've had them—do not cause breast cancer. They do make cancer harder to detect, however, so you should have more rigorous screening—such as an ultrasound along with your mammogram.

Note: Some new concerns have been raised about textured implants possibly causing a form of lymphoma, but not breast cancer. Additional research is ongoing.

Coffee: No link between coffee consumption and breast cancer has ever been found, and there even is some evidence that drinking coffee may have a protective effect.

Note: Artificial sweeteners have not been linked to breast cancer, but they have been associated with obesity and insulin-resistance (so have no more than two servings a day).

Here's What Does Matter

The good news is that there are many positive steps you can take to lower your risk for breast cancer. *Not surprisingly, they involve diet, exercise and other lifestyle choices, such as…*

• **Watching your weight.** Being overweight or obese is the single most preventable cause of breast cancer worldwide. Having more fat tissue raises your estrogen and insulin levels. Extra weight increases your risk by anywhere from 50% to 250%. The research is very clear that the risk for breast cancer is much higher if you are overweight postmenopause, although the exact reason for that is not known.

• **Lowering the amount of alcohol you drink.** Alcohol is the other big enemy of healthy breast tissue. All types of alcohol increase estrogen levels, and estrogen is a potent fuel for cancer cells. One drink a day increases your breast cancer risk by 10%…two drinks, by 30%…three drinks, by 40%—you can see where this is going. However, one drink a day does ostensibly provide heart-health benefits. To keep the heart-health benefits and minimize breast cancer risk, stick to no more than one drink a day (or seven over a week) and make it red wine with its breast-friendly resveratrol and anti-estrogen effect.

• **Colorizing your plate.** Aim for a meal that's 70% fresh fruits, vegetables and leafy greens. Fruits and vegetables are loaded with phytonutrients, plus anticancer and anti-inflammatory properties that directly target cell mutations and put the brakes on cancer development. They prevent and repair DNA damage, destroy harmful cells, inhibit blood supply to tumors and protect against cell damage from environmental toxins.

• **Going meatless more often.** Animal protein, including fish, can increase your risk for breast cancer. Think of it as a side dish, not the main star of your plate. Even egg consumption should be limited to two a week. In one large-scale UK study, a high intake of meat (red meat, white meat, processed meat, poultry) showed increases in breast cancer risk when compared with vegetarians. Red meat was particularly flagged—the study found a 41% increased risk. But even poultry increased participants' risk by 22%. Yes, fish contains omega-3s that generally are beneficial, but fish—like meat and poultry—causes the body to produce insulin-like growth factor-1 (IGF-1), which has the primary job of promoting cell growth. That's great when you are a child. Once you're an adult, you need some IGF-1 to repair cells after exercise, for example, but an excess is going to send cell production into overdrive, including production of cancer cells. (See the next page for surprising alternative sources of protein.)

To make matters worse, conventional meat in the US and Canada contains a growth hormone (zeranol) that has been banned in Europe for decades because of its link to early puberty, which increases breast cancer risk. In fact, zeranol has been shown in labs to turn healthy breast cells to cancer in only 21 days.

Note: Even if you choose organic or grass-fed meat, be careful how you prepare it. When meats are well-done or char-grilled, cancer-causing compounds can form on the surface. Women who consistently eat well-done hamburgers, bacon and steak have a 362% higher risk for breast cancer than women who consume meat cooked rare or medium.

• **Moving your body more.** Women who get just three to four hours a week of moderate-to-vigorous physical activity have 30% to 40% lower risk for breast cancer than women who are inactive. Work out more than four hours a week, and you'll enjoy a 58% decrease in risk. Activity reduces estrogen levels, improves insulin sensitivity and maintains weight loss.

• **Finding alternatives to hormone replacement therapy.** Decades of evidence show that hormone replacement therapy (HRT) can increase risk for breast cancer. According to the Women's Health Initiative, there are 25% more breast cancers in HRT users than nonusers. To relieve the symptoms of menopause, try topical vaginal estrogen and laser treatments for vaginal dryness. For hot flashes, try herbal remedies such as black cohosh, evening primrose oil and soy. Acupuncture, biofeedback and yoga also may be beneficial. If you do decide to try HRT or bioidentical hormone replacement therapy (BHRT), take the lowest possible dose for the shortest amount of time necessary.

• **Avoiding environmental toxins.** Minimizing your exposure to endocrine disrupting compounds (EDCs) such as BPA, phthalates and parabens, which lurk in many household products, can help lessen your breast cancer risk. Choose organic and locally grown foods when possible, filter all water sources, fill your home with houseplants that act as potted air purifiers and pass on personal-care products that list EDCs on the label.

• **Finding time for daily stress relief.** Acute or chronic stress impairs the immune system, which gives diseases the opportunity to flourish, so take 20 minutes a day to do something that centers you such as yoga or meditation.

Meatless Monday All Week Long

Trying to go meatless more often, but worried about getting enough protein? You know to eat beans and nuts, but here are five lesser known foods that are full of protein…

⅓ cup seitan* = 21 grams protein (avoid if you have celiac disease or are gluten-intolerant)

1 cup green peas = 8 grams protein

1 cup cooked wild rice = 6.6 grams protein

¼ cup dry steel-cut oats = 5 grams protein

½ cup cooked of either spinach, broccoli, brussels sprouts, organic corn, avocado = 2 grams protein

*Seitan is a popular vegetarian meat substitute made from wheat that has the look and texture of meat when cooked.

An Inside Look at BRCA-Related Cancer

Pamela N. Munster, MD, professor of medicine at University of California, San Francisco, where she is leader of the Helen Diller Family Comprehensive Cancer Center and coleader of the Center for BRCA Research. She is author of *Twisting Fate: My Journey with BRCA—from Breast Cancer Doctor to Patient and Back.*

In 2012, Pamela N. Munster, MD, was discussing a new breast cancer medication with a colleague when her phone vibrated. The voice on the other end told the BRCA expert that multiple "irregularities" had been detected on her own breast scan.

At age 48, Dr. Munster was diagnosed with an early form of breast cancer…subsequent genetic testing revealed she was BRCA2 positive, meaning that she was far more likely to develop breast cancer and ovarian cancer than the general population. She went from doctor to patient, undergoing treatment and recovery, to then see her father get diagnosed with a BRCA-related pancreatic cancer.

Here, she shares the details of her experience, along with important facts about the BRCA genetic mutation that could save your life or the life of someone you love.

The 411 on BRCA

Everybody has two copies of the BRCA1 and BRCA2 genes. Their everyday role is to produce special tumor-suppressing proteins that help to repair any DNA damage that occurs constantly as part of a normal process in all cells.

Problems can arise when either of these two genes is abnormal. A faulty BRCA gene can allow DNA damage to go unrepaired and give cancer more opportunities to develop. For reasons that are not yet completely clear, BRCA genes are particularly important in certain tissues causing specific cancers.

A woman with a BRCA mutation has a 60% to 80% lifetime risk of developing breast cancer, compared with 12% for the average woman. Her lifetime ovarian cancer risk is also higher—about 40% to 50% for those with a BRCA1 mutation and approximately 20% to 30% for those with a BRCA2 mutation, compared with less than 2% for the average woman.

An underrecognized problem: Men can carry BRCA mutations, too, driving their lifetime breast cancer risk up to 5% to 10% versus 0.1% for the average man. They are also seven times more likely to develop prostate cancer, often a very aggressive form and at an earlier age than usual.

A study presented at the 2017 Annual Scientific Meeting of the American Urological Association found that men with BRCA mutations are also at greater risk of developing multiple other types of cancer. Particularly, BRCA2 mutations are linked to skin, pancreatic, digestive tract and colorectal cancers. Women with BRCA2 mutations also are at increased risk for these cancers.

Criteria for Getting Tested

Many people think, *My mother didn't have breast cancer, so I don't have to worry.* But anyone with a BRCA1 or BRCA2 mutation, male or female, can pass it on to their daughters and sons, who will each have a 50% chance of inheriting the mutation, and the cancer doesn't necessarily need to be in an immediate relative for you to have a mutation. *Consider BRCA mutation testing if you…*

●**Have a relative, on either side, who was diagnosed with breast cancer before age 50,** had cancer in both breasts or was a male with breast cancer.

●**Have both breast and ovarian cancers in your family, on either side,** especially multiple people with breast cancer, or if you're of Ashkenazi Jewish descent.

●**Have any relative with pancreatic cancer or male relatives with prostate cancer at a younger age.**

●**Are adopted or have few close relatives and therefore an unknown or limited family medical history.**

It's never too late for testing. Once I tested positive, I knew it had to be from my dad or my mom. So I encouraged my then-78-year-old father to get tested. His own mother survived breast cancer in her 60s, so my mutation was likely passed down through him. He tested positive for the BRCA2 mutation.

One year later, he began complaining of unexplained abdominal pain. This vague symptom might be waved off in most patients, but knowing his BRCA status and increased cancer risk, I urged him to get a full workup. An MRI revealed pancreatic cancer, with a large tumor that was deemed inoperable. But because he received a chemo targeted to BRCA tumors, despite his age, his tumor shrunk by half, rendering it operable. He just surpassed his five-year survival mark.

Given the high lifetime risk for breast cancer in BRCA mutation carriers, prophylactic mastectomy or very close monitoring is suggested. When it comes to ovarian cancer, most women with a BRCA mutation will opt to have their ovaries removed once they have completed childbearing. If you're past menopause and have already gone through the changes that come from the loss of estrogen, the effects of the surgery may be more tolerable. Hormone replacement therapy may ease the transition for those undergoing the surgery in their 30s or 40s.

Be cautious with at-home tests. Last year, the FDA approved 23andMe's direct-to-consumer BRCA test. While advances have been made in this field, there can be perils. You may not want to find out potentially life-altering news for yourself and your family via mail without the counseling and support of a health-care provider who can put the relevance of your mutation into perspective or refer you to a clinic for screening and prophylactic surgeries if you indeed carry a mutation.

Also, many tests only screen for certain mutations—23andMe screens for three mutations in the BRCA1 and BRCA2 genes out of more than 1,000. These three variants are almost exclusively found in the Ashkenazi Jewish population. So if you are of another ethnicity, your results will likely come back negative even if you are, in fact, BRCA positive. I'm of Swiss-French ancestry, and my own 23andMe results showed no BRCA mutations.

Bottom line: Consult a specialist for a full screening if you want testing. Find one via the National Society of Genetic Counselors at NSGC.org/findageneticcounselor. Insurance covers testing if you meet certain criteria such as a family history of breast cancer.

Larks Have Less Risk

Women who prefer mornings (known as "larks") are 40% less likely to get breast cancer than those who are evening types (aka "night owls").

Theory: A woman's body clock may contribute, in unknown ways, to her breast cancer risk.

National Cancer Research Institute.

Childbirth Raises Breast Cancer Risk

A new study contradicts earlier ones that said childbirth reduces the risk for breast cancer. Childbirth does appear to reduce risk, but this benefit appears to develop only about two decades after a woman gives birth. Until that time, childbirth actually raises breast cancer risk—risk is highest about five years after a woman gives birth.

Hazel Nichols, PhD, assistant professor, department of epidemiology, University of North Carolina Grillings School of Global Public Health, Chapel Hill, and coauthor of an analysis of 15 prospective studies from around the world, published in *Annals of Internal Medicine*.

Don't Call It Cancer

Laura Esserman, MD, University of California, San Francisco, breast cancer specialist.

We Americans are "can do" people. We pride ourselves on fighting against the odds. But what if the odds already favor you?

That's often true with cancer. About one-third are so slow-growing that they pose little or no risk to general health or life. These include the breast cancer ductal carcinoma in situ…papillary thyroid cancer…and many prostate, bladder and cervical cancers. Aggressive treatment brings the risk for serious side effects with little-to-no benefit. Watchful waiting—working with your doctor to closely monitor the cancer—leads to better outcomes.

A simple name change helps a lot. When you call it 'cancer,' everyone's in a hurry. Patients rush into treatments that might have long-term negative consequences. So my colleagues and I propose the term IDLE—short for "indolent lesion of epithelial origin." ("Lesion" is an abnormal change in an organ… "epithelial" refers to an organ's lining.) IDLE dispenses with the word cancer and emphasizes that these are not aggressive killers—they're, well, idle or nearly so.

That name change could lead to smarter decisions and healthier lives. In an online survey, participants asked what they would do if they had "thyroid cancer" were twice as likely to opt for aggressive surgery than if they had a "papillary lesion" or "abnormal cells." So if you or a loved one is diagnosed with cancer, ask your doctor whether it's the kind that grows slowly or rapidly. If slowly, strongly consider conservative treatments. There are a lot of situations where less is more.

MRI for Breast Cancer: The Merits of Twice-Yearly Screening

Greg Karczmar, PhD, professor of radiology, member of the Committee on Medical Physics and the College, The University of Chicago...director of MRI research and coauthor of study titled "Intensive Surveillance with Biannual Dynamic Contrast-Enhanced Magnetic Resonance Imaging Downstages Breast Cancer in BRCA1 Mutation Carriers," published in *Clinical Cancer Research*.

Having a high genetic risk for breast cancer has led many women to at least consider a prophylactic mastectomy—having their breasts removed so that cancer can't develop. A new study suggests another far less drastic option...a new schedule for breast cancer screenings.

Current screening guidelines for people at high risk for breast cancer involve an annual breast MRI along with a mammogram. However, a review of several studies found that, with this level of surveillance, some patients' cancers were not found in their earliest stages and, for a group of them, the cancer had already spread to lymph nodes, making it more difficult to treat.

The new study: Researchers from the US and Brazil wanted to test a more aggressive screening schedule—a breast MRI every six months along with a yearly mammogram. They enrolled 295 women at high risk for breast cancer—the women either had a lifetime breast cancer risk of 20% or higher and/or had tested positive for the BRCA1 or BRCA2 gene mutation.

During the 12-year study (2004 to 2016), 17 breast cancers were found. Fifteen oc-

curred in women with a genetic mutation, primarily BRCA1. All of the cancers were found at an early stage, with tumors less than one centimeter in diameter, and before any had spread to lymph nodes. All these women were treated and were disease-free at the time the study was published in 2018.

Surprising finding: The mammograms did not add to the cancer diagnosis rate, and the researchers suggest that they can be eliminated in future studies. They conclude that high-risk breast cancer can be found at an earlier stage through breast MRIs at six-month intervals alone.

Will this study change the current guidelines? Not yet, but twice-yearly MRIs do make sense for women at the highest risk for breast cancer...and with several advantages over mammograms. Yearly mammograms have significant radiation exposure and they result in more false positives than MRIs. This means more callbacks and more biopsies to see whether or not there's cancer. MRIs do not use radiation and they're more accurate, so women need fewer unnecessary follow-up tests.

Because a second yearly MRI adds to screening costs, it may take more studies to get guidelines changed and have insurance companies pay for the second test. However, the researchers believe that twice a year MRIs will actually be cost effective. Finding an aggressive cancer at an early stage can save tens of thousands of dollars in treatment costs, not to mention the emotional toll that advanced cancer takes on patients. For these reasons, it's an expense people at high risk for breast cancer might be willing to pay for on their own.

Another factor that may help push through a change in the guidelines is new faster MRI technology. Called ultrafast dynamic contrast enhanced MRI (DCE-MRI), this is a scanning method that can be included as part of another type of MRI called abbreviated MRI. Compared with conventional DCE-MRI, which takes 60 to 90 seconds per image, the ultrafast version takes only three to four seconds per image for the first 60 seconds of scanning—for a total scan time of less than 10 minutes. Shorter procedures may reduce cost and be as effective as traditional MRIs for screening.

Researchers at The University of Chicago have already started another study involving high-risk women. It's comparing a yearly traditional MRI plus a DCE-MRI at six months to the conventional (full-length) MRI scan performed twice per year. In addition, for intermediate and normal risk women, the team is developing scanning methods that require much lower doses of the contrast dye used in these tests to address the concerns of the public and the medical community regarding potential negative effects of these agents.

Why Your Screening Mammograms Should Be in 3-D

Susan Harvey, MD, director of breast imaging in the Russell H. Morgan Department of Radiology and Radiological Science at Johns Hopkins Medicine in Baltimore.

While a 3-D mammography machine looks like a 2-D machine and compresses your breasts just as a 2-D does, there's a big difference. The top of the 3-D machine moves in an arc above each breast taking multiple images—think of each one as a thin slice—from many angles. A computer then takes all those thin slices and arranges them into a set of highly focused 3-D images for a radiologist to read. This imaging technology is called tomosynthesis.

The 3-D images make it easier to distinguish normal overlapping breast tissue from tumors, so it's harder for cancers to hide. That means not just better detection but also fewer false positives and fewer callbacks, when you're asked to come back because of a potentially abnormal finding. In other words, fewer scary moments waiting to get another test to know if something is wrong—though it's often a false alarm, who wants a day or even a few hours of anxiety while waiting to find out?

It's true that 3-D mammography exposes you to more radiation than 2-D does, but the extra amount is small and the total amount is small—and certainly less dangerous than having an early cancer go undetected.

Another advantage to 3-D: Because 3-D mammography is better than 2-D mammography not only at finding abnormalities but also at characterizing abnormalities, women are less likely to need follow-up biopsies, which are invasive. And if you are recalled after a 3-D mammogram, there's a greater chance than with a 2-D mammogram that a follow-up, noninvasive breast ultrasound will provide all the additional information needed.

In women with dense breasts, having a 3-D mammogram makes tumors easier to see.

Note: If you have dense breasts, you might also need a breast ultrasound as an extra screening, but you may be able to schedule both tests for the same day—and have both tests covered by insurance as wellness screenings if having dense breasts is listed in your medical records. Ask your insurance provider in advance.

Also: When 3-D first became available, most insurance companies wouldn't cover it. Now most do.

Don't Ignore Vaginal Bleeding

Vaginal bleeding after menopause can be an early sign of cancer. About 9% of women with postmenopausal bleeding are diagnosed with endometrial cancer, which is highly curable in its early stages. If you have bleeding, it's important to have an ultrasound or biopsy to rule out cancer.

Megan A. Clarke, PhD, MHS, is postdoctoral fellow in the division of cancer epidemiology and genetics at National Cancer Institute, Rockville, Maryland, and coauthor of a meta-analysis published in *JAMA Internal Medicine*.

After Breast Cancer: Are You Getting the Right Imaging Tests?

Benjamin L. Franc, MD, clinical professor of radiology and nuclear medicine at the Stanford School of Medicine in California and lead author of the study "Geographic Variation in Postoperative Imaging for Low-Risk Breast Cancer," published in *Journal of the National Comprehensive Cancer Network*.

If you are one of the three million breast cancer survivors, follow-up imaging tests are an important part of your long-term care. But a new study has found that many women may not be getting the right guidance from their doctors regarding how often and even what type of testing to get.

Researchers at University of California, San Francisco analyzed medical claims of 36,000 women with early-stage breast cancer over the first 18 months after breast surgery.

While guidelines for breast imaging, established by the National Comprehensive Cancer Network and other organizations recommend a yearly mammogram or, in some cases, breast MRI, at least nearly a third of women aren't getting this and possibly as many as a third more may be getting imaging they don't need—full-body imaging with more advanced tests using CT, MRI, PET or bone scan technology, which are not recommended, can be expensive and can expose patients to unnecessary radiation.

How could it be that so many women aren't following guidelines or aren't following them correctly? They may be getting different advice from their doctors who might not yet be following evidence-based guidelines. There may be other factors at work, too. Fear of cancer recurrence may cause some women to avoid imaging…and others to seek advanced imaging in the hopes of finding cancer recurrence as early as possible.

Important: While full-body imaging is good at finding early metastasis, study after study shows it doesn't improve survival or quality of life and it may also be dangerous. Since a recurrence might not occur for up to 20 years, unnecessary additional radiation exposure can really add up. There is also the chance that testing will pick up a cyst or nodule in distant parts of the body that is not cancer at all—such false positives can add to anxiety levels and lead to more unnecessary testing.

The guidelines do say that a full-body scan may be indicated if you have symptoms of recurrence. Most recurrences are found by patients between doctor visits. *Perform a breast self-examination every month and let your doctor know if you find any possible recurrence symptoms such as…*

- **A new lump**
- **A rash or skin change in your breast area**
- **New or worsening pain**
- **Development of a nagging cough or shortness of breath**
- **Yellowing of your skin or eyes**
- **Loss of weight, energy or appetite**

This list is not all-inclusive and you should share with your physician anything different that you notice about your body or how you feel.

Most women live long and full lives with a low risk of recurrence, so a sensible surveillance plan is what you need. Develop a plan with your doctor soon after surgery and stick to it.

Breast Cancer Drug Breakthrough

Patients with very hard to treat "triple-negative" breast cancer with the immune marker PD-L1—which disproportionately strikes young women—whose cancer had metastasized survived 10 months longer when the immunotherapy drug *atezolizumab* was added to standard chemotherapy. The new regimen is in clinical trial—ask your doctor about availability.

Leisha Emens, MD, PhD, is cofounder of Hillman Cancer Immunology and Immunotherapy Program at University of Pittsburgh Medical Center and coleader of the study published in *The New England Journal of Medicine.*

Screening for Ovarian Cancer May Save Lives (So Why Isn't It Being Done?)

John R. van Nagell Jr., MD, professor of obstetrics and gynecology and director of ovarian cancer screening at the University of Kentucky Markey Cancer Center in Lexington and lead author of "Survival of Women with Type I and II Epithelial Ovarian Cancer Detected by Ultrasound Screening," published in *Obstetrics & Gynecology.*

Ovarian cancer is the deadliest of all gynecologic cancers in the US. That's because symptoms rarely occur until it has reached an advanced stage. While it can be treated successfully at stage I or II, most women aren't diagnosed until stage III or IV, and at these later stages, the cure rate is as low as 10%.

What you may not know is that there is a test that may be able to detect ovarian cancer at an earlier stage than pelvic examination. It's called transvaginal ultrasound (TVUS). The problem is that national guidelines do not advocate TVUS screening—except for women at high risk for ovarian cancer—because there have been no randomized controlled US studies showing that its widespread use will improve survival. However, findings from a recently published 30-year study indicate that TVUS screening may detect ovarian cancer at an earlier stage than routine pelvic examination.

The study: Researchers at the Markey Cancer Center enrolled 46,000 women considered at risk for ovarian cancer—they were either age 50 and older (yes, that's all it takes

to increase a woman's risk) or age 25 and older with a family history of ovarian cancer. These participants were given a yearly TVUS screening and followed for 30 years to see if screening would affect stage at detection and patient outcomes. The researchers compared the participants' stage at detection and outcomes to those of unscreened women with clinically detected ovarian cancer who were referred to the cancer center during the same time period.

The findings: Seventy-one of the study participants were diagnosed with ovarian cancer over the course of the study. In two-thirds of these women, the cancer was found in stage I or stage II. By comparison, two-thirds of the clinically-detected patients had stage III or stage IV cancer at the time they were diagnosed.

Another finding: The 10-year survival rate for study participants with screen-detected ovarian cancer was more than 30% higher than that of unscreened women with clinically detected ovarian cancer.

So what's keeping ovarian cancer screening from being adopted? There will need to be additional well-conducted studies—even longer and larger than this one—showing that screening is cost effective and prolongs survival.

One barrier to "cost effectiveness" is that most tumors discovered by screening do not turn out to be cancerous. In the Markey study, among the women whose screening revealed ovarian tumors, only 25% were cancer. Although the procedure to remove the tumors has a low complication rate, needing to operate on four patients to find one cancer increases the cost of screening. Also, ovarian cancer is relatively rare—the lifetime risk among the general population of women is just over 1%.

Advances in genetic testing may soon be able to narrow down who can benefit most from TVUS screening. Screening is not recommended for women in the general population. However, women should have an open discussion with their doctor about their individual risk for ovarian cancer. For instance, if you have a mother or sister with a history of breast cancer or ovarian cancer, your lifetime risk could be up to 5%. If you tested positive for a BRCA1 cancer gene mutation, your lifetime risk could be 40% to 60% (in this situation, some women elect to have their ovaries removed to prevent cancer, a procedure that is often covered by insurance).

Even if you're not at high risk for ovarian cancer, be aware of its symptoms and talk to your doctor immediately if you experience one or more of the following...

- **Bloating**
- **Abdominal or pelvic pain**
- **Feeling full quickly while eating**
- **Urinary frequency or urgency**

Beware: Uterine Cancer Is on the Rise

Centers for Disease Control and Prevention, Morbidity and Mortality Weekly Report, "Uterine Cancer Incidence and Mortality–United States, 1999-2016," December 2018.
Cancer.net.

While many cancers, including lung and colon cancers, have been decreasing in the US, the opposite is true of uterine cancer.

New cases of this cancer (also called endometrial cancer because it starts in the endometrium, the lining of the uterus) are up 12% since 1999 and deaths are up by 21%!

What's going on? These trends follow the rise in obesity among women in the US. Women who are overweight or obese are two to four times more likely to develop uterine cancer than women who are at a healthy weight. The connection is the female hormone estrogen, which stimulates this cancer and is overproduced in fat cells. In fact, about 40% of uterine cancer cases are linked to obesity.

Other uterine cancer risk factors include having diabetes and eating a diet high in animal fat (two factors also associated with being overweight or obese), being over age 50 and having a family history of uterine cancer.

Black women are twice as likely to die from uterine cancer as women of other races. This may be due to a higher rate of obesity and being diagnosed at a later stage of the cancer than other women.

To lower your risk for uterine cancer, the Centers for Disease Control and Prevention suggests eating a healthy diet and being physically active in order to maintain a normal weight.

Because screening tests for uterine cancer are not done routinely, it's important to know the warning signs, most commonly vaginal bleeding after sexual intercourse, between periods or after menopause. This is often the first and most important sign that can lead to an early diagnosis—90% of women with this cancer have abnormal vaginal bleeding, so don't ignore it. Other signs include pain after sexual intercourse, lower-belly pain and pain after passing urine.

Note: The test called transvaginal ultrasound is available for screening women at high risk for uterine cancer. It is also used to help diagnose cancer in women who have symptoms.

Early diagnosis and treatment are the keys to survival. When treated at an early stage, survival rates after five years are 80% to 90%. Once this cancer has time to spread, the five-year survival rate drops to under 30%.

Breakthroughs in Lung Cancer

Timothy Burns, MD, PhD, assistant professor of medicine in the department of medicine, Division of Hematology/Oncology, at UPMC Hillman Cancer Center in Pittsburgh, where his laboratory focuses on discovering targeted therapies for lung cancer. His scientific papers on lung cancer have appeared in *Nature Genetics, Oncogene, Cancer Research, Molecular Cancer Research, Cancer* and many other medical journals.

Lung cancer kills more Americans—both smokers and nonsmokers—than colon, breast and prostate cancers combined.

But the good news is, treatment options are now extending the lives of many people affected by this formidable disease.

Latest development: Recently announced treatment breakthroughs provide new hope for people with non-small cell lung cancer (NSCLC)—the type of malignancy responsible for 85% of all lung cancers.

The New Heavy Hitters

•**Immunotherapy.** Some of the newest treatments for NSCLC are immune checkpoint inhibitors—drugs that energize the immune system to kill cancer cells by blocking one of two cancer-promoting proteins, PD-1 and PD-L1. These drugs include *pembrolizumab* (Keytruda), the immunotherapy treatment credited with saving the life of former President Jimmy Carter when melanoma spread to his brain…*nivolumab* (Opdivo)…*atezolizumab* (Tecentriq)…and *durvalumab* (Imfinzi).

Typically, these drugs are used only as second-line therapies for patients with advanced disease who haven't responded to other types of treatments, such as chemotherapy. But several studies presented at the 2018 annual meeting of the American Association for Cancer Research show that immunotherapy can work as a first-line therapy for people with advanced NSCLC, improving survival.

New scientific findings: A combination of the immunotherapy drug *pembrolizumab* and chemotherapy worked better than chemo alone as a first-line treatment for patients with metastatic NSCLC—69% were still alive after one year in the combo group, with only 49% alive in the chemo-only group, according to a one-year study published in *The New England Journal of Medicine.*

In a similar one-year study, patients with stage IV lung cancer were given either chemotherapy or two immunotherapy drugs—*nivolumab* and *ipilimumab* (Yervoy), which blocks CTLA-4, a protein similar to PD-1. Those treated with immunotherapy were 42% less likely to have their disease progress than those who received other treatment.

Meanwhile, research focusing on the use of immunotherapy without chemotherapy as a first-line treatment—reported at a recent meeting of the American Society of Clinical Oncology—also delivered positive results. The stage IV NSCLC patients getting pembrolizumab lived four to eight months longer than those getting chemo. Only 18% of the immunotherapy patients suffered severe side effects, such as inflammation of the lung, liver or colon, versus 41% of those in the chemo group.

Takeaway: With the impressive results of these studies, first-line treatment with an immunotherapy drug with or without chemotherapy is now the standard-of-care for most cases of advanced NSCLC. If a test of your tumor tissue shows that you have a high PD-L1 activity—and one-third of patients with NSCLC do—then single-agent immunotherapy might be the best first treatment for you with or without chemotherapy. Patients whose tumor does not express high levels of this marker still benefit from the combination of immunotherapy with chemotherapy in the majority of cases. Talk to your oncologist.

•**Gene-modulating drugs.** This type of therapy uses drugs to turn off one of several genetic mutations (oncogenes) that can drive lung cancer. As estimated 10% to 20% of NSCLC patients have the epidermal growth factor receptor (EGFR) mutation, which is treated with drugs such as *erlotinib* (Tarceva), *afatinib* (Gilotrif), *gefitinib* (Iressa) and *osimertinib* (Tagrisso). An estimated 5% have the anaplastic lymphoma kinase (ALK) mutation, which is treated with drugs such as *crizotinib* (Xalkori), *ceritinib* (Zykadia), *alectinib* (Alecensa) and *brigatinib* (Alunbrig).

These oral drugs are so powerful that they can, in rare cases, extend life by five years or more. However, the newer and more effective of these drugs—such as alectinib for ALK—has been used as a second-line therapy. Now this treatment paradigm is changing.

New scientific findings: In a study published in 2018, more than 500 NSCLC patients with an EGFR mutation got either osimertinib as a first-line treatment or the previous standard therapy (*erlotinib* or *gefitinib*). After 12 months, those taking osimertinib had a 54% lower risk for disease progression or death. In 2018, the FDA approved *osimertinib* for first-line treatment of metastatic NSCLC.

In a study of more than 300 metastatic NSCLC patients with the ALK mutation, the disease progressed or death occurred in 41% of those receiving *alectinib* (a newer more effective drug) compared with 68% receiving *crizotinib*, an older drug, after about a year and a half. The alectinib group also had fewer side effects. Patients receiving alectinib had control of their tumors for almost three years, on average.

Takeaway: If you are diagnosed with NSCLC, get tested to find out if you have a genetic mutation driving the disease. If you do, talk to your oncologist about the best gene-targeting drug for you—patients with these mutations often do not benefit from immunotherapy.

The Liquid Biopsy Option...

The gold standard for biopsies in NSCLC is a tissue biopsy—removing a portion of the tumor and testing it—to identify the specific type of cancer and genetic mutations that inform treatment decisions.

Problem: In many cases, a tissue biopsy isn't possible—for example, the position of the tumor in the lung or other organ may make it too difficult to biopsy, or the patient may have emphysema.

Solution: A liquid (blood-based) biopsy can be used when a tissue biopsy is not an option. The FDA approved liquid biopsy for lung cancer in 2016. A recent study published in *JAMA Oncology* suggests that combining liquid biopsies with tumor biopsies can improve the chance of finding a targetable mutation. Ask your oncologist

if this is right for you. FoundationOne and Guardant360 are the two most widely used liquid biopsies.

The Blood Pressure Medicine That May Increase Risk for Lung Cancer

Study titled, "Angiotensin Converting Enzyme Inhibitors and Risk of Lung Cancer: Population Based Cohort Study," led by researchers at McGill University in Montreal, Canada, and published in *The BMJ*.

When you're prescribed an ACE (angiotensin converting enzyme) inhibitor to reduce high blood pressure, you're likely to hear about side effects such as dry cough, headaches, dizziness and fatigue. According to new research, lung cancer may be a frightening addition to that list.

ACE inhibitors, such as Lotensin, Vasotec, Prinivil, Zestril, Accupril and Altace, are used by millions of people. They're not only very common and effective medications for lowering blood pressure, they're also prescibed for conditions including heart disease, diabetes, kidney disease and migraine headaches.

Concern over a link between them and lung cancer isn't new. But previous studies found mixed results. They also involved small numbers of participants who were followed for short periods of time.

This new study included almost one million patients who were newly started on a blood pressure drug. Within this group of patients, researchers compared the risk of developing lung cancer in patients on long-term ACE inhibitors with patients on an angiotensin receptor blocker (ARB), another type of high blood pressure medication. None of the patients had any cancer diagnosis at the start of the study.

Over the course of the decade-long study, just under 8,000 participants developed lung cancer, a rate of about 0.8%. Compared with patients on ARBs, patients on ACE inhibitors had a higher risk of developing lung cancer. This increased risk wasn't evident until after five years on the drug, at which point it was 22% higher. At 10 years, it was 31% higher. Surprisingly, the risk increase was the same for smokers and nonsmokers.

What's the connection between a drug designed to improve health and the deadliest cancer for men and women in the US? The researchers suspect that it may be the accumulation of a naturally occurring substance in the lung called bradykinin. Its role is to dilate blood vessels, which in turn reduces blood pressure. ACE inhibitors work by increasing bradykinin, but at the same time, bradykinin has been linked to the growth of lung cancer cells.

While the increased risk for lung cancer needs to be confirmed by other studies, if you're on an ACE inhibitor or your doctor suggests that you start one, discuss the lung cancer risk, especially as it goes up over time, and whether an alternative is a safer option for you. Complicating the picture is that taking ACE inhibitors long-term has been shown to lower the risk for breast cancer.

If appropriate for your situation, you might be able to reduce your blood pressure with lifestyle changes—and these don't carry any risks!

Aspirin for Colon Cancer

The US Preventive Services Task Force has recommended that aspirin be considered to reduce risk for colorectal cancer in people with advanced colon polyps, after an analysis found that it reduces the risk by 40%.

However: In a study of 84 patients ages 40 to 91, only 42.9% of patients with advanced colon polyps, determined by biopsy, were taking aspirin.

Note: Even if you have been diagnosed with colon polyps, daily aspirin increases bleeding risk. Ask your doctor for advice.

Charles H. Hennekens, MD, DrPH, senior academic advisor, Schmidt College of Medicine, Florida Atlantic University, Boca Raton.

Why You're Not Following Colon Cancer Screening Guidelines

Douglas A. Corley, MD, PhD, gastroenterologist at Kaiser Permanente, San Francisco Medical Center, research scientist at Kaiser Permanente, Northern California, clinical professor of medicine at University of California, San Francisco, and senior author of the study "Modifiable Failures in the Colorectal Cancer Screening Process and Their Association with Risk of Death," published in *Gastroenterology*.

Considering it's no secret that colon cancer screenings save lives, it's shocking to learn that a whopping 76% of deaths from the disease can be traced back to screening failures—on the part of patients.

According to a study of 1,750 people who died from colorectal cancer, researchers at the health organization Kaiser Permanente found that 34% didn't have any screenings at all, 33% didn't get tested as often as recommended, and 8% didn't do the needed follow-up after an abnormal test.

How can it be that people don't take advantage of tests proved to detect cancer early, when it's highly curable?

The list of deterrents is long. It takes time and planning and effort to do the prep, line up a friend or loved one to take you and take time off for the procedure. It's so much easier to put it off indefinitely even though the financial cost of the screening is covered by insurance.

Just Get Screened!

Some health-care centers around the country have started outreach efforts to get and keep patients up to date on screenings, both with reminders and colonoscopy alternatives that can be done at home. For instance, Kaiser Permanente patients are sent test kits by mail—and now more than 80% of its patients are up to date with screenings, as compared to the national average of 60%. What's more, the number of deaths from colorectal cancer among its patients has dropped by 50% in the 10 years since this program was started.

But you can't rely on your doctor or local hospital to nudge you into action. While colonoscopy is still the gold standard (and the only option for people at high-risk), if you don't have time for it, don't want to do the prep, or whatever reason you're putting it off, talk to your doctor about whether you can start with a home test. These tests, which have become more accurate over the years, involve collecting one or more stool samples and sending them off to a lab or doctor's office.

Important: If you test positive, you will need a colonoscopy to investigate, and it won't be considered a screening test, so you will be charged. If you have a high deductible and will end up paying for this out-of-pocket, you might want to rethink starting with a home test, since preventive colonoscopy screening is covered by insurance.

If you do opt for an at-home test, know that there are differences among the available tests (see next article).

Follow Up

Regardless of the type of test you have—at home or a colonoscopy—if results come back abnormal, follow up within eight to 12 weeks. You owe it to your health and to your loved ones to take this and all the important screening steps.

Another Option?

In 2016, the FDA approved a blood test that looks for a marker of colorectal cancer called mSEPT9. Not enough studies have been done to say that it is as accurate as the home tests, and it has a high false-positive rate—about

20% compared to less than 5% for fecal immunochemical test. However, some doctors feel it's a better-than-nothing option for people refusing all other first-round screening tests and worth discussing with your healthcare provider.

Colonoscopy Isn't the Only Way to Prevent Colon Cancer

Andrew M. D. Wolf, MD, an internist and associate professor of medicine at University of Virginia School of Medicine in Charlottesville. He is a member of the American Cancer Society's (ACS) Guideline Development Group and chair of the ACS's Colorectal Cancer Screening Work Group.

Colonoscopy has generally been considered the gold standard for detecting and preventing colorectal cancer. But it's not the only option.

What you may not realize: A handful of other tests—which are easier, cheaper and quicker—are now available and may encourage more people to actually get tested. *What you need to know…*

The Inconvenience Factor

The American Cancer Society (ACS) and other major health groups have urged Americans to regularly undergo colonoscopy. And with good reason. Colonoscopy can detect more than 90% of cancers and precancerous polyps that are larger than about one-half inch.

The problem is, more than one-third of Americans who should be screened for colorectal cancer haven't had screening—in part due to the onerous "prep" that includes fasting and drinking quarts of a foul-tasting liquid and often means spending hours on the toilet as your insides empty out.

Easier Tests

New guidelines from the ACS advise patients with average risk for colon cancer (that is, no family history, genetic syndrome, inflammatory bowel disease or personal history of radiation to the abdomen or pelvic area to treat a prior cancer) to undergo regular screenings starting at age 45. Previously, screening started at age 50, but the age has been dropped to 45 because in recent years the percentage of colorectal cancer cases involving younger adults has risen. The recommended tests include colonoscopy, CT colonography and sigmoidoscopy (discussed later)—along with a number of high-sensitivity stool tests.

Colonoscopy is most effective at detecting precancerous polyps, but for people who won't go for the procedure, stool-based tests (when performed regularly) can be almost as accurate as colonoscopy at detecting colorectal cancer.

Caveats: If you test positive on one of these tests, you'll still need to follow up with colonoscopy. And the tests must be repeated every one to five years, depending on the test. Colonoscopy is typically undergone every 10 years (more frequently if polyps are detected). *Other tests to discuss with your doctor…*

• **Guaiac fecal occult blood test (gFOBT).** This test uses a chemical (guaiac) to detect a blood component in stools. The presence of blood is a common sign of cancer. The test can detect 60% to 80% of colon cancers, though it is even more accurate if done every year, as recommended.

However, all stool tests, including gFOBT, are more likely than colonoscopy to miss precancerous polyps, which are less likely to bleed than cancer. This is why gFOBT should be repeated yearly—to catch the polyps that have turned into early-stage cancer and begun to bleed.

What it involves: You use an applicator stick to smear a bit of stool on a test card. You repeat this on two or three consecutive days, then return the cards to your doctor (or mail to a testing laboratory).

Pros: gFOBT only requires a stool "smear." The test usually costs $25 or less and is covered by insurance.

Cons: You must collect several smears… give up red meat for several days because the test can't differentiate dietary animal blood from human blood…and temporarily quit taking medications, such as aspirin or ibuprofen (Motrin), that can cause intestinal bleeding.

• **Fecal immunochemical test (FIT).** A more recent variation of the gFOBT, FIT uses an antibody to detect blood hemoglobin in a stool sample. It's about 80% effective at detecting cancers, though is even more accurate when repeated yearly, as recommended.

What it involves: Test kits vary by manufacturer, so read directions carefully. Typically, you stick a long-handled brush into a stool sample…transfer the sample to a special collection card…and mail it to a testing laboratory. The cost is about the same or slightly more than the gFOBT, and it's covered by insurance.

Pros: You only need a single stool sample…there are no dietary restrictions…and the test only detects human hemoglobin from the lower digestive tract, which reduces false readings from dietary sources and noncancerous causes of stomach/upper-intestinal bleeding.

Cons: Like gFOBT, the test usually misses precancerous polyps. Still, due to FIT's improved accuracy and convenience, most experts consider it to be a better test than gFOBT, but the latter remains available based on its low cost and track record of detecting cancers.

• **Cologuard.** This is the newest screening test. It combines blood-stool detection with the ability to detect DNA mutations often associated with colorectal cancers. Overall, Cologuard can detect about 92% of cancers—better than gFOBT and FIT. It also can detect more than 40% of "advanced" polyps (larger or with more precancerous features) compared with about 25% for FIT. The test is expensive—about $650, though it is covered by Medicare and most insurers.

What it involves: A small container is placed under the toilet seat to collect a complete stool, which is then sent to a testing laboratory.

Pros: Cologuard is done at three-year intervals rather than every year. It doesn't require preparation or dietary restrictions.

Cons: It has more false positives (about 13%) than other tests, which lead to more unnecessary follow-up colonoscopies.

The Other Options

• **Flexible sigmoidoscopy.** Like colonoscopy, it utilizes a flexible, camera-tipped tube to examine the lower part of the colon (the sigmoid colon) and the rectum. Repeated every five years, it provides some of the same benefits as colonoscopy but doesn't require sedation. Most insurers cover it.

The downsides: Sigmoidoscopy won't detect polyps/cancers in the upper half of the colon. Also, the lack of sedation, while considered safer, means the procedure is more uncomfortable than colonoscopy.

• **CT colonography,** also known as virtual colonoscopy, is an imaging test that is comparable to colonoscopy at detecting advanced adenomas and cancers. It is noninvasive, and sedation isn't required.

However, CT colonography requires a bowel prep, and you must drink a contrast dye. Medicare and many private insurers do not cover CT colonography. CT scans produce radiation exposure, but newer technology has lowered the amount of radiation considerably.

Finally, an Early Warning Sign of Pancreatic Cancer

Study titled "Pancreatic Cancer Following Acute Pancreatitis: A Population-based Matched Cohort Study" by researchers at Karolinska Institutet in Stockholm, Sweden, published in *The American Journal of Gastroenterology.*

The greatest challenge with pancreatic cancer is that the only chance of a cure is with early diagnosis and surgery...

Cancer Drug Gets FDA Nod

A breakthrough cancer drug received accelerated FDA approval. *Larotrectinib* (Vitrakvi) is the first primary tumor-agnostic therapy—it attacks malignancies that have specific genetic characteristics regardless of where the cancer is in the body. In three separate studies, 122 patients with 24 cancer types, including breast, pancreatic, lung and thyroid (with an NTRK gene fusion) that had not spread to other parts of the body but could not be safely surgically removed, had an overall response rate—meaning tumors shrank either partially or completely—of more than 80%.

Ulrik Lassen, MD, PhD, head, department of oncology, Rigshospitalet, Copenhagen.

yet for 90% of people with this deadly disease, when symptoms occur, it's too late for surgery to help.

Now scientists are finding that a specific pancreatic condition could serve as an early warning system—acute pancreatitis.

Pancreatitis is an inflammation of the pancreas. It can be an acute (short-lived) episode, which depending on the cause can turn into a long-term, chronic disease. With acute pancreatitis, symptoms start suddenly and include abdominal and back pain, nausea, vomiting and fever.

Doctors have known that pancreatitis increases the risk for pancreatic cancer, but the new research suggests that acute pancreatitis could be the first sign of it...and presents an opportunity to proactively test for it.

The study: Swedish researchers followed about 50,000 patients newly diagnosed with acute pancreatitis. They matched them with a group of close to 140,000 people free of pancreatitis and followed them over an average period of five years. During this time, there were 769 cases of pancreatic cancer... and 70% of the cases were in the people who had had acute pancreatitis.

Even more important was the finding that the risk for pancreatic cancer was highest in the first two months after acute pancreatitis. In fact, the risk was close to 200 times higher. The researchers believe that this very high likelihood suggests that pancreatic cancer may already be present during the first episode of acute pancreatitis.

It's important to note that most cases of acute pancreatitis are caused by either gallstones or heavy use of alcohol, and that the pancreatic cancer risk is associated with drinking, not gallstones. Alcohol abuse is a shared risk factor for pancreatic cancer and pancreatitis (so is smoking).

If you or a loved one is diagnosed with acute pancreatitis, talk to your doctor about doing an imaging study to look for pancreatic cancer, preferably an endoscopic ultrasound (EUS). EUS is done by placing a flexible scope down the throat and through the stomach. Sound waves from the tip of the scope are used to form images of the pancreas. EUS is close to 100% accurate at finding pancreatic cancers smaller than 25 millimeters. Removing a tumor at this stage gives the best chance for long-term survival. Talk to your doctor about any need for future imaging tests if the results of the first one are negative.

Diagnosing pancreatic cancer during an episode of acute pancreatitis could lead to successful surgery. Missing an early diagnosis could mean missing the chance for surgical treatment…and survival.

Device Fights Brain Tumors

A wearable device applied to a patient's shaved scalp slows the growth of glioblastoma (an aggressive brain tumor) by delivering continuous, low-intensity electric currents to brain tissue. The FDA-cleared Optune device is used in addition to chemotherapy. Median survival among patients using the device is about five months longer than for those who do not use the device—and significantly more of the treated group were alive up to two to four years afterward.

Roger Stupp, MD, chief of neuro-oncology and medical director, Malnati Brain Tumor Institute, Northwestern University Feinberg School of Medicine, Chicago.

Power Up to Fight Cancer

Rebecca Shannonhouse, editor, *Bottom Line Heath.*

You probably know that people who exercise are less likely to develop various types of cancer. But for those who have cancer, physical activity can be even more important. It increases strength, eases treatment side effects, improves quality of life—and even helps cancer patients live longer.

The problem is, oncologists and other frontline caregivers don't always have the resources to steer patients to suitable exercise programs.

Good news: Just about every community in the US has a YMCA, and many team with the Livestrong Foundation (a nonprofit organization that supports cancer survivors) to provide the "Livestrong at the YMCA" program, which offers strength, balance and cardiovascular conditioning.

The 12-week programs, at 245 Ys in 41 states, require a doctor's OK and are free or low cost. The small groups, which meet twice weekly for 75 to 90 minutes, are led by YMCA-certified instructors and include quality-of-life and functional assessments, along with fitness training.

Positive results: Participants report having less cancer-related fatigue, improved cardiovascular endurance and better quality of life.

If you or a loved one has been diagnosed with cancer or treated for the disease in the past, check Livestrong.org/ymca-search for a Y program near you.

Melanoma: The Major Good News

Marianne Berwick, PhD, distinguished professor, department of internal medicine, University of New Mexico School of Medicine, and former chief, Division of Epidemiology, Biostatistics and Preventive Medicine, University of New Mexico Comprehensive Cancer Center, both in Albuquerque.

Many adults grew up during the sun-loving era of the 1950s, '60s and '70s.

Now: It's believed to be partially responsible for the quadrupling of melanoma cases over the past several decades. More than 9,000 Americans die from the disease each year.

Patients and doctors also are paying more attention to skin changes that might be cancer—and spotting melanoma earlier.

Major good news: Early-stage melanoma is usually cured by lesion-removing surgery. The five-year survival rate for early-stage melanoma is 99%. But even stage III melanoma, cancer that has spread to nearby skin or lymph nodes, has a five-year survival rate of 63%. Stage IV melanoma, in which cancer has metastasized or spread to other sites in the body, has a five-year survival rate of 20%—but even for these advanced cases, new therapies designed to contain or reverse the disease are extending lives. *Here's what's new…*

Diagnosis

Examination of all the skin on your body by a savvy dermatologist at least once a year—and a biopsy of any suspicious moles—is still the best first-line of defense against melanoma. Be alert to the "ABCDE" warning signs for melanoma (see the next page). Bring any skin changes to your doctor's attention immediately (even if it isn't time for your yearly skin check).

Diagnostic danger: Melanoma is tough to diagnose, particularly in its early, or "thin," stage, when the mole is less than one-millimeter thick.

My advice: If your doctor tells you that you have melanoma, ask to have your biopsy slide sent to another pathologist for a second opinion. Check first with your insurance provider to see if that's covered and if you need preauthorization.

Also important: Most people think of melanoma as a brown or black spot that is changing. But amelanotic melanoma is pale and reddish and has a poor prognosis because it's usually detected after it has spread.

What to do: Alert your doctor to both dark and light unusual skin changes.

New option: If you have a suspicious lesion, you may be able to avoid surgical biopsy. Ask your doctor about having genetic testing instead, such as the Dermtech Pigmented Lesion Assay (PLA). It is highly accurate in distinguishing malignant melanoma from benign nevi, and may be covered by your insurer.

New Therapies

New therapies are brightening the previous grim outlook for advanced melanoma.

For example, several recently approved oral drugs inhibit a genetic mutation called BRAF that drives approximately 40% to 60% of melanomas. These drugs, which slow the growth of tumors and extend life, include *vemurafenib* (Zelboraf) and *dabrafenib* (Tafinlar).

A new class of drugs called MEK inhibitors—*trametinib* (Mekinist), *cobimetinib* (Cotellic) and others—inhibit the MEK protein, which helps speed the growth and spread of melanoma tumors.

New development: Combining dabrafenib and trametinib more than doubles average survival for advanced melanoma from five months to 11 months. Unfortunately, these drugs do have side effects, ranging from headaches and fatigue to kidney and heart problems—and even, ironically, basal cell carcinoma, another type of skin cancer. Also, although they can slow and shrink tumors and extend life for months, even years, the cancer eventually returns.

What to do: Make sure your oncologist tests your tumor for genetic mutations.

Immunotherapy—drugs such as *pembrolizumab* (Keytruda), *nivolumab* (Opdivo) and *ipilimumab* (Yervoy) that stimulate the immune system to fight cancer—is another new way to treat advanced melanoma. But the drugs work only in a small percentage of patients, control cancer for a limited time, are very expensive and have a range of debilitating and even deadly side effects.

New development: Combination immunotherapy—such as the immunotherapeutic drug Keytruda with cellular therapy, which uses immune cells such as interleukin or interferon—is showing better results in clinical trials. FDA-approved interferon and interleukin-based treatments for melanoma include *aldesleukin* (Proleukin), *interferon alfa-2b* (Intron A) and *peginterferon alfa-2b* (Sylatron).

Fewer Surgical Complications

Once melanoma is diagnosed, a sentinel-lymph-node biopsy can determine whether it has spread to nearby lymph nodes. Often, all lymph nodes in an area are removed if cancer is found in the sentinel lymph node. However, removing all the lymph nodes in an arm or a leg can cause lymphedema—permanent, painful swelling of the limb that limits activity and can lead to frequent infections.

New scientific finding: Less extreme surgery is just as effective, according to a study conducted at 63 medical centers and reported in *The New England Journal of Medicine*.

Details: 1,900 patients with melanoma that had spread to at least one lymph node either had all their lymph nodes in the area of the affected node immediately removed…or had only the affected lymph node or nodes removed, while the other nodes in the area were tracked with ultrasound. If melanoma occurred in a new node, the other lymph nodes were removed. After three years, the two groups had the same survival times.

But patients who had all their lymph nodes removed had four times the risk for severe swelling in the affected arm or leg.

ABCDE Warning Signs of Melanoma

Asymmetry…irregular Borders…more than one or uneven distribution of Color…Diameter larger than one-quarter inch…Evolution, such as changes in color and/or size.

New Hope for Bladder Cancer

Brant Allen Inman, MD, MS, a urologist, associate professor of surgery at Duke University School of Medicine and a member of the Duke Cancer Institute, all in Durham, North Carolina. He specializes in diagnostic tests/therapies for bladder cancer and other genitourinary malignancies.

After years without any significant treatment advances or new prevention strategies, bladder cancer is finally getting its due.

Recent developments: The FDA approved five new drugs in 2016–2017 for the treatment of metastatic bladder cancer. It's an important development because these cancers are often deadly, with a five-year survival rate as low as 15% when the cancer is advanced.

Even though the prognosis for people diagnosed with early-stage bladder cancer has been good for quite some time—up to 95% are alive after five years when the cancer is confined to the inner layer of the bladder wall—a late-stage diagnosis now has more treatment options than ever before. In some cases, a new treatment option can double survival time.

What's more, research is uncovering additional steps that can help prevent bladder cancer from recurring after it's been treated—strategies that also will help protect people from developing this malignancy in the first place.

Prevention Is Best

Even though bladder cancer does not get as much public attention as certain other types, it is the sixth most common cancer in the US (and the fourth most common among men), with about 81,000 new cases diagnosed every year.

The good news is that most bladder cancers (about 75%) are non-muscle invasive—that is, they're limited to the lining of the bladder…are usually diagnosed early…and respond well to treatment.

One distinguishing characteristic of bladder cancer is its recurrence rate. More than half of all people treated for this malignancy will have a recurrence. For this reason, it's crucial for anyone with bladder cancer to do everything possible to prevent a recurrence.

Smokers are four to seven times more likely to develop bladder cancer than nonsmokers. The toxins from cigarette smoke are excreted from the body in the urine—and spend many hours concentrated in the bladder, where they can trigger cancer-causing changes. *Other ways to help prevent a bladder cancer diagnosis or recurrence…*

• **Eat more kale.** Cruciferous vegetables (such as kale, broccoli, cauliflower and cabbage) are high in isothiocyanates, chemical compounds that inhibit the ability of cancer cells, including bladder cancer cells, to proliferate. Men who consumed cruciferous vegetables more than five times a week were 51% less likely to develop bladder cancer than those who ate them less than once a week, according to the Health Professionals Follow-Up Study.

• **Stay hydrated.** People who drink more water urinate more frequently, which reduces chemical concentrations and exposure times from cigarette smoke (including secondhand smoke), workplace chemicals (such as polyaromatic hydrocarbons and dyes), air pollution, etc.

Important exception: Research has shown that people who drink water from private wells that may be contaminated with arsenic are at increased risk for bladder can-cer. Water that contains high levels of nitrate, a by-product of fertilizers and animal feedlots, has been linked to higher rates of bladder cancer in postmenopausal women.

Take note: If you drink well water, get it checked!

Catch It Early

After prevention, early detection is, of course, the best way to avoid bladder cancer deaths.

An annual urine test may be worthwhile if you're at high risk—for example, you're already having symptoms (discussed below)…you are exposed to workplace toxins that increase your risk…you're a smoker…and/or you have a personal or family history of bladder cancer.

Important: About 80% to 90% of patients who are diagnosed with bladder cancer will have visible traces of blood in the urine. Blood can appear for many reasons, including urinary tract infections (UTIs) or prostate problems. However, if you see blood in your urine, I advise that you assume it might be cancer and see a physician or possibly a urologist.

Other red flags: Frequent trouble urinating…feeling pain or burning while urinating…and feeling that you need to urinate right away, even when the bladder isn't full. Particularly in women, bladder cancer may be misdiagnosed as a recurrent UTI. A urine culture (not just an in-office urinalysis) is needed to diagnose UTI correctly.

Drug Breakthroughs

The recently FDA-approved checkpoint inhibitors target proteins that weaken the immune system. In doing so, the drugs—*pembrolizumab* (Keytruda), *avelumab* (Bavencio), *durvalumab* (Imfinzi), *nivolumab* (Opdivo) and *atezolizumab* (Tecentriq)—intensify immune activity against tumor cells.

An older form of immunotherapy, called intravesical therapy, uses a bacterium (BCG) that's instilled into the bladder. This approach inhibits cancer progression and can reduce the risk for recurrences by about 40%. BCG causes an inflammatory reaction that leads to the recruitment of other immune cells to the bladder, which helps eradicate bladder tumors and helps prevent them from recurring.

Depending on the stage of the cancer, checkpoint inhibitors are an important advancement because they can help patients who didn't do well with BCG or other treatments—or who improved initially but later suffered a cancer recurrence.

The drugs aren't a cure, but they can double the survival time in some cases of metastatic cancer that has not responded to chemotherapy. This means the average survival time of six months is increased to 10 to 12 months.

Another potential benefit: It's hoped that checkpoint inhibitors will control cancer well enough that removal of the bladder, which has been required in those who haven't responded well to other treatments, can be delayed or avoided altogether—but this is still being studied.

Downside: Immunotherapy drugs can increase levels of inflammation throughout the body. Many of these inflammatory reactions are minor and can be managed with topical creams or by stopping the drug temporarily for a couple of weeks. However, in some cases, the reactions can be severe and, in very rare cases, even fatal. When the reaction is more severe, the drug is stopped and the overactive immune system is suppressed by giving steroids and other immunosuppressive drugs.

Massage for Cancer Patients

Susan G. Salvo, EdD, LMT, instructor, Louisiana Institute of Massage Therapy, Lake Charles. SusanSalvo.com

I s it safe to continue getting massages after a cancer diagnosis?

There's a widely held misconception that massage causes cancer to spread. In fact,

the National Comprehensive Cancer Network recommends massage, as long as precautions are observed.

Research has shown that massage can improve sleep and reduce pain, anxiety, depression and fatigue in cancer patients. It also can decrease side effects related to chemotherapy, radiation and surgery. In research, participants received a 30-minute massage once daily, biweekly or weekly.

Precautions: Your massage practitioner should have training in oncology massage. For a referral, ask your doctor or check the Society for Oncology Massage at S4OM.org.

Also, tell your therapist your goals for therapy…the type of cancer you have (as well as tumor sites and metastases)…the treatments you've received, including side effects…locations of any implanted devices, such as a port for chemo…and any restrictions made by your doctor.

Insurance may cover the cost of massage for cancer patients.

Getting Your Sex Life Back on Track After Cancer

Sharon L. Bober, PhD, director of the Sexual Health Program at Dana-Farber Cancer Institute and senior psychologist and assistant professor of psychiatry at Harvard Medical School, both in Boston.

W hile you're undergoing treatment for cancer, sex is likely not at the top of your mind. But once the treatments are—thankfully!—behind you, while you're getting the rest of your life back on track, you might yearn for the sexual intimacy and pleasure you used to have. You may have new challenges post-cancer, but there are many solutions.

Unfortunately, most patients are left in the dark about the sexual side effects of their cancer. Health-care providers don't bring up the topic while discussing treatment options—partly because they don't want to embarrass their patients, and partly because they're focused on more serious health concerns. Patients also may feel too embarrassed to mention sex. And for patients older than age 50—especially those without a partner—oncologists may assume that sex is no longer important.

So it's up to you to start the conversation. For instance, you might say, "I'm having a lot of discomfort and things have really changed in my sex life. Can I talk to you about it or can you tell me who I can talk to?"

Here are some common sex challenges that cancer survivors face…

•**You just survived a life-threatening illness**—now you feel guilty for even complaining about something as "trivial" as sex. Many patients believe that a nonexistent sex life is the price they have to pay for surviving cancer. Nothing could be further from the truth! Sexual health is essential to quality of life and an important contributor to your whole health. And intimacy with a loving partner can help you heal by releasing feel-good hormones, including oxytocin, that ease anxiety.

•**Your genitalia just aren't the same.** Chemo and hormone treatments can dry out the vagina and cause it to atrophy, making sex, masturbation and gynecological exams painful. Radiation, surgery and chemo can cause erectile dysfunction in men, even if their cancer was not directly related to their genital area, such as prostate or bladder cancer.

For women: Using a vaginal moisturizer on a regular basis can bring better long-term relief than lubricants. Lubricants temporarily relieve vaginal and vulvar dryness and reduce friction. Vaginal moisturizers provide longer-term relief for dryness, itching and irritation—and also can restore the health of the vaginal lining.

You may need to apply a moisturizer more often than is recommended on the box for the most effective relief—at least three to five times a week is ideal, applied at bedtime for the best absorption.

Good options: Replens, Hyalo Gyn, PrevaLeaf Oasis…or pure coconut oil. Ask your health-care provider to recommend what would be best for you.

For men: While doctors are quick to solve erection problems with a prescription for a phosphodiesterase-5 (PDE5) inhibitor such as *sildenafil* (Viagra), there are other options. Penile injections—sometimes called intracavernosal injection therapy—are more effective than taking PDE5 pills. While the idea may seem daunting, men are often glad to hear that there is another option when the "little blue pill" doesn't work. Vacuum erection devices that increase blood flow into the penis to help achieve an erection and penile rings to help maintain one are other options.

For both women and men: A pelvic-floor physical therapist can help restore sexual function with massage, dilators and exercises to build up pelvic-floor muscles, loosen tight muscles and stretch and desensitize scar tissue.

Bonus: These therapies also can reduce urinary and fecal incontinence, a common side effect of cancer therapies. If there isn't a specially trained pelvic-floor PT near you, a regular physical therapist may know where you can find one…or may know some exercises that can help.

•**You've tried having sex, but it's just not the same.** Sexual pleasure depends on more than the mechanics of intercourse. Think about ways to achieve intimacy and pleasure without the pressure of reaching an orgasm…or even penile penetration of the vagina. Do what you did when you were dating—hug, cuddle, touch and kiss.

Explore using toys, such as a vibrator, or try new foreplay techniques—experiment with what feels good. Starting slowly, taking your time and expanding your repertoire are all key. A satisfying sex life won't happen overnight. But the journey can be enjoyable, too!

•**You're willing to get help from a professional, but you have no clue what kind you need or where to find one.** Online resources can provide useful information to help you recover your sexual health on your own…or point you toward a trained professional who can assist you. Will2Love.com is a site founded and run by medical doctors and psychologists that focuses on sexual health for cancer survivors. It's a self-help program that you can do at home and lists psychologists who provide phone counseling.

You also can find providers who specialize in sexual medicine at the International Society for Sexual Medicine, ISSM.info. And there are online forums filled with men and women who are going through the same issues you are at Breast Cancer.org…the American Cancer Society's Cancer Survivors Network, CSN.Cancer.org/forum…and FORCE (Facing Our Risk of Cancer Empowered), FacingOurRisk.org/index.php.

Sometimes, all it takes is talking to the right person—perhaps a urologist, a social worker, a nurse or a fellow patient—to rediscover the intimacy you once had.

If It's Your Spouse Who Had Cancer…

When your love life was fine, you probably didn't talk about sex. But now that it's not going as well, while you don't want to stir up negative emotions, it's important to bring the topic into the open for discussion. Framing concerns, fears and wishes using "I" statements instead of "you" can keep the conversation from sounding accusatory.

Example: "I know you feel self-conscious about your body, but you are as beautiful/handsome to me as ever, and I've never stopped wanting you. Can we talk about this?"

Pick a good time and a safe, neutral place to talk, even if you have to schedule it. (For instance, don't launch into this topic when the two of you are getting into bed.) You might be happily surprised at how relieved your partner is to talk!

Skin Creams OK

Patients undergoing radiation have long been told not to use skin cream in the hours before treatment due to a belief that it increases the amount of radiation absorbed by the skin. Recent tests showed no difference in the surface dose of radiation when lotion was applied to a material similar to human tissue just before radiation therapy.

Exception: Thick layers of cream (more than 3 mm, or about the thickness of two stacked pennies) did increase the radiation dose.

If you are undergoing radiation treatment: Ask your doctor about using a product such as an unscented petroleum-based topical ointment.

Brian C. Baumann, MD, assistant professor of radiation oncology, Washington University School of Medicine, St. Louis.

Rose Geranium Remedy

Cancer patients with nasal symptoms caused by treatment get relief with a nasal spray of rose geranium oil mixed into sesame oil. Almost all patients undergoing chemo or other drug regimens reported significant reduction of nasal side effects including pain, sores and bleeding when they used the spray. Ask your doctor to prescribe a spray of medical-grade sesame and rose geranium oils, which can be filled by a compounding pharmacist.

Elizabeth Cathcart-Rake, MD, is chief fellow in hematology/oncology at Mayo Clinic, Rochester, Minnesota. Her research was published in *BMJ Supportive & Palliative Care*.

Injection Stops Chemo Pain

Preclinical animal study: A single injection of a naturally occurring protein

(AIBP) may stop the severe, lingering pain from chemotherapy—without the risk for addiction from opioid painkillers.

Cell Reports.

Head and Neck Cancer Treatment: The Right Timing Is Survival

Allen Ho, MD, director, Head and Neck Cancer Program, associate professor of surgery, Cedars-Sinai Medical Center, Los Angeles, and lead author of study titled "Quantitative Survival Impact of Composite Treatment Delays in Head and Neck Cancer" published in *Cancer*.

When you're diagnosed with head or neck cancer, a lot of information will be thrown at you all at once. There is so much to take in, specialists to talk to, treatment decisions to make. Should you schedule surgery immediately? When should you start radiation? How long should all these treatments take? A recent study has found lifesaving answers to these questions.

The study: Researchers at Cedars-Sinai Medical Center in Los Angeles examined the medical records of 15,064 head and neck cancer patients in the US who underwent surgery and a full course of radiation for their cancer. *They looked at these key treatment intervals to see what effect they had on patient survival…*

 • **The time from diagnosis to the day of surgery**

 • **The time from surgery to the start of radiation**

 • **The time from the first to the last radiation treatment**

The findings: What impacted survival rates was the length of time between surgery and the start of radiation as well as the length of time between the first and last radiation treatment.

Typically, radiation starts between 14 and 40 days after surgery. For every day beyond 40 days, the risk of death went up progressively each day until 70 days post-surgery, at which point this risk leveled off. The five-year survival rate dropped progressively from 66.5% for those who started by day 40 down to 50% for those who started after day 70 or later.

When radiation wasn't completed within the usual 40 days (about six weeks), the risk of death increased each day up to 55 days, at which point, again, this risk leveled off. The five-year survival rate dropped progressively from 59.9% for those who finished radiation on time to 50.8% for those who needed 55 days or more.

The researchers also looked at the total treatment—from the day of surgery through the completion of radiation. Survival was greatest when this took up to 84 days. However, as the span increased to 123 days or more, five-year survival dropped from 70% to 47.9%.

Why does time become more of a factor after surgery than before? Surgery disrupts blood flow, which disrupts oxygen supply to cancer cells that remain after surgery. Radiation uses oxygen to kill the cancer cells. With less oxygen, radiation is less effective—and cancer cells have more opportunity to grow. The researchers noted that when there were delays once radiation started, cancer cells that were not yet destroyed were possibly more resistant to radiation.

Minimize Delays

There are common reasons for delays, both before the start of radiation and during this treatment. For instance, if there are complications with the surgery or if you don't recover as quickly as expected, the radiation treatments will likely need to be postponed.

Once you start radiation, if side effects such as dehydration, mouth ulcers and swelling become serious, you could need a treatment break—usually a minimum of two days to recover.

One way to minimize the likelihood of such delays is to develop a treatment plan with built-in contingencies that will still allow you to complete surgery and radiation within the optimal time. Head and neck cancer treatment often involves seeing many specialists, including a surgical oncologist, a radiation oncologist, a medical oncologist, a dentist (because radiation can affect your teeth), a speech and swallow therapist and a nutritionist.

The one delay that did not impact survival rates was the interval between diagnosis and surgery, so take the time you need to meet with everyone on your team and plan out every step of your treatment, including how all possible setbacks will be handled. Start by scheduling radiation treatments as soon after surgery as possible to improve radiation's ability to destroy microscopic disease.

Another key step is to optimize your health as much as you can before surgery. Continue to eat well to maintain your weight and strength in the days before radiation since food may not taste good once you start that treatment and you may not have much of an appetite. Also, get needed sleep and find ways to exercise.

Step Up to Defeat Cancer Fatigue

A recent study of advanced cancer patients undergoing treatment found that increased daily steps and stairs climbed correlated with less fatigue and pain and fewer hospitalizations.

Takeaway: Fitness trackers, which record steps and other data, may help doctors assess how treatment is affecting a patient's health and daily functioning.

Andrew Hendifar, MD, medical director for pancreatic cancer, Cedars-Sinai Samuel Oschin Comprehensive Cancer Institute, Los Angeles.

"I'm Scared My Cancer Will Come Back"

Kathleen Ashton, PhD, a health psychologist at Cleveland Clinic who works with breast cancer patients and patients at risk for breast cancer, and a faculty member of Lerner College of Medicine, both in Cleveland.

You made it through cancer treatment. You should be feeling free and happy, but you can't stop feeling like there's a sword hanging over your head. For many, if not most, survivors, fear of cancer coming back is a persistent concern. It can affect quality of life for many years after treatment, and for some, the fear becomes severe and disabling.

The risk of recurrence varies widely between types of cancer. For each type of cancer, the stage, cell type, treatment and genetic makeup of the patient also affect risk of recurrence. For some common cancers like colon, breast and prostate cancers, the overall risk is about 20% to 30%, but for others, such as bladder cancer and lymphoma, it can be twice as high, so it's normal for patients to have worries.

But for some, normal worries build into significant fear and anxiety...into a condition that even has its own name, FOCR—fear of cancer recurrence. Some people are at higher risk for FOCR than others, such as those whose cancer has a high recurrence rate, such as ovarian, lung and brain cancers. Another risk factor is having a history of anxiety or depression before cancer.

How to Recognize FOCR

People with FOCR are unable to escape worry and anxiety. Similar to people with PTSD, they may avoid anything that reminds them of cancer, including skipping follow-up appointments and cancer surveillance testing—the very things that could help protect them. *Other clues to watch for include...*

- **Sleep problems**
- **Racing thoughts**

- **Constant tension or anxiety**
- **Irritability**
- **Loss of interest in the future**
- **Feeling that life is out of control**

Obviously, FOCR will affect your quality of life. If you have symptoms, let your doctor know so it can be diagnosed and, most important, treated.

Take Action to Manage FOCR

Step one to manage FOCR is a cancer survivorship plan, which should be set up with your cancer team soon after treatment. This is a must for any cancer survivor, so if you've been putting it off or have one but aren't following through, it's time for a reboot. *A survivorship plan includes…*

- **An honest discussion about the realistic risk for recurrence**
- **The type of surveillance testing you will follow**
- **Signs and symptoms of recurrence to look for**
- **A plan for what happens if recurrence occurs**
- **Lifestyle strategies to reduce the risk of recurrence**

If you've been afraid to verbalize any of these issues (maybe you feel talking about them makes recurrence loom even more), you might be surprised to learn that, for many survivors, having a plan actually reduces unreasonable fears of recurrence.

Feeling that life is out of your control is one of the hardest things cancer survivors live with. Taking back some control with lifestyle changes that reduce your risk of recurrence can be empowering. *For many cancer survivors, these include…*

- **Losing weight if you are overweight or maintaining a healthy weight**
- **Eating a healthy diet**—and, in particular, eating lots of vegetables and avoiding sugar and refined carbohydrates
- **Getting daily exercise**
- **Getting enough sleep**
- **Avoiding alcohol**
- **Not smoking**

Self-help strategies can also help. You might practice a formal stress reduction method such as meditation or guided relaxation or join a cancer recovery support group.

It can be difficult to cope with FOCR alone. Treatment from a mental health provider can help you conquer fears of recurrence. *Effective treatments include…*

- **Cognitive behavioral therapy,** a form of psychotherapy that helps you recognize unhealthy or unreasonable thoughts and behaviors and replace them with healthy coping strategies and an action plan.
- **Mindfulness and exposure therapies,** psychotherapies that teach you to be present with your thoughts. You may learn to face your fears without judgment and reduce the power of fearful thoughts over time.

Talking about cancer recurrence and planning for a healthy survivorship will control FOCR for most people, allowing for an active recovery and a full life.

Chapter 4

DIABETES BREAKTHROUGHS

Negative Personality Traits Up Diabetes Risk

All those "Negative Nellies" out there may have more to worry about than frown lines. Researchers digging into data from the Women's Health Initiative (WHI) recently identified an association between personality traits (such as negativity, pessimism and hostility) in postmenopausal women and a higher risk of developing type 2 diabetes.

The good news is, a sunnier disposition, including optimism, may help protect against diabetes. *Here's what the researchers found—and what's being recommended…*

Study details: Nearly 140,000 postmenopausal women who did not have diabetes completed a self-administered questionnaire that assessed their personality traits and their health behaviors, such as diet, exercise, smoking and drinking alcohol. Over the next 14 years, 19,240 (about 14%) of the women developed diabetes.

Those who scored highest for hostility (highest quartile) had a 17% increased risk of developing diabetes compared with those in the lowest quartile for hostility.

Those who scored highest for negativity had a 9% increased risk of developing the disease compared with those with the lowest negativity scores (lowest quartile).

For unknown reasons, the link between hostility and diabetes risk was not as pronounced in women who were obese compared with women who were not—though obesity remains a major risk factor for the disease.

Now the positive side: The study participants with positive personality traits characterized by high optimism, low negativity and low hostility had a 12% lower risk of developing diabetes compared with those who were least optimistic.

"Personality traits remain stable across one's lifetime," explains JoAnn Pinkerton, MD, executive director of The North American Menopause Society. For that reason, Dr. Pinkerton says, this new finding could help doctors identify women who may be at a higher risk for diabetes so that they can tailor prevention and treatment strategies to each woman's personality.

Takeaway: If you're a postmenopausal woman—especially if you have risk factors for diabetes, such as being overweight or

The study "Personality Traits and Diabetes Incidence Among Postmenopausal Women" was published in *Menopause*, the journal of The North American Menopause Society.

obese…low physical activity…and/or a family history of the disease—discuss with your doctor whether your personality may be putting you at even greater risk. Knowing where you stand is the first step to protecting your health!

The Diabetes Risk Factors That Aren't on Your Radar

Aaron Price, LICSW, clinical social worker and lecturer at the Joslin Diabetes Center in Boston, an affiliate of Harvard Medical School. Joslin.org

Study titled "Excess Mortality in Finnish Diabetic Subjects Due to Alcohol, Accidents and Suicide: A Nationwide Study" by researchers at the universities of Helsinki, Eastern Finland and Tampere, published in *European Journal of Endocrinology*.

According to a sweeping study done in Finland, deaths from alcoholism—both directly from diseases such as cirrhosis or from accidents related to drinking, such as falling while under the influence—and suicide are higher among people with diabetes than the general public, and even more so for people taking insulin.

The study: Researchers followed more than 200,000 women and men with diabetes over a seven-year period and compared their mortality rates to a similar number of people free from diabetes.

The findings: Surprisingly, women with diabetes, including those on only oral medication, had a risk for death related to alcohol use that was 10 times higher than the general population (for men with diabetes, that rate is seven times higher than the general population). In addition to increasing the risk for fatal accidents and suicide—roughly twice the number for men and slightly more than 50% higher for women, excessive drinking impairs self-care and can worsen diabetes itself. It's also linked to severe hypoglycemia (low blood sugar), which can be fatal. Though the researchers can't explain exactly why alcohol has a deadlier impact on women

with diabetes than men with diabetes, they suggest that it could be because women in general experience greater levels of depression than men do.

The Overlooked Part of Diabetes Care

Diabetes brings with it a wide range of emotions. Fear over complications can trigger anxiety and depression. You might feel guilty that you're not managing it as carefully as you think you should. The CDC estimates that in any 18-month period, 33% to 50% of those with diabetes are suffering from "diabetes distress."

Alcohol isn't the answer, but what is? *These three tweaks to your diabetes management style can help…*

• **Clarify the areas of self-care you need to improve on,** and create a clear plan to meet them. That may sound daunting, but you can make it easier on yourself by breaking down the steps into manageable pieces. Let's say that you should check your blood sugar four times a day, but you can't reach that number on a steady basis. Start with one or two daily checks, and tie them to existing lifestyle habits to make them easier to remember. For example, check your blood sugar every morning before you walk the dog and every evening after you eat dinner. After twice-a-day becomes rote, gradually add in more checks, ideally attached to other existing habits.

Important: Working with a diabetes coach can help you establish vital habits.

• **Let your family and friends become your partners in care.** There are many lifestyle changes to make when you develop diabetes, and few of them are easy. Rather than try to tough it out yourself, allow family members and friends to help you stay on track. Maybe one person can exercise with you every morning, and another helps cook meals with you every evening. As a bonus, you'll strengthen your relationships in the process.

•**Get professional support.** If you find that you're feeling down more days than not and certainly if you're drinking too much (more than one drink per day) or having thoughts of suicide, reach out to your doctor or a licensed mental health professional. A therapist who has been through the Mental Health Provider Diabetes Education Program, a joint program developed by the American Diabetes Association and the American Psychological Association, is specially trained to help people overcome their struggles with diabetes. You can find a practitioner near you through the search function at the American Diabetes Association website.

Magnesium-Rich Foods Could Reduce Diabetes Risk

Scientists tracked roughly 200,000 people for 28 years. Those who reported getting the most magnesium had a 15% lower risk for type 2 diabetes than those who reported getting the least. Good sources of magnesium include whole grains, leafy greens, nuts and beans.

Study by researchers at Harvard T.H. Chan School of Public Health, Boston, published in *Diabetes Care*.

The Diabetes Danger Most Doctors Miss

George L. King, MD, chief scientific officer at the Boston-based Joslin Diabetes Center. He is author, with Royce Flippin, of *Reverse Your Diabetes in 12 Weeks*. Joslin.org

Most of the nearly 30 million Americans who have type 2 diabetes are not even aware that cardiovascular problems pose a huge risk for them.

Even more troubling: Your doctor may be facing a knowledge gap, too—for different reasons. A new generation of prescription diabetes medications now is available, and these drugs are particularly effective at helping people with type 2 diabetes control their blood sugar while simultaneously reducing their risk for cardiovascular disease. (One botanical supplement may have similar benefits—see page 80.) But the proper use of these medications can be so complicated that your doctor may not be making the right choice for you.

New Heart-Friendly Diabetes Drugs

For many years, there were only three types of drugs—not counting insulin—to help people with type 2 diabetes control their blood glucose levels. Metformin typically was prescribed first (and still is)—it's effective, safe and affordable. It has not been shown to increase or decrease cardiovascular risk.

When metformin wasn't enough to control blood sugar, sulfonylureas often have been prescribed in addition. They are effective—sometimes too effective, leading to dangerous low-blood-sugar episodes. More disturbing, some studies have found that long-term use of sulfonylureas are associated with an increased risk for heart disease. Similarly, thiazolidinediones, introduced in the 1990s, have been shown to increase the risk for heart failure.

What's new: In the past decade, and especially in just the past few years, a host of new, heart-friendly diabetes drugs have appeared. Most notable are the glucagon-like peptide-1 receptor agonists (GLP-1 agonists, for short) and sodium–glucose cotransporter 2 inhibitors (SGLT2 inhibitors). Both types have been shown in large studies to not just control blood glucose levels but also reduce the risk for heart failure—and reduce mortality in people with type 2 diabetes.

Other new diabetes drugs include dipeptidyl peptidase-4 inhibitors (DPP-4 inhibitors), which don't increase cardiovascular risk, and colesevelam and bromocriptine, both of which may reduce cardiovascular risk but have significant side effects. Each of these is a different type of drug, and the complexity is leading to some not-so-smart prescriptions and danger for patients.

The Doctor Knowledge Gap

Metformin remains the "first-line" type 2 diabetes drug. But what should be prescribed when, together with lifestyle changes, it's not enough? Unfortunately, some doctors will not come up with the best answer to that question.

Type 2 diabetes typically is treated by primary care physicians, some of whom are not well-versed in the latest research…or who lack the time to figure out which of the drug options is best-suited to a particular patient. Don't blame your doctor—selecting type 2 diabetes drugs has very quickly become very complicated. Doctors must not only sort through an ever-widening range of drug options with various (and different) side effects, but they also must consider each patient's blood glucose levels, cardiovascular condition, other prescribed medications and, increasingly, financial situation.

Example: New joint guidelines from the American Diabetes Association and the European Association for the Study of Diabetes, recommend the use of GLP-1 agonists or SGLT2 inhibitors as the second drug after metformin for patients with type 2 diabetes who have cardiovascular disease. But while metformin and sulfonylureas can cost less than $10 for a 30-day supply, these newer drugs can run $400 or more per month for patients who must pay out of pocket…and might have hefty co-pays. There are many medical caveats, too—such as not using SGLT2 inhibitors in a patient with a certain degree of kidney failure…and how to ramp up the dosage of a GLP-1 agonist to decrease potential side effects.

What Diabetes Patients Should Do

Do not assume that the glucose-control drugs your doctor has prescribed are necessarily the best drugs for you. *In particular…*

• **If you take a drug other than metformin to control blood glucose**—and especially if you take three or more glucose-control drugs—ask your doctor to explain why he/she selected each of these drugs.

• **If you have a history of heart attack or stroke and are taking multiple drugs to control your blood glucose**—but are not taking a GLP-1 agonist or SGLT2 inhibitor—ask your doctor whether one of these might be appropriate for you.

• **If your doctor cannot explain why he chose the drugs you are taking in a way that you can understand** and that sounds reasonable, ask for a referral to an endocrinologist who specializes in the treatment of diabetes.

The Growing Power of Lifestyle

The new diabetes medications give doctors new tools to tailor treatment to an individual's most important risks, including cardiovascular risk. But it's never a good idea to take an additional drug to control your blood sugar if you can do so through lifestyle changes instead, which are more powerful and healthier than any drugs. Fortunately, most of the lifestyle changes that help control blood sugar also protect your heart. Even small changes—such as getting up from your desk and walking around for five minutes every hour—can be very helpful. *My recommendations…*

• **Work up to walking 10,000 steps a day.** You can track this on your phone or with a fitness watch or pedometer.

• **Get 60 minutes of more vigorous exercise every other day**—evenly split between aerobics (such as treadmill jogging) and strength training.

Good news: Those jogging "steps" count toward your 10,000.

• **At mealtime, follow the two-one-one formula**—two portions nonstarchy vegetables (especially dark, leafy greens)…one portion whole grains, legumes or starchy vegetables…and one portion protein-rich food (fish, poultry, lean beef, tofu). For dessert, fruit is best.

• **Get seven or eight hours of sleep a night.**

I know the power of these lifestyle changes from personal experience. About 25 years ago, when my father was age 72, he developed diabetes and was promptly placed on three medications. He took them, but at the same time he began walking an hour a day and eating as I describe above. A year and a half later, while he still technically "had" diabetes, he no longer needed any medication to control it. That's why I have been following this lifestyle myself ever since.

Vitamin D Lowers Diabetes Risk

Healthy adults whose blood levels of 25-hydroxyvitamin D, a marker for vitamin D, were more than 30 ng/mL had one-third the risk for diabetes, and those with levels above 50 ng/mL had one-fifth the risk. Currently, the recommended minimum level is 20 ng/mL. Your doctor can order a test of your vitamin D level and, if needed, recommend supplementation.

Cedric F. Garland, DrPH, is an epidemiologist at University of California San Diego School of Medicine and coauthor of a 12-year study published in *PLOS ONE*.

Pecans Head Off Type 2 Diabetes

Pecans may help head off type 2 diabetes. When people ate a typical American diet—low in fruits and vegetables and high in calorically dense foods—for four weeks,

those who consumed 1.5 ounces of pecans daily (a little less than one-half cup) had lower diabetes risk markers than those who did not eat the nuts. Risk markers included insulin levels and insulin resistance.

Study by researchers at Tufts University, Boston, published in *Nutrients*.

Ketogenic Diet Helps Prevent Diabetes Better Than Exercise

Ketogenic diet helps prevent diabetes better than exercise by stopping metabolic syndrome from turning into diabetes. In a study of people who ate a standard American diet with or without exercise…or a ketogenic diet with a focus on fish, lean meat, poultry, low-carb vegetables, cheese, avocados and other specified foods…those who stuck to the ketogenic diet for 10 weeks had the greatest improvement in metabolic-syndrome symptoms.

Study of adults diagnosed with metabolic syndrome by researchers at Bethel University, St. Paul, published in *Diabetes & Metabolic Syndrome: Clinical Research & Reviews*.

The New, Ultimate Diabetes Screening

Michael Snyder, PhD, researcher, chair of Stanford University's department of genetics and director of the Center for Genomics and Personalized Medicine, Stanford, California, and coauthor of the study titled "Glucotypes Reveal New Patterns of Glucose Dysregulation," published in *PLOS Biology*.

Think you don't have diabetes just because your last blood sugar test said so? Think again! A small but potentially groundbreaking study at Stanford University reveals that annual blood sugar tests—even the vaunted "A1c" test—tell you what's going

71

on in your body only at the moment you had the test.

That can be a problem because, as the study revealed, your blood sugar actually could be spiking to levels throughout the day that would classify you as one of the 30 million adults in the US with undiagnosed, full-blown type 2 diabetes or as one of the additional 84 million adults with prediabetes, diabetes waiting in the wings.

To better understand spikes in blood sugar levels, the researchers recruited 25 men and 32 women, ages 25 to 76, nearly all with no known prior history of diabetes or prediabetes. Interestingly, as part of their screening for participation, two were found to already have diabetes and 14, prediabetes.

Each participant wore a continuous glucose monitor, or CGM, for up to four weeks. (A CGM system includes a tiny sensor that's inserted just under the skin on one side of the abdomen, and it checks blood sugar levels every five minutes around the clock, transmitting data wirelessly to a nearby smartphone or receiver.) Blood sugar levels were recorded as study volunteers worked, slept, ate, hung out with friends or cared for their families...in other words, during all their normal day-to-day activities.

Some of the results were startling. Many participants who did not have diabetes based on initial screening experienced frequent blood sugar surges that put them into the prediabetic or even the diabetic range. The researchers also noted that blood sugar ranges were much higher in some participants than in others in response to specific foods. Other studies have shown that over time, high glucose spikes in people can damage organs including the pancreas, liver and heart.

What Wearing a CGM Can Tell You

While a CGM is traditionally recommended for people with diabetes as an alternative to frequent finger pricks to track blood sugar, for people without diabetes, wearing the device once a year may be a great way to see whether you're in the danger zone for developing the disease, says study coauthor Michael Snyder, PhD. For your first time, you might wear the sensor for three or four weeks, he says, while keeping a journal of everything you eat and noting which foods trigger spikes. By cutting back on these foods, it may be that you can help delay or even prevent the onset of full-blown diabetes. In successive years, wearing a CGM for just one week would enable you to catch any changes and make any needed adjustments, says Dr. Snyder.

To get started, you'll need to ask your doctor for a CGM prescription, instructions on how to use it (it causes only a brief sting as the sensor is inserted) and a follow-up appointment to discuss the readings. You might be met with skepticism at first, but this example of personalized medicine can give you far greater insights into your health than a single test and offer the opportunity to prevent a lifelong condition that comes with serious complications, including heart disease. While insurance won't pay for a CGM for someone without diabetes, Dr. Snyder believes that these devices will soon become inexpensive and direct-to-consumer, giving people easy access to monitoring their glucose levels.

Hot Baths Can Reduce Diabetes Risk

Hot baths can reduce blood sugar and chronic inflammation in a similar way that exercise can. Study subjects sat up to their necks for an hour in 102°F water each day for two weeks.

Implication: People unable or unwilling to exercise might be able to reduce the risk for diabetes and other inflammation-related ills. Ask your doctor whether hot baths are safe for you.

Christof Leicht, PhD, is a lecturer in exercise physiology at Loughborough University in the UK and leader of a study of overweight, sedentary men published in *Journal of Applied Physiology*.

Insulin Storage Danger

When sensors were placed near insulin in the refrigerator or a diabetes bag (used for carrying insulin during the day) of 388 patients, 79% of the insulin was stored outside of the recommended temperature range. Insulin stored in the refrigerator was out of the recommended range of 36°F to 46°F two-and-a-half hours a day, on average, during the 49-day monitoring period.

Important: Because temperature deviations are known to affect insulin's blood glucose–lowering effect, always place a thermometer near insulin in the refrigerator—and in a diabetes bag—to ensure its potency.

Katarina Braune, MD, resident physician, department of paediatric endocrinology and diabetes, Charité Universitaetsmedizin, Berlin, Germany.

Sleepy After Dinner?

Joel Fuhrman, MD, family physician and nutritional researcher in Flemington, New Jersey, and author of *The End of Diabetes* and *Fast Food Genocide*. DrFuhrman.com

Falling asleep right after dinner could be a sign of diabetes. But after-dinner (postprandial) sleepiness also can occur because you're not getting enough sleep at night or you're overeating at dinner. A rush of calories into the digestive tract, especially after a heavy meal, increases blood flow to the digestive organs and away from the brain, resulting in increased sleepiness.

Also, if you're eating the standard American diet (aka SAD), it is low in antioxidants and phytochemicals. Eating this way can lead to a buildup of free radicals and other toxic metabolites that can, over time, contribute to a host of health problems, including diabetes, heart disease and depression. An unhealthy diet may also be high in refined carbs, which are quickly digested, giving you that sugar rush and subsequent crash.

My advice: Keep dinner small and simple by having a large vegetable salad, a bowl of vegetable-bean soup (or bean dish) and one fresh fruit for dessert. Beans, which are a "good" carbohydrate, rank low on the glycemic index (a measure of how much a food raises your blood sugar) and are considered among the most "diabetic favorable" foods. Any fruit—fresh or frozen—is a vast improvement over a conventional baked or sugary dessert. If you want to add an animal product or heavier starchy foods, do so with lunch.

Most people won't feel sleepy after a nutritious veggie-rich meal, but if you do, you should talk to your doctor about diabetes.

Lose This Much Weight

Losing 15% of your weight starts diabetes remission, reports Gerald Bernstein, MD, FACP.

Recent finding: The pancreas's insulin-producing beta cells began functioning normally again when people lost 15% of their weight (about 30 pounds for a 200-pound person), reversing their type 2 diabetes. It's not yet known how long this benefit will last.

Gerald Bernstein, MD, FACP, is director of the diabetes management program at The Gerald J. Friedman Diabetes Institute in New York City.

Don't Ignore Your Feet

David G. Armstrong, DPM, MD, PhD, a podiatric surgeon and professor of surgery at Keck School of Medicine of University of Southern California in Los Angeles. He is also founder and cochair of the International Diabetic Foot Conference (DFCon.com), an international symposium on the diabetic foot, and lead author of "Diabetic Foot Ulcers and Their Recurrence," published in *The New England Journal of Medicine*.

Feet are easy to ignore...unless they hurt. That's one big reason many people with diabetes are at risk for losing their feet—

their disease has robbed them, to a large extent, of what doctors call "the gift of pain."

Here's what happens: Diabetes damages nerves, which can lead to a loss of feeling. This means that an ill-fitting shoe or an ingrown toenail can start a silent cascade of injury, leading to a foot ulcer (open sore or wound) and infection.

Many people with diabetes also have poor blood flow, and that can allow an infection to fester—raising the risk that an unnoticed cut or blister could lead to the loss of toes, a foot or even an entire lower leg. Such amputations happen nearly 75,000 times each year in the US.

Even worse danger: Once a person with diabetes has a foot ulcer, his/her chance of dying in the next 10 years doubles. If the foot ulcer leads to amputation, the five-year risk for death is 70%.

But those tragic complications don't have to happen to you. *Here are five simple steps to help prevent foot ulcers and limb loss…*

STEP #1: Watch your blood sugar—and more. If you maintain good control of your blood sugar, your heart and kidneys will thank you—and so will your feet. Of course, you need to take your medications, watch your diet, and if your feet are still healthy, use them to stay active—walking is good preventive medicine for your whole body.

Warning: If you already have nerve damage in your feet, talk to your primary care doctor or foot doctor (podiatrist) about the right dose of walking for you. There may be times when you have to stay off your feet to save them.

STEP #2: Be smart about your shoes and socks. You need to wear both—whether you're inside or outside your house. (If you've lost sensation in your feet, don't walk around the house barefoot! At least wear house slippers.)

In choosing your socks, start with a clean, lightly padded pair with no irritating seams. Choose well-fitted, supportive shoes with plenty of room for your toes (no pointy-toed shoes!)—and get in the habit of checking inside for foreign objects before slipping them on. Even though high heels aren't recommended, women with diabetes may want to wear moderate heels (no more than two inches) for special occasions.

Buying tip: It's widely known that you should shop for shoes late in the day, when your feet may have swelled a bit, but this is vital for people with diabetes so that they don't buy shoes that are too tight. And stay away from cheap plastic and vinyl shoes—they may be less expensive, but they don't breathe enough, which causes your feet to perspire, increasing the chance for a blister to develop.

If diabetes has already caused changes, such as neuropathy and especially a previous blister or wound on your feet, talk with a podiatrist about the best shoes and inserts for you. These supportive shoes can be pricey (more than $100), but insurers often cover at least one pair per year—though you may want more so that you can allow your shoes to air out for a day between wearings.

Also: See your podiatrist at least once a year to make sure your feet are healthy and you're wearing the right shoes.

STEP #3: Knock your socks off! You need to do this every day to get a good look at your feet. Carefully examine the tops, the soles, the heels—and between your toes, where moisture and friction can lead to trouble. Use a mirror (or ask a family member to help if needed).

Goal: Get to know your feet so well that you will notice changes from day to day. Any new redness could signal trouble. Look for swelling, calluses, sores, blisters or ingrown toenails, and let your primary care physician or podiatrist know about these warning signs.

Important: There's one other time to strip off your shoes and socks—each and every time that you see your primary care doctor (not just your podiatrist). Take off your socks as soon as you reach the exam table. That way, both of you will remember to look at and talk about your feet.

STEP #4: Watch out for hot spots. If areas of your skin heat up, that can be a sign of inflammation. If you detect that heat early enough, you may be able to head off an ulcer.

Helpful: Consider doing your foot check in the morning before you've been walking on your feet all day. But if that doesn't work for your schedule, just be sure you do your foot check regularly.

Do not be surprised if your doctor asks you to take the temperature of your feet in several spots each day—looking for areas of one foot that are a few degrees warmer than the same areas of the other foot. This can be done with an inexpensive thermometer that can be purchased online, such as Advocate's Non-Contact Infrared Thermometer or Equinox Digital Non-Contact Infrared Thermometer.

Also: If you and your podiatrist are game, you can try out newer heat-sensing socks. These can be paired with your smartphone or other devices to send alerts to you. One such product, Siren's Diabetic Socks, is expected to hit the market soon. You can preorder these socks at Siren.care or 888-459-5470.

STEP #5: Pamper those puppies. Dry skin is more easily damaged, so after washing your feet in warm (not hot) water, apply a rich moisturizing cream. Keep toenails trimmed, straight across—and if that becomes difficult for you, ask your health-care providers for nail-trimming help. Make sure to ask your podiatrist before going to a nail salon. *Also, avoid these missteps…*

• **Do not put moisturizer between your toes**—excess moisture there can promote infection. Use talcum powder or cornstarch in those areas.

• **Do not warm your feet with hot-water bottles or heating pads**—you might not feel when it's too hot. Wear warm socks instead.

• **Do not use acids or chemical corn removers,** which could damage the skin and lead to foot ulcers. See a podiatrist for help.

• **Do not attempt "bathroom surgery" on corns, calluses or ingrown toenails.** Consult a podiatrist.

• **Do not smoke.** Quitting is one of the best things you can do to improve blood flow—to your feet and everywhere else. Do not give up trying if you have not quit yet.

Fasting for Diabetes

People with type 2 diabetes who ate 500 to 600 calories on two nonconsecutive days each week (and their normal diet on other days) for 12 months had similar blood sugar control as those who ate a calorie-restricted diet (1,200 to 1,500 calories) every day. Intermittent fasting is effective at controlling diabetes, especially for those who do not like restricting calories every day.

Important: Talk to your doctor before starting any new diet if you have diabetes.

Peter M. Clifton, MD, PhD, professor of nutrition, School of Pharmacy and Medical Sciences, University of South Australia, Adelaide.

Diabetes: The High-Fiber Fix

Liping Zhao, PhD, Eveleigh-Fenton Chair of Applied Microbiology in the department of biochemistry and microbiology at the Rutgers School of Environmental and Biological Sciences, The State University of New Jersey in New Brunswick, and lead author of the study "Gut Bacteria Selectively Promoted by Dietary Fibers Alleviate Type 2 Diabetes" published in *Science*.

What if you could eat to beat diabetes? You can. New research shows that people who are willing to more than double the fiber in their diets from 16 to 37 grams per day can better control diabetes. It needs to be a high amount of diverse types of fibers, and getting nearly 40 grams may sound like a tall order, but it's actually not that hard—and it could make a radical difference in your blood sugar level.

Why It Works

Common thinking about why fiber is good for people with type 2 diabetes is that fiber slows down your digestive system. That means less of a sugar spike after eating, important when your body doesn't make enough insulin to handle a high sugar load. Fiber also makes you feel full on less food, and that can help with weight loss, an important goal for many people with diabetes. This means that the benefits are from the physical properties of fiber themselves rather than from improving glycemic control.

But when researchers followed two groups of people with diabetes eating different amounts of fiber, they found that people who ate nearly 40 grams of diverse fibers a day actually regained their own glycemic control back to a higher level than the group that ate only 16 grams—a win-win-win for the 37-gram eaters. The high-fiber-intake group showed a steady increase of insulin secretion and insulin sensitivity, borne out with rigorous medical tests such as the oral glucose tolerance test (OGTT) at the end of each month on the new diet for three consecutive months. This demonstrated that the high-fiber diet actually led to better glycemic control and does not just reduce the sugar load of your diet and make you feel full. Something more fundamental happened.

How that works: By studying the gut bacteria, or gut biome, of the participants, the researchers found that intake of diverse fibers selectively increased a group of bacteria that digest fiber and produce a type of substance called short-chain fatty acids. Higher levels of these acids, acetic and butyric acids, were linked to an increased production of the hormone GLP-1, known to increase insulin secretion.

Interestingly, production of these acids also reduced the pH of the gut, which makes it a less favorable environment for other not-so-good-for-you bacteria, such as producers of indole and hydrogen sulfide, two smelly and toxic compounds that can inhibit GLP-1 production. Endotoxin producers, which can induce inflammation and damage insulin receptors, were also reduced, leading to high insulin sensitivity of all body cells of the patients.

Think of it this way: Picture cultivating a tall tree so that it forms a tight canopy that creates a special environment within the forest. This group of fiber-utilizing gut bacteria are the tall trees of our healthy "gut forest." Eating enough fibers to grow your tall tree gut bacteria may be critical to your health.

In a nutshell, more diverse fibers means more insulin and higher insulin sensitivity, explains lead study author Liping Zhao, PhD, of Rutgers University. Dr. Zhao believes that feeding those short-chain fatty acid-producing bacteria more fibers will not only help people manage type 2 diabetes, it also may help reduce the risk of developing type 2 diabetes, important for people diagnosed with metabolic syndrome or prediabetes.

Fixing Your Fiber Shortfall

Here's a bit of hominid history you may or may not want to share at your next dinner party. According to Dr. Zhao, studies of fossilized feces from our ancient ancestors shows that they may have eaten 200 to 400 grams of fiber every day! The point being, our modern diets are truly puny in fiber compared with what our bodies might have evolved for. Today, the average American eats only about 16 grams of fiber per day, not nearly enough to get fiber's diabetes-fighting (or many other) benefits.

To get 37 grams of fiber into your diet each day without overeating, you're going to want to choose foods that provide the most grams per serving. When you read nutrition labels, focus on the number of grams rather than the percentage of the recommended daily amount, because that's based on the lower guideline of 25 grams per day. *Here are some of the foods highest in various fibers…*

• **Beans** (15 grams in 1 cup of cooked black beans)

- **Split peas** (16.3 g in 1 cup cooked)
- **Lentils** (15.6 in 1 cup cooked)
- **Fruits, especially those with edible skins** (8 g in 1 cup raspberries, 5.5 g in a medium pear)
- **Vegetables** (10.3 g in 1 medium artichoke, steamed, 8.8 g in 1 cup cooked green peas and 5.1 g in 1 cup cooked broccoli)
- **Whole grains** (5 g in ½ cup rolled oats uncooked, and 6 g in 1 cup cooked pearl barley)
- **Nuts and seeds** (5.2 g in 1.5 ounces almonds, 5.6 g in 2 tablespoons of flaxseed)

Note: If you're wondering if fiber supplements are an easy way out, they're not. You not only need a steady amount of fiber across the day, but you also need the very diverse mix of fibers available through food.

Important: Work with your certified diabetes educator or endocrinologist on the best way to increase your fiber intake as part of your blood sugar management.

On the Horizon

The future of fiber and the gut biome may be personalized nutrition. Since everyone's biome is different, tests will measure which bacteria in your gut respond best to which high-fiber foods and in what quantity. With this information, you will be able get your gut biome into top shape. These tests are already being studied, says Dr. Zhao.

Common Diabetes Medications Are Linked to Infection

Common diabetes medications are linked to a dangerous infection called Fournier's gangrene SGLT2 inhibitors, which include Jardiance and Invokana, reduce blood glucose by stimulating its excretion in the urine. When sugary urine leaks and remains on the skin in the groin area, the tissue can become irritated and infected. Always practice good hygiene, but if you have redness or swelling of the genitals, call your doctor. These symptoms can worsen quickly and lead to serious problems such as blindness, kidney damage and heart disease.

Gerald Bernstein, MD, is director of the Diabetes Management Program, Friedman Diabetes Institute, Lenox Hill Hospital, New York City.

Medicare Now Covers Diabetes Prevention

Angela Forfia, senior manager of prevention with the American Association of Diabetes Educators, Chicago. DiabetesEducator.org

As of April 2018, Medicare started covering the cost of certain diabetes-prevention programs for participants diagnosed with prediabetes. Nearly half of Americans age 65 or older have prediabetes, meaning that they are at significant risk for type 2 diabetes. Unfortunately, most people who have prediabetes do not realize they have it.

Diabetes-prevention programs provide education…personal counseling on lifestyle changes that can prevent or delay type 2 diabetes…and access to support groups with the goals of increasing physical activity, improving eating habits and achieving modest weight loss—weight loss of just 5% to 7% often can dramatically reduce type 2 diabetes risk. According to the Centers for Disease Control and Prevention (CDC), these programs can reduce the odds of developing type 2 diabetes by 71% among people over age 60 who have prediabetes.

Medicare's coverage is provided for free to Medicare enrollees who qualify. (Many private health plans also cover diabetes-prevention programs.)

What to do: Use an online screening tool to determine whether you are at risk for prediabetes.

Example: "Risk Test Hedgehogs (Hedgehogs on Vacation)" is a 60-second prediabetes screening video available on YouTube.

If you could be at risk, ask your healthcare provider for a prediabetes blood test. If your doctor tells you that your blood test results meet the criteria for prediabetes, ask whether he/she knows of a Medicare Diabetes Prevention Program (MDPP) in your area. If not, locate diabetes-prevention programs in your area through the CDC's database (NCCD.CDC.gov/ddt_dprp) and contact one to ask whether it is a Medicare program. Even if no program in your area is covered by Medicare, consider paying out of pocket—it is better than getting diabetes.

Blood Sugar–Testing Devices Go High-Tech

Elena Toschi, MD, insulin pump specialist and type 1 diabetes researcher at Joslin Diabetes Center and instructor in medicine at Harvard Medical School, both in Boston. Joslin.org

Are you ready to make endless finger-sticks and insulin injections things of the past?

High-tech devices can help you manage diabetes with less pain and better blood sugar control.

Continuous Glucose Monitors (CGM)

Good for: People who need tight glucose control with intensive insulin therapy or don't always know when glucose levels change.

If you rely on 10 or more finger pricks a day or are having a hard time regulating your blood sugar, the newest CGMs can really simplify your life. And you'll have more accurate monitoring, with the equivalent of close to 300 checks per day with minimal finger sticks.

A tiny sensor, inserted under the skin of your belly or upper arm, reads the glucose level in tissue fluid every few minutes and sends it wirelessly to a monitor, smartphone or tablet computer. You can read the results directly on your monitor and use your smart-phone or computer to keep track of your glucose levels.

A "stand-alone" CGM can be used with an insulin pump or without—the monitor tells you when your blood sugar is out of range, and then you can do your own insulin injections based on your diabetes management plan. Some models send out an alarm tone to alert you when your glucose level is too low or too high. These benefits make CGMs useful for people with type 1 diabetes and those with type 2 diabetes who need frequent insulin.

More advantages: You can wear the sensor and transmitter during most everyday activities, including showering and sleeping. A CGM also can relay readings to your doctor's office. *To consider…*

• **Abbott FreeStyle Libre.** This sensor goes on your arm and can stay in place for 10 days. You scan a mobile reader over the sensor to see your glucose reading. A cloud-based software management system allows you to view reports, see trends and change settings. Unlike most CGMs, the FreeStyle Libre does not require finger-stick checks or calibrations. One drawback is that it does not send out alarms.

• **Dexcom G5 Mobile.** This CGM sends glucose results to a receiver and your mobile device. Alarms and alerts warn of high or low glucose limits that you set in advance. This CGM does need to be calibrated with a finger stick every 12 hours. It can be worn for seven days and can be a stand-alone CGM or part of a closed-loop system with the Tandem Diabetes Care t:slim insulin pump (more on this later). You can share your data with your doctor or caregiver. The FDA has recently cleared the Dexcom G6, which is factory-calibrated—no need for finger sticks.

• **Medtronic Guardian Connect.** This CGM is practically a mind reader, with a feature that alerts you an hour before you may hit either your high- or low-glucose limit. The sensor relays readings only to a smartphone app.

Also, you'll need to do twice-daily finger sticks to calibrate it, and when used as a stand-alone and not in concert with a MiniMed system insulin pump (see next page), you'll need to check your glucose level with a finger stick before making a treatment decision.

Cost: There are up-front costs ranging from under $100 for the Abbott reader to $600 or more for the other CGMs listed, plus batteries and sensors. Insurance coverage varies and is changing all the time, so check with your carrier.

Note: Medicare recently started covering some CGMs.

Combination CGM and Insulin Pumps: Hybrid Closed-Loop Systems

Good for: People who need many insulin injections every day and/or need to adjust insulin dosing based on their blood glucose level, meal type and physical activity.

A computerized insulin pump delivers insulin through a catheter inserted under your skin. The newest pumps and CGMs have been programmed to work together in what's called a hybrid closed-loop system.

The CGM reads sensor glucose levels and sends readings to the pump. Then the pump adjusts the amount of insulin to deliver. You'll still need to monitor your glucose level and perform finger pricks to confirm that the CGM is working correctly, plus make manual adjustments to account for meals and high blood glucose levels. Taking a training program at a clinic or diabetes center will help you become a pro at using it.

Hybrid closed-loop system options typically require a finger stick calibration several times a day, and the glucose-monitoring sensor can be worn for up to seven days at a time. Some are wearable while bathing and even swimming. *To consider…*

•**Tandem Diabetes Care t:slim.** This insulin pump can function as a pump alone or can work with the Dexcom G5 Mobile. You can pick different tones that signal when blood glucose falls below or rises above levels you set.

•**Medtronic MiniMed 670G System.** The latest model of the MiniMed has an Auto-Mode feature that automatically adjusts basal

insulin delivery based on your glucose values and recent insulin delivery. It automatically stops insulin delivery if glucose gets too low.

Cost: The cost of an insulin pump itself is in the thousands, with a monthly cost for supplies. Many insurance companies do cover insulin pumps, but there may be co-pays and deductibles. Medicare may cover it with certain requirements.

Insulin Pens Get Smarter

If you don't need the level of insulin management a pump provides but still need insulin injections, the pen format is an advancement over a syringe and vials. You can load a cartridge in a reusable pen or use a single-use throwaway model.

Insulin pens are becoming smarter, too. For example, the reusable Companion InPen with Bluetooth technology and connectivity to Apple Health offers tracking and timing of insulin doses over time and even gives insulin temperature checks—the pen will send a message to your phone to remind you if you miss a dose and if your insulin gets too warm or too cold. An InPen itself lasts for one year, but you'll need to replace its insulin cartridge weekly or monthly.

A New Health Risk for People with Type 2 Diabetes: Low Iron

Milton Fabian Suárez-Ortegón, PhD, Usher Institute of Population Health Sciences and Informatics, University of Edinburgh, Scotland, UK, coauthor of study titled "Decreased Iron Stores Are Associated with Cardiovascular Disease in Patients with Type 2 Diabetes Both Cross-sectionally and Longitudinally," published in *Atherosclerosis*.

When you have diabetes, lowering your heart disease risk by watching your blood pressure and weight is critical.

But there's another risk factor that needs to be on your radar, and it's a surprising one: your iron level.

Researchers came to this finding after analyzing data from two different studies on heart disease in people with type 2 diabetes, one done in Spain and the other in Scotland—different populations in many ways, including their diets and levels of alcohol consumption. Yet both groups showed the same pattern of increased risk of heart disease when their iron levels were low. In fact, people with diabetes and low iron were 217% more likely to develop heart disease than those with normal levels of iron.

We don't know whether people with diabetes who increase their iron levels by taking supplements or changing their diets can reduce their risk of heart disease. More research is needed to confirm the link and learn the exact mechanism. But Milton Fabian Suárez-Ortegón, PhD, one of the researchers, said that in the meantime it makes sense for people with diabetes and their doctors to be aware of the finding because, at the very least, an iron deficiency can be a marker of other conditions and can lead to anemia if levels drop extremely low. Remember that simply having diabetes can have as big an impact on your heart and blood vessels as having a heart attack. So, doing everything you can to protect your heart is very important.

Prevent a Deficiency

All men and postmenopausal women need at least 8 mg of iron a day; all other women need 18 mg. You may be able to get all you need from your diet. Meat, seafood (particularly oysters and mussels), poultry and liver are particularly good sources because they contain both hemeand nonhemeiron (heme is the easier of the two types for the body to absorb). Plant foods, notably cooked spinach, lentils and beans, quinoa, and nuts including hazelnuts pistachios and cashews, deliver a good amount of iron but only the nonheme type. (They have plenty of other nutrients, though, so keep eating them!) In fact, eat-ing a food high in vitamin C or one of the iron-rich meats or seafoods along with these plant-based foods will increase the amount of iron your body extracts. Calcium, on the other hand, can interfere with iron absorption—you can lessen this effect when your meal includes a variety of foods.

Yes, you can get iron from a supplement, but it's hard to know how much supplemental iron will be safe and effective without results from blood tests. (Too much iron can cause side effects such as an upset stomach and constipation, and can interfere with absorption of medications.) Your best bet is to check with your health care provider before supplementing on your own.

This Supplement Fights Diabetes and Protects Your Heart

Michael Murray, ND, a leading authority on natural medicine. He has authored or coauthored more than 30 books featuring natural approaches to health, including *Bottom Line's Encyclopedia of Healing Foods* and *The Encyclopedia of Natural Medicine*. Doctor Murray.com

Expensive drugs are not the only option for people with type 2 diabetes to control blood sugar and protect cardiovascular health. A natural supplement called berberine can provide both of these benefits as well.

The supplement, derived from goldenseal root and other plants, activates an enzyme that makes the body more sensitive to insulin, thus helping to control blood sugar. A 2015 statistical review of 27 clinical trials concluded that berberine can control blood sugar as effectively as the go-to diabetes drug metformin.

Bonus: Like the diabetes drugs called GLP-1 agonists and SGLT2 inhibitors, berberine is good for the heart. It reduces high blood pressure, improves the ability of blood vessels to dilate and helps prevent heart failure.

Side effects—uncommon and usually mild—can include nausea and stomach upset.

What to do: Before you take any supplement, discuss it with your medical doctor or naturopathic physician to rule out any possible interactions with another medication.

Example: Berberine can interfere with the effectiveness of certain antibiotics and other drugs. A typical dose is 500 mg two to three times daily before meals, but discuss the right dosing for you with your doctor. If berberine works, your doctor might be able to reduce the dose of one or more of your diabetes drugs.

Artificial Pancreas Breakthrough

An artificial pancreas, which consists of an automated insulin pump and continuous glucose monitor, has been used in patients with type 1 diabetes.

Recent finding: The device, which automatically detects blood sugar levels and delivers insulin, may also help people with type 2 diabetes who are hospitalized.

The New England Journal of Medicine.

8 Ways to Save Money on Insulin

Sandra Arévalo, MPH, RDN, CDE, a certified diabetes educator, director of nutrition services at Montefiore Community Programs in New York City and spokesperson for the Academy of Nutrition and Dietetics and the American Association of Diabetes Educators.

If you rely on insulin to manage diabetes, the ouch may be more in your wallet than at your injection site. Even with insurance, you could be laying out hundreds of dollars each month. And no, it's not your imagination. Insulin prices have been steadily rising.

Because of cost, one-third of people on insulin aren't taking it as directed, according to a study in *JAMA Internal Medicine*. This can have disastrous consequences as patients put themselves at short-term risk for dangerously high blood sugar...not to mention the long-term risks for eye, kidney, heart and nerve damage.

1. Review your insulin needs with your doctor. While there's no generic insulin available yet, some brands have been on the market longer and therefore cost less. The long-lasting once-a-day injections are more convenient, but twice-a-day drugs are typically cheaper. Have a frank discussion with your doctor to explore whether a lower-cost insulin regimen will work for you.

2. Know your health insurance plan's drug formularies. This will tell you the price tier for each type of insulin. Formularies are different from one insurance company to another, so if you're on Medicare or are self-insured, be sure to compare the drug prices for different plans during the annual open enrollment period. It may pay to switch plans.

3. Ask about drug programs that help with costs. Your doctor or diabetes educator may have coupons or rebate forms for insulin from the drug companies that manufacture them. However, if they're only for newer drugs, these medications could still be pricier than older ones, even with the discount. Do the math before deciding. All the insulin manufactured in the US comes from just three companies, and they all—Eli Lilly, Novo Nordisk and Sanofi—offer some level of assistance to people who meet their eligibility requirements.

4. You may be eligible for free or low-cost insulin programs from independent assistance programs such as Needy Meds, Partnership for Prescription Assistance, Rx Assist, and Rx Hope. The Charles Ray III Diabetes Association provides meters, strips and other supplies to those who cannot afford them, freeing up some of your budget for insulin.

5. Shop around to compare costs. Prices can vary considerably from pharmacy to pharmacy. Your neighborhood drugstore may charge more (or less) than the chain at the strip mall. Prices can vary even between outlets of the same chain of stores. So take the time to call around and get quotes before you fill your next prescription—and don't forget to include the pharmacy at the discount shopping club you belong to. You also may be able to save money if you use the mail-order pharmacy connected to your insurance plan—buying one 90-day supply is cheaper than three separate monthly refills.

6. Sign up for pharmacy rewards programs. Some national chains offer shopping benefits after you fill a certain number of prescriptions. While the rewards aren't applicable to the cost of medications, you can use them to cut the bill for your other drugstore items. Also look for various discounts offered when you buy online, such as savings when you sign up for auto shipments. These discounts will apply to testing supplies, not the insulin itself. But saving on items such as test strips will reduce your total diabetes medication outlay. There are also independent medication discount plans that offer savings at thousands of pharmacies across the country without any paperwork.

7. Reduce your need for insulin. If you haven't already gotten serious about diet and exercise, doing so now could still have a profound effect on your diabetes. Remember that the more junk food you eat, especially food with refined carbs such as cookies, cake, muffins and sugary beverages, the more insulin you need to control blood sugar. Work with a nutritionist and a fitness trainer to develop a life plan for better blood sugar control.

Note: Never change your medications without consulting your doctor.

8. Consider joining a drug trial. Some research studies include free insulin and supplies for participants. You can find open trials at the National Institute for Diabetes and Digestive and Kidney Diseases. Another, less involved option is to sign up for focus groups where participation is compensated with free supplies. Ask your health-care team members if they know of these in your area.

Stay tuned for more insulin options. That the US supply of insulin is controlled by just three companies helps explain escalating prices for a drug that's nearly 100 years old. (*Note*: There are numerous lawsuits currently being brought against them on the public's behalf.) Biosimilars, which are close but not identical drugs, are coming to the insulin market in March 2020 as part of the FDA's response to sky-high insulin prices. It's unclear how much (or how soon) this new competition will lower prices, but the goal is for it to ultimately make a difference. Talk to your doctor about switching to a biosimilar when one is available.

The Upside of Diabetes

The partners of more than 180,000 people newly diagnosed with diabetes were significantly more likely to change their health behaviors for the better when compared with people whose partners did not have the disease. Specifically, partners of people with diabetes were about 50% more likely to take a weight-management class. They also were more likely to participate in glucose, lipid and blood pressure screening and get a flu shot.

Julie Schmittdiel, PhD, research scientist, Kaiser Permanente, Oakland, California.

Questions to Ask When Choosing a Certified Diabetes Educator

National Certification Board for Diabetes Educators, Joslin Diabetes Center, American Association of Diabetes Educators. BottomLineHealth.com

Your doctors don't have time to work with you on your specific blood sugar concerns—but there is someone who does. A certified diabetes educator (CDE)

will learn about your specific case of diabetes and your preferences for managing it…help you make the most important day-to-day lifestyle and treatment decisions…and guide you to more effective actions that you might never have thought of. *Before hiring a CDE, ask these questions to make sure this is the right person to guide your diabetes management…*

When were you last certified? To properly use the designation "CDE," a healthcare provider must have met the eligibility requirements of the specialty's governing board—the National Certification Board for Diabetes Educators—and passed an exam covering all aspects of managing diabetes. A CDE must then renew the credential every five years. This requires accruing a minimum of 1,000 hours of practice as a diabetes educator as well as keeping up-to-date on the latest research and treatments for diabetes care. If a candidate's certification is more than five years old, it suggests that he/she may not be as experienced or as knowledgeable as you would want.

What is your background? CDEs usually have been trained in at least one other type of health care. Many have already been registered nurses (RNs), registered dietitians (RDs) or exercise physiologists (BS or MS in exercise physiology and certified by the American College of Sports Medicine), to name just a few. Knowing the background of the CDEs you're considering will help you find the best match for your unique needs, and whoever you hire should also be able to tell you how his background will specifically benefit you. For instance, if planning meals, counting carbs and losing weight are key issues for you, a CDE who is also a registered dietitian should outline nutrition changes he will likely suggest.

What will diabetes counseling sessions with you be like? Some diabetes educators work one-on-one with patients. Others provide group counseling and/or classes at hospitals, diabetes centers or doctor offices. To help you decide on the best format for you, ask for an overview of how a candidate operates and what he will cover. Ask his opinion of the benefits of private versus group classes and which you are most likely to benefit from and why. The answers should be specific. Topics should include diet, exercise and glucose monitoring, all of which should be geared to your immediate needs. If you choose to work with a CDE one-on-one, find out whether he is available at a time and place that is convenient for you and can be flexible if your schedule changes.

How will you work with my doctor? You want a CDE who will share your progress with your doctor and work with that doctor if the CDE sees that adjustments to your treatment plan are needed.

How will you involve my family in my care? Managing diabetes is easier with support at home. A good CDE recognizes this and will have ideas for you to increase the amount of support you get from those who live with you or who you see very often. He should also welcome close family members at your sessions or classes.

What will I learn beyond the basics? Ask your CDE what he can do for you beyond getting you set up with everyday diabetes management tools such as a blood glucose meter. A CDE should be able to tell you how he plans to help you reduce your risk for setbacks and cope with challenging situations, such as attending holiday dinners and birthday parties. The suggestions should seem practical to you even if they might sound a bit challenging at first.

How will you keep me motivated? An important part of the CDE's job is to keep clients actively on track with a diabetes management plan. The CDE you choose should be able to articulate the seven self-care behaviors developed by the American Association of Diabetes Educators, which range from healthy eating to healthy coping, and outline a plan to help you adopt them. How often you should meet depends on your needs, but generally after the initial meeting, you should meet at least once a year plus whenever there is a change in your treatment, living conditions (such as moving to assisted living or a teen going away to college) or if any health complications arise.

How will we know I'm making progress? A good CDE will outline how he will assess your progress, including reviewing your blood glucose monitoring readings and explaining the results of tests such as the A1C to you in a way you can understand. A CDE should say that he will work with you on achieving goals, such as avoiding wide blood glucose fluctuations, but never promise a quick-fix because diabetes management takes time and every patient is unique.

Do you take my insurance? Most CDE sessions are covered by Medicare or private insurance (you may need a referral from your doctor). If you don't want to end up paying out of pocket, ask up-front whether the CDE you're considering is covered by your plan.

Diabetes Link to Pancreatic Cancer

Recent-onset diabetes may signal higher risk for pancreatic cancer, warns V. Wendy Setiawan, PhD. The risk is three to four times higher in the first three years after a diabetes diagnosis in people over age 50, compared with those who don't have diabetes. While pancreatic cancer risk is low, if you've been recently diagnosed with diabetes and have pancreatic cancer risk factors, such as family history, ask your doctor

about monitoring for early signs of the lethal cancer.

V. Wendy Setiawan, PhD, epidemiologist at Keck School of Medicine, University of Southern California, Los Angeles, and coauthor of a study published in *Journal of the National Cancer Institute*.

Surprising Eye Protector

People with diabetes who took the diabetes drug metformin were only half as likely to develop age-related macular degeneration (AMD) as those not taking the medication.

Theory: The drug's inflammation-fighting properties may also help guard against AMD.

American Academy of Ophthalmology annual meeting.

Easier Eye Screening

Vision loss can be prevented by early detection of diabetic retinopathy, a type of damage to the retina caused by high blood sugar.

Problem: About half of people with diabetes don't get annual eye exams.

New: The FDA has cleared a device (IDx-DR) that allows primary care doctors to screen their diabetic patients for retinopathy to determine whether the patient should be referred to an ophthalmologist.

Malvina Eydelman, MD, director, division of ophthalmic and ear, nose and throat devices at the FDA, Silver Spring, Maryland.

Chapter 5

EMOTIONAL RESCUE

Don't Let Fear About Your Illness Get the Best of You

Nothing instills more fear than a diagnosis of cancer or another life-challenging illness. Will your health continue to deteriorate? Will treatments disfigure your body? How will you find the energy to cope with insurance…household responsibilities…and endless rounds of doctor visits and follow-up tests?

Even if the treatments for a serious diagnosis are successful and you (finally!) get a clean bill of health, the fearful feelings won't necessarily stop. You'll always wonder whether you might hear the dreaded words, "Your disease has come back."

Eye-opening research: Among cancer patients—including those who eventually have a full remission—30% to 50% experience some degree of distress, an extreme form of psychological stress. Up to 32% of cancer survivors experience post-traumatic stress disorder (PTSD), compared with just 1% to 4% of the general population.

How do you push through the crushing fear and helpless uncertainty? To learn more,

we spoke with Michael E. Ryan, PsyD, a psychologist at Henry Ford Cancer Institute who cares for patients and disease survivors.

What are patients' biggest fears? For those with cancer, the fear of a recurrence is huge. Even those who have been cancer-free for years admit that they often worry the disease will come back and they'll have to go through the same grueling process all over again, or this time they won't be so lucky.

But cancer patients aren't alone in harboring these worries. No one with a chronic or life-threatening illness, whether it's heart failure, Alzheimer's disease or Parkinson's disease, feels completely secure. Every exam (especially imaging scans) and follow-up tests can trigger intense "scanxiety," the fear that the other shoe is about to drop. They think about death and mortality—and what will happen to their loved ones should their lives be cut short.

Some people deal with anxiety by avoiding uncomfortable thoughts. Others worry about everything—that every bruise, rash or ache

Michael E. Ryan, PsyD, a psychologist and clinical director of Supportive Oncology Services at Henry Ford Cancer Institute in Detroit. She uses evidence-based methods for assessing patients and intervention techniques to help them cope with the emotional and social challenges that arise from serious illnesses.

means that the disease has come back. It can be difficult to strike a balance between symptoms that need further medical evaluation and ones that are just part of normal life.

I reassure my patients that their anxiety will tend to lessen over time—but initially it's going to be high.

Isn't it normal to be afraid? It's more important to ask about the degree of anxiety, fear and depression. Everyone deals with stress, but not everyone develops a disorder that requires medication or therapeutic management. Some people have the ability to remain reasonably upbeat and optimistic, regardless of the diagnosis.

Others do need help. Some people experience depression or a traumatic response to a diagnosis and treatment, which can cause symptoms such as anxiety, insomnia, nightmares, memory loss, poor concentration, etc.—long after the initial diagnosis. Up to 58% of cancer patients experience clinical depression, and between 6% and 23% experience anxiety disorders, according to research published in *Seminars in Oncology Nursing*.

How can someone tell the difference between "average" and severe stress? It's normal to feel anxious, worried, down or discouraged when you discover that you have a serious illness. This begins to improve for most people once treatment has started and they know what to expect or as they get further out from remission. They regain a sense of control.

It's reasonable to be concerned, however, when you realize that all you think about is your illness—and that stress/anxiety are interfering with your ability to enjoy a good quality of life. You might lose interest in activities that used to give you pleasure…feel perpetually angry, depressed or morose…or notice that your personal relationships have become strained (or nonexistent).

Some people cope well with adversity, but others struggle. At our cancer center, we routinely assess patients for stress, anxiety and depression…and we repeat the assessment every six months during treatments.

Are there personal characteristics that predict who will do well/poorly after a frightening diagnosis? We've found that people who perceive that they have good social support—from friends, a spouse, a faith group, etc.—tend to have fewer negative emotions than those who are more isolated or feel they have poor support.

I tell patients that this is a time in their lives when they should reach out to others. You can't always generalize because some people are naturally more solitary and reclusive, but nearly everyone can benefit from some kind of support.

Practically every community has support groups for cancer patients and cancer survivors. Such groups also exist for other serious illnesses, including heart disease and multiple sclerosis.

In general, I worry more about patients who live alone and don't have a close network of friends/loved ones. Inadequate social support often increases risks of not being able to follow through with necessary treatments.

Does stress increase the risk for a cancer recurrence? We know from laboratory studies that animals that are well cared for respond to treatments better, have slower disease progression and a better response to treatment than animals with high levels of stress.

A study in *Annals of Oncology* that looked at breast cancer patients found that those who took beta-blockers (blood pressure drugs that also block the effects of stress hormones) were more likely to survive their cancer treatments.

Regardless of the medical condition a person is coping with, stress can lead to poor lifestyle behaviors that do affect survival—things like not exercising, smoking, getting poor sleep, eating junk food, etc.

What advice do you give for managing anxiety? It's different for everyone. In general, the most important step is to do anything besides sitting alone and dwelling on your fears. See your friends…take daily walks… join a book club…or take up yoga.

Of course, you should also take advantage of professional resources—psychologists, social workers, hospital programs, etc. In many large hospital systems, these services are often available right where you have other medical appointments for convenience. Behavioral health services often are covered by insurance for a typical co-pay, but check with your insurer.

There are also many free programs available through local medical centers and the community—either in person, over the phone or online. A social worker, if available, can help identify resources and assess the supportive care services that are needed.

I also stress remaining well-informed. Talk to your doctor about your condition and the main treatments. Ask for printed materials or reputable online resources. Independent online searches can provide both good and bad sources of information. Be sure to stick with reliable websites, such as the National Institutes of Health and groups that focus on specific chronic illnesses such as the American Heart Association or American Cancer Society.

Talk to other patients in a support group. Information is empowering, even when things seem discouraging. However, not everyone thrives on more information, and it can increase sadness and anxiety, which is not helpful. For these individuals, it makes sense to perhaps discuss their illness and treatments only with their doctors.

You don't want to let cancer or any other disease always take center stage. You need to inject joy in your life—whether it's spending time with your grandkids or spending an afternoon in nature. It's important to acknowledge that not every moment will be perfect, but there are often opportunities to find moments of happiness.

Is Being a Perfectionist Making You Sick?

Gordon L. Flett, PhD, professor, department of psychology, director, LaMarsh Centre for Child and Youth Research, York University, Canada, and coauthor of *Perfectionism: A Relational Approach to Conceptualization, Assessment, and Treatment.*

Thomas Curran, PhD, assistant professor, University of Bath, England, and lead author of study titled "Perfectionism Is Increasing Over Time: A Meta-Analysis of Birth Cohort Differences from 1989 to 2016" published in *Psychological Bulletin.*

Center for Collegiate Mental Health 2015 Annual Report, Penn State University.

What's wrong with needing to be a 10 out of 10 in every way all the time? For starters, you're setting yourself up for failure and a lot of heartache because perfection is actually an impossible goal...a quest that can hurt relationships and harm your body and mind. And the quest for perfection is on the rise.

The Problem with Perfectionism

Perfectionists are never satisfied with almost perfect and are self-critical for not being flawless. Their constant pursuit for perfection (instead of excellence) is a source of chronic stress, according to Gordon L. Flett, PhD, a leading researcher on perfectionism.

There are actually three "flavors" of perfectionism, each of which can hurt you in a different way...

Self-oriented perfectionism: Demanding perfection from yourself.

Other-oriented perfectionism: Expecting those around you to be perfect.

Socially prescribed perfectionism: The belief that others expect perfection from you.

While perfectionists act in ways that create or perpetuate stress by striving excessively or, if they are other-oriented, provoking fights with others, they don't react well to stress. Their coping style is focused on emotion—for instance, you might get angry at yourself for making a mistake that you cannot stop thinking about—and that avoids seeking support and help from others. At times, this avoidance comes in the form of chronic procrastination in dealing with tasks and problems.

The constant stress of perfectionism is linked to burnout—a combination of emotional and physical exhaustion. Other problems include sleep disturbances, headaches, arthritis and fibromyalgia, the complex disorder that causes widespread (and hard-to-treat) pain.

Psychological issues are common too, such as anxiety, chronic worry and depression. According to the National Eating Disorders Association, self-oriented perfectionism is one of the strongest risk factors for developing an eating disorder such as anorexia nervosa or bulimia.

Perfectionists are more prone to suicidal thoughts and attempts than nonperfectionists. But even in the absence of suicide, research has also shown that perfectionism is associated with premature death linked to other causes, possibly due to stress and depression.

A Growing Emotional Epidemic

A 2017 research review led by Thomas Curran, PhD, at University of Bath in England, was the first to look at perfectionism across generational lines by analyzing data from numerous studies of college students conducted at different periods of time, from the late 1980s to 2016. Collectively, the studies reflected more than 40,000 American, Canadian and British students in all. Each of the studies analyzed had participants complete the Multidimensional Perfectionism Scale, a test for generational changes in perfectionism that "scores" according to a percentile.

The findings: The most recent generation of college students scored higher in each type of perfectionism than earlier generations of students. Taken from a baseline average score of the 50th percentile, between 1989 to 2016, self-oriented perfectionism rose 10%, socially-prescribed jumped 32% and other-oriented grew by 16%.

Note: Many people hold high levels of one, two or even all three types, but for most, one form will dominate.

Why the increase? Young college-educated adults now believe that people are more harshly judged than they used to be and that being perfect will result in getting the desired approval from others.

According to a separate report done by the Center for Collegiate Mental Health at Penn State University, students on college campuses are also reporting more symptoms of anxiety, depression and social anxiety than previous generations.

#Flawless?

Today's society values excessively high standards of performance and approval from others. This promotes a desire to be flawless or at least appear to be, according to Dr. Curran. The look of perfection depicted in old media, such as the pages of magazines and in advertising, has now expanded to new media platforms that people are exposed to nearly every waking minute. Instagram, Facebook and Snapchat fuel perfectionism by emphasizing unrealistic ideals and creating an inescapable visual culture where flaws and deficiencies are scrubbed out, reinforcing the message that imperfection is to be frowned upon and avoided.

There is no "cure" for perfectionism. It sits on a spectrum and all people have higher or lower levels of certain tendencies. *But there are ways to break free…*

• **Give yourself a break.** Fight your natural tendency to be self-critical and show yourself some compassion instead.

• **Stop focusing on outcomes.** If you take a class or take up a new skill, enjoy the process of learning instead of stressing over how you're doing compared with others in the class or wondering how fast you can master the new skill.

• **Set realistic and manageable goals.** You don't have to be a tennis ace to be successful on your club's team, for instance.

Important: If you think that your perfectionism is out of control, it's time to seek mental health care. Dr. Flett says that interpersonal-based therapy can be effective. An interpersonal approach is appropriate when people try to be perfect to compensate for unmet interpersonal needs, such as the need to be loved and to matter to others. But be prepared to make a long-term commitment to treatment, especially if you've been a perfectionist for years. Old thoughts and habits are hard to break.

If you can't or won't reduce your level of perfectionism, the focus of therapy may shift to helping you cope with it and finding more adaptive ways to respond when life is inevitably not perfect.

Depression During Perimenopause: A Commonly Missed Diagnosis

"Guidelines for the Evaluation and Treatment of Perimenopausal Depression: Summary and Recommendations," from The North American Menopause Society, National Network on Depression Centers Women and Mood Disorders Task Force, and International Menopause Society, published simultaneously in *Menopause* and *Journal of Women's Health*.

Hot flashes, night sweats and sexual dysfunction are synonymous with menopause and perimenopause—the three- or four-year period just before menopause. Such symptoms often emerge for the first time as a woman's hormone levels begin their life-changing decline.

An underrecognized threat: A woman's risk for depression also increases during perimenopause. Unfortunately, depression in perimenopausal women often falls under the diagnosis radar because these symptoms tend to get lost amidst other menopause-related changes.

Good news: A task force of clinicians and scientists recently published the first-ever guidelines for recognizing and treating perimenopausal depression. The new guidelines have been endorsed by the International Menopause Society.

For many women, perimenopause creates a "perfect storm" of responsibilities and stressors. While undergoing the initial hormonal changes, many women also are juggling child and/or parent care, increasing career demands and/or other significant life changes.

Women who have previously suffered from depression may experience these stressors more intensely when they accompany the hormonal changes of perimenopause. Even women who have no prior history of depression are at increased risk during perimenopause, although the reasons are not entirely clear.

According to the guidelines, perimenopause should be viewed as a "window of vulnerability" for the development of depressive symptoms, and clinicians are encouraged to look for signs of psychological distress in perimenopausal women. Red flags for triggers that can lead to depression include bereavement (women may experience more losses of loved ones during this time than in previous years)…and body changes associated with reproductive aging (such as weight gain and vaginal dryness).

Takeaway: Because each woman experiences perimenopause differently, it's important to schedule regular doctor's visits and discuss any symptoms with the physician.

The most appropriate treatment will depend on the woman's particular distress. For example, if she has low energy due to poor sleep caused by night sweats, hormone therapy may help. If a woman has a history of depression and perimenopause is making it worse, an antidepressant might be most effective. Cognitive behavioral therapy—with or without medication—may be the best choice if a woman finds herself ruminating over family and career burdens. The new guidelines are intended to customize depression treatment for women during this time of her life.

Stay Happy All Year

Norman E. Rosenthal, MD, clinical professor of psychiatry at Georgetown University School of Medicine, Washington, DC. He is the psychiatrist who first identified seasonal affective disorder and is author of *Winter Blues: Everything You Need to Know to Beat Seasonal Affective Disorder*, now in its fourth edition. NormanRosenthal.com

Summer, sadly, doesn't last forever. Some of us feel the onset of seasonal affective disorder (SAD), the condition that gives people depressed moods every fall and winter. SAD is no laughing matter—it can make a big chunk of the year a terrible time for sufferers and can hurt their relationships, job performance and overall health.

Not everyone who gets SAD in the fall and/or winter feels sad. Depression is the best-known symptom of SAD, but people who have relatively mild SAD may not become depressed. As a result, they might fail to realize that they have SAD and never seek treatment. But even mild cases can have serious consequences. Mild SAD can produce a decline in energy and productivity and an increase in appetite (especially for carbohydrate-rich foods), easily resulting in unhealthful weight gain.

What to do: If your energy levels are consistently down or your appetite up during times of year when you do not get much sunlight, you might have SAD—so try a do-it-yourself SAD treatment for a few weeks and see if these symptoms fade. To do this, get outside in sunlight for 30 to 60 minutes each day, even if you must bundle up against cold temperatures to do so...or use a light-therapy lamp for 30 to 60 minutes each day. (More on light-therapy lamps and other SAD treatments below.) Try to get your light (whether from the sun or a light-therapy lamp) in the mornings—that's when research suggests light is most effective at staving off SAD.

Size matters if you buy a light-therapy lamp. You can find light-therapy lamps online and in stores for as little as $30, and almost all of them claim to produce the 10,000-lux light intensity that's recommended and effective for treating SAD. What the lower-end lamp makers tend not to mention is that their lamps might deliver 10,000 lux only if you position your eyes an inch or two from the light, which is impractical and uncomfortable.

What to do: Select a light-therapy lamp that produces 10,000 lux from a lit surface that measures at least 12 inches by 18 inches. Light-therapy lamps this size tend to remain effective over a significantly longer distance.

Examples: Carex Day-Light Classic Bright Light Therapy Lamp, 10,000 lux up to 12 inches away (Carex.com, recently about $115 at Amazon.com)...Sunbox SunRay II, 10,000 lux up to 23 inches away ($359 at Sunbox.com).

Fall/winter SAD treatments need not increase skin cancer risks. It turns out that it isn't the sunlight that reaches our skin that wards off SAD. It's the sunlight that reaches our eyes. When the eyes receive bright light, it triggers the release of mood-regulating neurotransmitters such as serotonin that seem to combat SAD. That means you can apply sunscreen to keep your skin safe when you head outside without increasing your risk for SAD. It also means that you can successfully treat SAD with a light-therapy lamp that filters out

How Baths Can Heal

Patients with depression who took twice-weekly hot baths (104°F/40°C) for 20 minutes followed by 20 minutes wrapped in blankets with hot water bottles significantly lowered their depression scores in eight weeks. Because depression, body temperature and sleep are known to be linked—and the daily rise and fall of body temperature is out of sync in people with depression—hot baths may relieve depression by resetting body temperature and circadian rhythm.

Bonus: The patients liked the therapy—only two out of 22 dropped out, compared with 13 who dropped out of a control group of 23 who exercised instead.

Study by researchers at Medical Center–University of Freiburg, Germany, published in *bioRxiv*.

potentially dangerous UV rays, as most do. (Though for other health reasons, it's good to let some sun reach your skin—see below.)

Caution: Do wear sunglasses outside on bright days if you are not trying to treat SAD…or when you spend more than an hour in bright sunlight during a day. Excessive amounts of bright light can increase cataract risk.

Exercise and mind-set can help treat winter SAD, too. Light therapy is the best-known treatment for SAD, but if light alone doesn't do the trick, there are other treatments you can try. Exercising causes the body to release SAD-combating neurotransmitters such as serotonin just as bright light does. And a professor at University of Vermont has shown that cognitive behavioral therapy, a form of talk therapy that modifies negative thoughts, can be helpful, too.

What to do: Don't just go outside for 30 to 60 minutes of sunlight in the winter—exercise outside for at least part of this time. If you struggle to drag yourself out of bed in the morning for exercise and sunshine, make plans with a friend or personal trainer to exercise together. Adding another person increases the odds that you will follow through.

When you catch yourself engaging in negative self-talk in the fall/winter, counter with positive responses.

Example: You think, I'm so lazy. Immediately question this by reviewing things that you have done that weren't lazy…and then think, Let's see what I can do today.

If none of this cures your SAD, ask your doctor about cognitive behavioral therapy with a qualified therapist and about pharmaceutical treatments or supplements—prescription antidepressants can be effective for SAD.

There is a summer version of SAD, but it isn't like its winter cousin. Winter SAD typically brings depressed moods, low energy and an increase in appetite…but there's also a summer version of this condition. Summer SAD, also called reverse SAD, generally produces agitated moods, insomnia, loss of appetite and, in some cases, suicidal ideas. This might explain why there are more suicides in the summer than in the winter in the US, even though winter is the time of year that most people tend to associate with bleak moods. Another difference—while winter SAD is caused by insufficient exposure to sunlight, the cause of summer SAD is less clear-cut. It could be too much sunlight…hot temperatures…or some combination of the two.

What to do: If you regularly experience agitation, insomnia, decreased appetite and/or suicidal thoughts during weeks when you spend lots of time in the summer sun or in hot weather, cut back on time in bright sunlight…take cool showers, baths or swims midday…turn up the air-conditioning…make sure that your bedroom is very dark when you go to bed and until you wake up—add blackout shades/curtains if necessary. If symptoms persist, discuss what you are experiencing with a medical doctor or therapist.

Considering Therapy? "Group" Might Be Best for You

Molyn Leszcz, MD, professor of psychiatry at University of Toronto and Mount Sinai Hospital, Toronto. He is president-elect of the American Group Psychotherapy Association and coauthor of the textbook *The Theory and Practice of Group Psychotherapy, 5th edition.* His research has been published in *International Journal of Group Psychotherapy, American Journal of Psychotherapy* and other professional journals.

When you think of psychotherapy, you probably imagine yourself sitting on a comfy couch alone with a compassionate professional with whom you share your innermost thoughts and feelings. But there's another approach that's just as effective for most of the problems that drive people to therapy—and it offers certain advantages that the more traditional one-on-one approach lacks.

If you're seeking professional help for depression or anxiety…a recent or long-ago trauma…drug or alcohol abuse…or troubled relationships, group therapy (often known simply as "group") is worth considering.

Getting It Together

Just like individual therapy, there are different kinds of therapy groups. Some use methods such as cognitive behavioral therapy (CBT) to help participants change dysfunctional thoughts and behaviors, while interpersonal or psychodynamic groups promote insight into members' feelings about themselves and others.

They are not support groups, which are generally narrower in scope and bring together people who share a stressful situation like recent divorce, a traumatic life experience or a serious medical illness for mutual encouragement and the exchange of coping strategies. A psychotherapy group is designed to accomplish more—it will not only help a member get over a divorce, for example, but also help him/her to understand why the marriage failed and to work toward a healthier future relationship.

Strength in Numbers

Therapy groups ideally have five to 10 members and are led by a therapist specially trained in this kind of work. Most groups meet every week for an hour and a half to two hours. Some go on indefinitely with members joining and leaving or graduating over time, while others gather the same people for a set term of weeks or months.

Key distinction: Group therapy isn't just psychotherapy with the therapist's attention divided multiple ways. The group becomes a social microcosm in which members talk about their actual impressions of one another in the group sessions—ideally with compassion and authenticity. For example, if one participant talks about her relationship difficulties, others in the group offer insights into the possible reasons—a lack of empathy, perhaps, or a tendency to devalue any relationship.

It's the therapist's responsibility to set the ground rules (including confidentiality and mutual respect) and boundaries on what constitutes appropriate, helpful and effective feedback within the group. The group is a living laboratory offering the benefit of multiple perspectives and honest feedback. And because a trained therapist is on hand, it's a safe space to try out new ways of behaving and relating.

Group can be therapeutic for another important reason. We are naturally social creatures who need to feel that we belong and are valued. As loneliness continues to increase—with health risks that are comparable to smoking and obesity—group therapy offers an antidote. You get to know fellow members thoroughly, and they get to know you. The group confers a sense of belonging that may translate to the world at large.

Additional benefit: Even though we generally seek therapy for help with our problems, group also offers the opportunity to help others—an empowering boost to self-esteem.

Is Group for You?

Groups have proven to be as effective as individual therapy for most psychological problems and emotional disorders—and for some people, group offers even more benefits.

Exception: In cases where there are intense concerns about privacy and trust—due, for example, to an early-life trauma—a person might start with individual therapy and then add or shift to group.

Easy on the pocketbook: Insurance that covers individual therapy generally covers group, too. Because group costs, on average, about one-half as much as individual therapy, it is an appealing choice if you're paying out of pocket.

Initially, many people prefer individual to group therapy, often because groups—at work or growing up, for example—haven't been kind to them. They fear belittling, exclusion or even bullying. But in a group run by a trained therapist, that won't happen. The therapist will ensure a safe, respectful environment for all.

And while members of a group are expected to participate actively, there's no pressure for them to speak at every session or whenever called upon—or to disclose more about themselves than they want to.

Finding a Group

If you're considering group therapy, referrals from health professionals can be helpful. Start by calling the therapist who leads the group. Find out what the group will be like and what kind of people will be in it, and make sure the therapist has specialized training in group work.

Good resource: The American Group Psychotherapy Association maintains a directory of therapists who meet its standards, which include appropriate training. Go to AGPA.org and click on "Find a Certified Group Therapist."

There are also more than 20 local group therapy associations across the country that are affiliated with AGPA. (At the site, click on "About Us," then "Affiliate Societies.") These are a great resource for finding a well-trained and qualified group therapist in your area.

New opportunity: Groups that meet online via such digital media as Zoom or Skype. This can be especially helpful for people in isolated areas where mental health facilities are scarce or to bring together individuals isolated in their communities.

Be Kind to Yourself...for Better Health

Study titled "Soothing Your Heart and Feeling Connected: A New Experimental Paradigm to Study the Benefits of Self-Compassion," by researchers at University of Exeter and University of Oxford, both in England, published in *Clinical Psychological Science*.

"Think kind thoughts and call me in the morning" may seem like an odd prescription, but it's gaining traction as an effective way to improve your health.

Past research has shown that negative thoughts about yourself (and others) are linked to weakened immunity and increased risk for serious health problems ranging from heart disease to dementia.

But could more compassionate thoughts have a positive impact on health?

To find out, researchers at the Universities of Exeter and Oxford conducted a new study that adds to a growing body of evidence suggesting that kinder, gentler thoughts can indeed offer important mental and physical benefits.

Study details: The researchers divided 135 college students into five groups—each receiving different 11-minute audio recordings that conveyed a range of negative, self-critical messages versus positive, self-compassionate messages.

Not surprisingly, the group that heard instructions to think critically about themselves had increased heart rates and higher sweat responses—both markers for feelings of threat and distress. By comparison, the group that was encouraged to adopt thoughts of "loving kindness," in which they focused kind and soothing thoughts on a loved one and on themselves, had a positive physical response—their heart rates and sweat responses slowed by two or three beats per minute, on average.

"These findings suggest that being kind to oneself switches off the threat response and puts the body in a state of safety and relaxation that is important for regeneration and healing," explains study lead study author Hans Kirschner, PhD, a graduate fellow at the University of Exeter.

This research, published in *Clinical Psychological Science*, gives insight into why people with recurrent depression, for example, seem to benefit from mindfulness-based cognitive therapy that teaches them to become more self-compassionate, according to the study authors.

Caveat: Because the research included only healthy participants, it does not prove that people with depression would benefit from a single self-compassion exercise, as used in the study. However, the researchers believe that a more self-compassionate way of thinking, in general, could be "quite transformative" for many people.

More research is planned to investigate the physiological responses and mood improvement that individuals with recurrent depression may derive from self-compassion practices.

To give self-compassion a try: Notice negative thoughts you have about yourself throughout your day…and replace them with a more positive, self-compassionate message. Even though this may not be easy at first, it will likely become more natural with daily practice.

How to Support Someone with Cancer

Alan Wolfelt, PhD, founder and director of Center for Loss & Life Transition and author of *Healing a Friend or Loved One's Grieving Heart After a Cancer Diagnosis.* CenterForLoss.com

You'd never consciously abandon a friend who has cancer, and yet that's the message many people inadvertently send…either by not reaching out at all or by changing the topic to something less threatening whenever the friend brings up his/her illness. Of course, you want to be supportive—it's just that you feel helpless or unsure of what to say. Some people blurt out platitudes ("This is all part of God's plan") or share their own cancer stories (or those of people they know), none of which is helpful.

If you find yourself in this situation—and most of us will someday—the most compassionate thing to say first is actually simple and straightforward: "I'm so sorry to learn this. I want you to know that, if you want to talk, I am here for you."

Then take these steps to be part of the support network that's so vital to everyone facing cancer…

• **Acknowledge your helplessness.** It's OK to be at a loss for words after your initial expression of sorrow. What's important

Healing Chicken

Farm favorite = therapy animal. In parts of the US, chickens have been embraced as therapy animals for people experiencing anxiety, isolation and loneliness.

Psychology Today.

is to take your cues from your friend, and that starts with listening to find out what he needs.

• **Reach out repeatedly.** Maybe your friend didn't respond to your initial e-mail or phone call because he was feeling overwhelmed. Don't give up! Let him know you're thinking of him with a text, an e-mail, a card or a phone call every other week. Is he your best friend? Then reach out more often—at least once a week. One of the trickiest parts of being a cancer companion is knowing when to reach out and when to stay away. While you do need to respect boundaries and overt requests to be left alone, remember this mantra—when in doubt, reach out. People who are struggling often need time and space to go into exile. Grief and coming to terms with mortality invite interior struggles and demand this alone time. But remember—if you do end up "bothering" him, chances are your efforts to be present will far outweigh any inconvenience you may cause.

• **Lend a hand.** When you do call, be straightforward and ask, "What do you most need help with right now?" Then follow through, whether it's cleaning his house, doing laundry, shopping for groceries, buying birthday gifts for a loved one or transportation to doctor appointments. And keep offering every so often, even if your friend turns down your request the first time, realizing it can be hard for him to admit needing such help at first. It may help to be specific—for instance, if you know she has children who need to be shuttled to soccer practice, offer to drive them. It's easier for your friend to say, "Yes, thank you," than to try to figure out what to ask for.

• **Squelch your inner cheerleader.** It's important to frequently ask "Is there anything you'd like to talk about?"—and then let your friend guide the conversation. If he's feeling pessimistic, don't try to "talk him out of it" by telling him that he's got a great doctor or that the odds are in his favor. The last thing he needs is a cheerleader. That's because you need to match his emotional tone or he'll feel disconnected from you. If he needs to befriend sadness, let him be sad. If you project that you can only accept happy emotions, he cannot be authentic with you and will often not want to be in your presence. Instead, simply allow him to express his fears, grief and any other emotions he's going through. Your empathetic reaction can make him feel hopeful again. When words seem inadequate, simply remind yourself that a great way to support your friend is: Mouth closed, ears open, presence available. Empathy is being in tune with what someone feels, not trying to change it.

• **Get comfortable with long pauses.** It's easy to feel uneasy when conversation tapers off. But if your friend doesn't want to talk—or is too distressed to speak or simply isn't really a talker—stay silent until he's ready to open up. Remember that just your being there is meaningful for your friend. Often, it means listening and overcoming the need to say something in return. How do you "listen" to silent types? By simply spending time with them. You might play cards, watch a movie or fold laundry together…and find that communication—verbal or nonverbal—happens naturally.

One thing that may help your friend communicate more easily is the EmPat Project—special "cancer" emojis created by artist Nina Beaty when she was undergoing treatment for lung cancer. Available through a free, downloadable app that you can add to text messages, these emojis rely on cute, funny drawings to telegraph a person's thoughts and moods. They're excellent shortcuts for saying "I'm overwhelmed" or "I'm having a good day" without having to overexplain.

The bottom line: It's not always necessary to talk, but always keep your ears open, and be available and present. Your friend will quickly realize that he can count on you to be part of his support system.

After a Suicide Attempt: Keeping Your Loved One Alive

Heidi Bryan serves on the National Suicide Prevention Lifeline Consumer Survivor Subcommittee, is a trained facilitator for suicide bereavement support groups and the coauthor of *Now What Do I Do? A Guide for Suicide-Attempt Survivors.* HeidiBryan.com

Most people who attempt suicide are not likely to die…at least not the first time. But they are likely to try again. The biggest risk comes within the first three months of a suicide attempt, but risk remains elevated throughout their depression recovery, which can be years long.

It's common for people close to someone who attempted suicide to say that they didn't see it coming. Loved ones tend to put blinders on, says Heidi Bryan, a member of the National Suicide Prevention Lifeline Consumer Survivor Committee. But once a suicide attempt has occurred, what you do and don't do, and what you say and don't say, matter—a lot—she says.

Bryan speaks from the heart and from experience. She has battled depression most of her life. Not only is she a suicide-attempt survivor, she also lost her brother to suicide in 1995.

A suicide attempt is traumatic for everyone involved, the depressed person and everyone who loves him or her. But you don't have to stand by and feel helpless, says Bryan.

Know that some people will be resistant to your intervening and that there's only so much you'll be able to do to persuade them to get help or cooperate, says Bryan. But it also has been her experience that when you show empathy—recognize the severe emotional pain that he is in, know that he didn't really want to die but wanted to end his pain—and approach him with compassion, the majority of suicide-attempt survivors will be cooperative. When feeling understood and having a sense of collaboration, they also have ownership of their life and aren't just being told what they need to do. This goes a very long way for someone who just attempted suicide.

First, make your home safer. Remove all guns. Just locking them up isn't enough. If you don't want to permanently get rid of them, see whether a friend or family member who lives elsewhere can safeguard them for you. At the very least, store ammunition separately from any gun, and keep both under lock and key. Only you should know where the key is kept.

Some people attempt to overdose with drugs. That's why you don't want to the attempt survivor to be in charge of his/her medications. Hide or lock up over-the-counter medicines, too, especially Tylenol, Bryan says.

Though people often think of Tylenol as safe, teens tend to use it to try to commit suicide, and overdosing with it can cause severe liver damage. It's in a lot of households and often overlooked as being potentially dangerous.

Do the same with liquor, pesticides and other poisons, razors, knives and rope. It can be difficult for you to live this way, but think of it as a small sacrifice to make sure that your home is a safe zone, Bryan says.

If the suicide-attempt survivor doesn't live with you, to make his environment safe, go with him to his home and remove as many access to means—items that could be used to attempt suicide—as possible.

If someone was hospitalized after a suicide attempt, it's recommended that he not go home to an empty house for the first few weeks. Have him stay with you or stay (or have someone stay) with him temporarily. If being with him around-the-clock isn't possible, maybe during the day is doable, supplemented with one or two check-in calls in

the evening until his suicidality subsides. See if you can form a safety network of friends and relatives to support the person during the initial period of crisis.

Try to keep your emotions in check. It's understandable if the suicide attempt left you angry or upset. But lashing out with statements such as, "What were you thinking?" or "How could you do this to me?" aren't helpful and could be very harmful, Bryan says, causing your loved one to withdraw rather than share what made him want to end his life.

Say thoughtful and kind things. How would you treat someone who had just had a heart attack? Reach out to your loved one with the same type of concern, Bryan says. Help him focus on reasons for living and making life more positive and meaningful. Unsure of how to take the first step? Bryan suggests saying this your loved one: "You may not feel loved, but you have to know that you are. Trust me to know that I'm right about this. So let's work together to get you feeling better. And always remember, you are not alone. I am here for you."

Educate yourself. Learn the warning signs of suicidal thoughts so that you can tell whether you need to step in before your loved one tries again. Sleeping too much or too little and losing interest in favorite pastimes are well-known signs of depression, but talking about being a burden to others or saying that life has no purpose are the kind of statements that often lead to suicide. For more signs, go to SuicidePreventionLifeline.org.

It can be painful and frightening for you to acknowledge that your loved one could be on the verge of another suicide attempt, but don't ignore any signs. Face them head-on.

Try this: Sit down with your loved one, and through loving conversation, identify three to five negative emotions that he's wrestling with. These might include, for example, anger, feeling overwhelmed or trapped. Determine a scale he can use to describe their severity—for instance, one is mild and five is bubbling over. Then have a daily check-in—ask whether the levels of these emotions are rising, and if they're nearing the top of the scale, agree that it's time for intervention, such as more intensive mental health therapy.

Walk the line between concern and smothering. Yes, you want to keep a watchful eye on your loved one and be in a position to take action to prevent another suicide attempt if needed, but you don't want to be constantly hovering—that will make him feel trapped and aggravate the situation, Bryan says. You and your loved one need to determine how much space feels right. It may take some trial and error, but don't give up.

While the majority of suicide-attempt survivors, when approached with empathy, compassion and collaboration, will respond positively to working together, that's not the case for everyone. If your efforts are met with a response such as, "Leave me alone," there isn't much you can do but leave him alone for a period of time. You might express concern about doing that and then wait for an opportunity to talk with him, Bryan says. He will need to process what happened. You can only do your best—the rest is up to the attempt survivor.

Fill out a "safety plan" together. This is a written plan that details a series of progressive steps he can take to address suicidal thoughts. First, list his specific warning signs that suicidal thoughts are starting to grow, such as the emotions listed above. Experiencing these are the signal to take action.

The next section of the plan lists at least three self-soothing steps that he can do himself to distract his mind from these thoughts. These can be as simple as meditating, journaling, cleaning out a drawer, holding ice cubes in his hand and letting them melt, or petting a dog. There should also be a list of external resources—a change in scenery, so to speak—such as going for a walk, to a movie or to a coffee shop to distract himself and stop the thoughts if the initial distractions don't work. You might also suggest that he try an app with a mood journal, distraction techniques and other resources, says Bryan, who recommends the free app MoodTools-Depression Aid for iOS devices.

The safety plan next lists at least three people he can call to talk to about his feelings—family or close friends—when self-soothing doesn't work.

It must include numbers for a crisis center such as the Suicide Prevention Lifeline at 1-800-273-TALK (8255), for a text such as Crisis Text Line at 741741 (patients can text with a trained crisis counselors), and for his doctor to contact for help.

The plan should also detail at least one thing that's important to him and makes life worth living so that he can look at this on his safety plan and be reminded of it when life looks bleak, Bryan adds.

Deal with your feelings, too. It may not be an easy conversation to have, but you and other family members should openly discuss what happened and everyone's feelings about it. You might all benefit from therapy, not just the person who attempted suicide, because you all need support, says Bryan. Make sure that the professional you choose is a good fit for everyone, is knowledgeable about specific treatments and practices that can help prevent suicide attempts and has an approach to care that suits your needs.

You can find even more resources at…

- **ReportingOnSuicide.org**
- **PleaseLive.org/after-attempt/**
- **SpeakingOfSuicide.com/**

And the online booklet, *A Journey Toward Health and Hope* from the Substance Abuse and Mental Health Services Administration (store.samhsa.gov).

Relax with Nature Sounds…Year-Round

If you find chirping birds, rustling winds, babbling brooks and other sounds of nature pleasing, a new study explains why.

Recent finding: When brain scans and heart monitoring were performed on study participants, nature sounds improved heart rate by activating the part of the nervous system that promotes relaxation, while artificial sounds, such as ticking clocks and hair dryers, caused the brain to operate in ways linked to anxiety and depression.

What to do: Get out for a walk in the woods, by the beach, etc., whenever possible.

Cassandra Gould van Praag, PhD, research associate, University of Oxford, UK.

A Common Depression Treatment May Be a Disaster If You're Left-Handed

Daniel Casasanto, PhD, associate professor of human development and psychology at the College of Human Ecology of Cornell University and coauthor with Geoffrey Brookshire, PhD, of a study titled "Approach Motivation in Human Cerebral Cortex" published in *Philosophical Transactions of the Royal Society B*. Casasanto.com

When you're a leftie living in a right-handed world, you know that certain common things just don't work for you—like a "regular" pair of scissors, which works only in the right hand. But you probably don't know that there are certain medical treatments that not only won't work for you…they may be dangerous for you just because you are left-handed. And even some doctors may not realize this.

These treatments are not for some exotic condition, either—they are used for depression and anxiety. Several non-invasive "brain stimulation" technologies are now available to treat depression and anxiety that haven't responded well to other therapies, and they are becoming more widely used. They employ magnets or electrical currents to increase activity in the part of the brain in the left hemisphere that is strongly linked with happiness and other positive emotions…and to decrease activity in the area of the right hemisphere responsible for negative emotions such as sadness, fear and distrust. But this one-size-fits all approach could actually harm lefties by worsening their depression and anxiety.

Why? Most research done on brain stimulation has involved only right-handed people. Yes, stimulating the left side of the brain is correct for right-handed folks, but not for left-handed ones because the two distinct emotional centers are reversed in a leftie's brain.

To study the idea of reversing the location of therapeutic brain stimulation for left-handed people, researchers at Cornell University recruited 30 healthy individuals whose "handedness" ranged from strongly right-handed to strongly left-handed. Pain-free electrical current was applied to the frontal cortex of each participant for 20 minutes a day for five days of testing. The researchers found that when righties were stimulated on the left sides of their brains, they said that they experienced an increase in positive emotions, and so did lefties who were stimulated on the right sides of their brains. In contrast, when righties were stimulated on the right side…or lefties stimulated on the left side, they experienced an increase in negative emotions.

Surprising finding: The study also showed that brain stimulation might be a waste of time for people who are ambidextrous, meaning they neither identify as a strong leftie or strong rightie…a person who may, for example, write with his right hand but buckle a belt with his left or vice versa. This is because such people's brain emotion centers are spread out over both brain hemispheres and can't be precisely targeted by a current.

Research involving participants with mental health disorders is needed to validate the findings, but if they hold, these results could change the way depression and anxiety are treated. Special left-handed approaches might also be developed for other types of brain conditions such as stroke or brain injury.

In the meantime, if your health-care provider suggests brain stimulation and you're left-handed or ambidextrous, share these findings and have a candid discussion with him/her about whether you're truly a good candidate for the procedure.

Lavender Might Work Better Than Drugs for Anxiety

Sniffing lavender for anxiety may be as effective as taking a drug, reports Hideki Kashiwadani, PhD. In a recent animal study, the scent of linalool, an alcohol component in lavender, induced an antianxiety response in mice similar to that of antianxiety medications. The effect has not yet been tested on humans, but it could prove to be very similar.

Hideki Kashiwadani, PhD, is a physiologist and neuroscientist at Kagoshima University, Kagoshima, Japan, and lead author of a study published in *Frontiers in Behavioral Neuroscience*.

Apps to Help Your Mental Health Can Backfire

Lisa Parker, PhD, postdoctoral research associate at University of Sydney, Australia, and lead author of the study titled, "Mental Health Messages in Prominent Mental Health Apps," published in *Annals of Family Medicine*.

Search "anxiety" or "depression" in the Apple App Store or Google Play store, and dozens of self-help mental-health apps appear. But do they work?

The truth is, few have been rigorously tested—and many encourage expectations that actually may harm mental health. So finds an analysis of the marketing used to promote 61 top-rated mental-health apps available in the US, UK, Canada and Australia. *Results…*

• **Many apps invoked vague scientific authority** with phrases such as "clinically proven" but didn't cite any research.

• **Apps often framed mental-health problems as present in everyone and characterized normal, healthy responses to stress as abnormal.**

• **Many encouraged frequent and excessive self-monitoring—which can make certain mental-health conditions worse.**

To be sure, some apps have been shown to be beneficial. Researchers cite another large-scale study published in *World Psychiatry* that found that there is evidence that some smartphone apps can help improve moods and reduce depressive symptoms.

Examples: The meditation app Headspace ($12.99 per month)…SuperBetter (free), which helps users confront tough challenges and reduce symptoms of anxiety and depression…and PTSD Coach (free), an app to help with post-traumatic stress disorder developed by the Departments of Defense and Veterans Affairs. All are available for both iOS and Android.

But even evidence-based apps still may encourage constant checking, which can undermine mental health. It's fine to use a meditation app such as Headspace on your own, but apps designed to treat depression or anxiety are best used along with a therapist. A self-help app should be just one part of your support system for mental health.

Relax Yourself Instantly

A furrowed brow or tight expression makes you tense overall. To quickly relax your body and your mind, relax your face—starting with your forehead.

Bottom Line research.

Anxiety Is Not "All in Your Head"

Anxiety can produce a range of physical symptoms, such as a racing heart…shortness of breath…constant exhaustion…sleep issues including inability to fall asleep or stay asleep, or waking up feeling drained rather than rested…muscle aches…gastrointestinal distress including stomach pain, constipation or diarrhea...sweaty palms...shaking and trembling...difficulty swallowing...getting colds frequently because of a depressed immune system. If you notice these symptoms, especially several of them, see your doctor. Consider cognitive behavioral therapy or other antianxiety treatments.

Self.com.

The Extreme Dangers of Widowhood

Felix Elwert, PhD, the Romnes Professor of Sociology and Population Health Sciences at University of Wisconsin-Madison. His research on "the widowhood effect" has been published in *American Journal of Public Health*, *American Sociological Review* and other leading professional journals.

Judith and Gerson Leiber were married for 72 years. She was a handbag designer...he was an artist. According to their *New York Times* obituaries, she was 97, and he was 96 when they died of dual heart attacks—just a few hours apart, in 2018.

The story would be astonishing...if it were not so familiar. Spouses who die in quick succession often make the news, whether they were famous in life or not.

Singers June Carter and Johnny Cash died within four months of each other—she from heart surgery complications and he from diabetes. The parents of football star Doug Flutie died of heart attacks less than an hour apart, according to their son. Such stories could be dismissed as mere coincidences. But social scientists say there's something real at work here.

They call it "the widowhood effect"—the increased risk for death we face when a spouse dies. That risk is elevated by more than 50% in the first month after the death, according to the largest studies on the phenomenon.

To learn more, we spoke with Felix Elwert, PhD, a sociologist and leading authority on widowhood.

How strong is the evidence that the widowhood effect is real?

It's one of the strongest findings we have on the connections between social factors and health. The link between marriage and death was first noticed back in 1858 by William Farr, a pioneering social scientist.

More recently, it's been confirmed by numerous large studies using varying methodologies. These studies have sorted out whether the link is merely an association—explained, for example, by the fact that spouses often share health-threatening habits or circumstances, including advanced age—or a matter of cause and effect. The evidence is strong that this is indeed a cause-and-effect relationship, at least in part. Losing a spouse does increase your risk for death in the near future.

How big is the risk and how long does it last?

As mentioned earlier, the risk spikes at least 50% above the normal death rate in the first month after the spouse's death. It then declines but remains higher than normal for years afterward. The overall increased risk approaches 20% over three or more years.

Do men and women have differing levels of risk?

Many people are surprised to learn that the biggest studies find no meaningful differences in death rates between recently widowed men and women—though conventional wisdom assumes men get more health benefits from marriage and thus face greater risks when a spouse dies.

However, the reasons for increased death rates vary between bereaved men and women, based on research by sociologist Linda Waite and colleagues at University of Chicago. In the case of an older man, for example, the loss of a spouse often means the loss of a primary caregiver—the person who cooks his meals, arranges his social life and makes sure he takes his pills and keeps his doctors' appointments.

Women may be better equipped to do those things for themselves but may suffer more for financial reasons—because in most older heterosexual couples, it's still true that men earn more than women over a lifetime. When men die, there's typically a reduction in pension and Social Security benefits to the surviving spouse.

Does grief itself play a role?

The sharp spike in deaths immediately after a spouse dies certainly suggests that the strain and shock of that loss, both of which are key elements of grief, do play roles. The days and weeks after a death can be especially stressful and disorienting. It is reasonable to assume that those disruptions can have all kinds of negative effects on health. But we do not have the psychological data to know to what extent those stresses make a direct contribution to deaths we see among widows and widowers.

Is there any group at decreased risk— and, if so, what could we learn from them?

In at least one ethnic group, African-Americans, researchers have failed to find the widowhood effect. That has led to speculation about what might protect black men and women. One factor could be that elderly African-Americans are much more likely than whites to live with other adult relatives—40% versus 20%. That may help the recently bereaved stay socially connected, which in turn can have health benefits.

We also know that African-American wives are more likely to work and African-American men are more likely to help out around the house than their white counterparts. This means that each spouse may be less specialized in his/her marriage roles and more able to cope when a spouse dies.

Does the spouse's cause of death have any influence—that is, are you more at risk if your spouse died of cancer than if he/she died from Alzheimer's?

The increased risk is seen after a spouse dies from almost any cause, ranging from cancer to a car crash to heart disease. There are two exceptions, though—there's no apparent increase in death among those whose spouses die of Alzheimer's disease or Parkinson's disease.

One theory is that deaths from Alzheimer's or Parkinson's have less impact because they are expected for years in advance. Another is that people with these conditions stop contributing to their spouses' health and well-being long before their deaths—meaning any adverse effects have already occurred.

Are people who lose a spouse likely to die in any particular way—from heart attacks, for example?

While the media tend to focus on serious conditions such as "broken heart syndrome"—a life-threatening heart problem sometimes seen in grieving people—research finds that deaths from all causes rise after the loss of a spouse.

There are, however, especially large increases in deaths from sudden events such as accidents as well as those from infections and certain chronic conditions, such as diabetes, that require careful daily management, according to our research published in *American Journal of Public Health*.

There's no single explanation for these deaths, but the pattern suggests that the widowhood effect in these cases is driven by the loss of social connection and daily support that had been provided by the spouse. For example, a spouse could call the ambulance if the other falls and breaks a bone, but a widowed person might well die of the same fracture because help is delayed.

Anxiety: Don't Get Stuck in This Hidden Trap of Grief

Claire Bidwell Smith, LCPC, a Los Angeles–based licensed therapist specializing in grief. Her latest book is *Anxiety: The Missing Stage of Grief*. She also is author of *The Rules of Inheritance* and *After This: When Life Is Over Where Do We Go?* ClaireBidwellSmith.com

Most of us do not like to think about grief. But when we do, what often comes to mind are the well-known "stages of grief"—denial, anger, bargaining, depression and acceptance—coined by the late Elisabeth Kübler-Ross.

Never mind that the Swiss-born psychiatrist originally intended her stages to describe the experiences of people facing their own deaths, not grieving someone else's. Or that she eventually made clear that not everyone goes through all the stages or in the same predictable order.

The missing stage: What's become increasingly clear is that one extremely common and often debilitating stage of grief is not included. That stage is anxiety.

One landmark study published in *American Journal of Psychiatry* found that the onset of generalized anxiety disorder is strongly associated, especially after age 40, with the unexpected death of a loved one. Beyond that, there's little research on how many people become anxious—or more anxious—after a death, yet it's something grief counselors see all the time.

●**It makes sense.** When someone close to you dies, one of your worst fears comes true. You are reminded that your own life will end some day, that bad things happen and that you are not always in control.

And maybe you were anxious already. Nearly one in five adults has suffered from anxiety in the past year, and nearly one in three has experienced an anxiety disorder sometime in their lives, according to the National Institute of Mental Health.

If you are one of those people, you may be especially vulnerable to renewed or intensified anxiety when a loved one dies. You may feel constantly worried, fearful, restless, jittery and irritable and may experience physical symptoms, such as a pounding heart, shortness of breath, muscle tension and sleeplessness.

For some people, the first undeniable sign is a panic attack—a sudden sense of impending doom that can be accompanied by rapid heartbeat, sweating, nausea, shaking, choking and a fear that you are going crazy or are about to die.

People often say that anxiety symptoms "come out of the blue." But here's what's often going on—a buildup of suppressed stress and emotion has finally found a way to get your attention. You can try in vain to push the feelings back down…or deal with them—and work past the anxiety. *Here are some of the most effective ways to do that…*

STEP #1: **Tell your story.** If you are fortunate, you will have a safe friend or family member who is willing to listen to your story—including your regrets and fears—without judgment or advice.

Many people find it helpful to see a professional grief counselor or attend a bereavement support group. Many hospitals and hospice organizations offer them, and finding one near you is likely just a Google search away. Many groups are organized by age or type of loss (for example, the loss of a spouse, parent or child or a loss due to suicide). Online grief forums can sometimes be valuable as well.

STEP #2: **Hear (or read) others' stories.** While it can be difficult at first, many people eventually find comfort in hearing or reading about the losses others have experienced. It can help you to feel less alone and less anxious. You can find that fellowship in a support group and by reading about others' experiences in online forums and books.

Some good memoirs to consider include: *Wild* by Cheryl Strayed (who lost her mother)…*The Year of Magical Thinking* by Joan Didion (who lost her spouse)…*Her* by Christa Parravani (who lost a sibling)…and *Truth & Beauty* by Ann Patchett (who lost a friend). There are many more. If reading is difficult for you at this time, consider listening to an audio version of the book.

STEP #3: **Release yourself through writing.** Many people are filled with regrets and a sense of guilt after a significant loss. Maybe they were not there when their loved one died. Or they think they said the wrong thing to the dying person.

One way to deal with such feelings: Write a letter to your deceased loved one. Apologize, if you feel the need, or say goodbye in the way you missed out on before. Some people also write letters to themselves—forgiving themselves, with kindness and compassion, for any perceived mistakes.

You can use writing to probe any feeling—including those you might be reluctant to admit to others (such as relief that a loved one who was suffering has died). Get a beautiful blank journal and try to use it for even just five to 10 minutes each day for as long as you feel the need. You can start by just writing what you are feeling—something like "I'm lonely" or "I'm scared," and then just keep writing for 10 minutes. If you're intimidated by the thought of writing out your feelings, you can dictate your feelings into your smartphone.

STEP #4: **Consider using cognitive behav-ioral therapy (CBT) techniques.** CBT is a short-term treatment often used for anxiety. It is a practical approach that helps people recognize and change thoughts and beliefs that contribute to their distress. While some people need the help of a therapist, there are CBT techniques you can try on your own. *The Anxiety & Worry Workbook* by the renowned American psychiatrist Aaron T. Beck, MD, is an excellent resource for this, as well as apps you can use on your smartphone.

Among the things you might try: Writing a list of your anxious thoughts (like I'm afraid I might have cancer)…noting the physical symptoms (such as a rapid heartbeat) and cognitive symptoms (such as an underlying fear that you will die just like your loved one did)…and observing the way you behave as a result (avoiding doctor appointments or seeking reassurance online).

Becoming aware of such links is a step toward breaking these negative patterns. But this can be hard—if you feel your anxiety is out of control and interfering with your life, be sure to seek professional treatment.

STEP #5: **Try meditating.** Like CBT, meditation is, at its core, a technique for helping you notice your thoughts—and break free from those working against you. Your mind may be humming with worries about the future, but you can learn to live in the present. It can be as simple as taking a few minutes each day to sit and focus on your breath moving in and out of your body, letting your thoughts come and go without judgment.

Skeptical? Just give it a chance. You might start with a class or workshop or get a good guidebook, such as *Wherever You Go, There You Are: Mindfulness Meditation in Everyday Life* by professor and meditation teacher Jon Kabat-Zinn, PhD.

STEP #6: **Start planning your own death.** It might sound counterintuitive to think about your own death when you're grieving the loss of someone dear to you. But remember this—the root of anxiety is uncertainty. Planning for your eventual death can help set your mind at ease…and lessen the anxieties of those we leave behind.

So get your own affairs in order—write (or update) your will…decide on a health-care proxy…create an advance directive…make your funeral wishes known…and let your friends and family members know what you would like them to have when you are gone. This can be scary, so take your time and enlist the support of a professional and/or friends and family members. But facing your fears can help you put them in their place and get on with life.

Natural Help for Bipolar Disorder Treatment

Andrew L. Rubman, ND, naturopathic physician and founder and medical director, Southbury Clinic for Traditional Medicines, Southbury, Connecticut. Study titled, "Evaluating the Effect of Coenzyme Q10 Augmentation on Treatment of Bipolar Depression: A Double-Blind Controlled Clinical Trial" by researchers at Hamadan University of Medical Sciences, Iran, published in *Journal of Clinical Psychopharmacology*.

Could preventing depressive episodes be as simple as getting a daily dose of a dietary supplement? A new study has found that a powerful antioxidant and anti-inflammatory agent has a place in the complex treatment of bipolar disorder, characterized by manic highs and depressive lows.

Researchers in Iran have found that CoQ10 can help improve mood. They divided 69 patients with bipolar disorder into two groups—one group took 200 mg of CoQ10 a day in addition to their mood stabilizers and antidepressants...the other group added a placebo. After eight weeks, the CoQ10 group had greater improvement of depression symptoms than the placebo group.

The finding makes sense: CoQ10 is vital to every cell's energy-producing process. More energy means less fatigue and feeling down.

Important: CoQ10 alone may not be the answer to treating bipolar disorder and you should never take any supplements or substitute supplements for medication without consulting your health-care provider. It certainly can be a helpful complement to your treatment even if prescriptions are working well. (On the other hand, some doctors have successfully used CoQ10 to effectively treat certain cases of diagnosed bipolar disorder that are characterized primarily by depression without typical prescription drugs—don't be surprised if your provider is willing to give it a try as a solo therapy.)

How to Supplement with CoQ10

Organ meats such as liver and kidneys are great sources of CoQ10 but not quite daily food choices people are likely to make. You'll find it in smaller amounts in beef, sardines, mackerel and peanuts, but not enough to get a significant amount in your system. That's why supplements are usually needed.

Once your doctor prescribes CoQ10, keep in mind that it's better to take 100 mg twice a day than a single 200 mg dose. Dividing the amount suggested by the study into two doses could prevent gastric upset, which is a rare but possible side effect. Also, more isn't better when it comes to CoQ10—more than 200 mg a day is often unnecessary and could invite more side effects.

Warning: If you also take a blood-thinner, some evidence suggests that CoQ10 may offset the blood-thinning effect of *warfarin* (Coumadin). Though other studies have not found this effect, if you decide to take CoQ10, ask your doctor to test your blood-clotting time to see if it has any effect on you.

More About CoQ10

If you take statins to reduce cholesterol, taking CoQ10 can help you avoid some of the more unpleasant side effects of those drugs, notably muscle pain and weakness and possible tendinitis. CoQ10 use has also been linked to migraine relief and even high blood pressure reduction.

Don't Just Manage Your Anxiety...Make It Work for You

Alicia Clark, PsyD, psychologist and author of *Hack Your Anxiety: How to Make Anxiety Work for You in Life, Love, and All That You Do.* AliciaClarkPsyD.com

Who hasn't felt butterflies in his/her stomach or even a sense of dread before an important event like a job interview? Anxiety is uncomfortable, so our first reaction is to try to make it stop—we fight it, run from it or simply aim to ignore it. But if you embrace it instead, you can turn all that negative energy into a positive.

Anxiety is a natural response to facing some type of challenge. Much like a baby's cry, anxiety is loud and grating and lasts until you find a solution. For instance, you may feel on edge and jumpy when facing a deadline and yet these very feelings can give you the focus and energy to complete your work...if you reframe your thinking and tap into anxiety as a resource. You want to control it instead of letting it control you. *Here's how...*

STEP 1: **Identify the source of your anxiety.** What are you afraid of or worried about? To channel it, you first need to name it and identify it—don't turn away from it, and don't get scared it will hurt you.

STEP 2: **Ask yourself if the anxiety** is over something reasonable and rational or is it just noise and irrational? *Example…*

- Rational anxiety—you're anxious because your plane is late and you might miss your connection.

- Irrational anxiety—you're anxious because the plane is late, so there must be something horribly wrong and the plane will go down in a fiery crash.

STEP 3: **Take action.** When your anxiety is irrational, make it rational. First, look at the evidence. What makes you think the plane will crash because it's late? Just because a plane could possibly crash doesn't mean it's probable. Think of the thousands of planes that take off and land every day without incident. You might even Google "how safe is it to fly" to put your mind at ease. If you feel like your anxiety is crossing over into panic, practice deep diaphragmatic breathing—you can't panic while doing this.

Even if your anxiety is rational as in the example above, wasting time worrying about being late isn't using anxiety to your advantage. You want to channel that energy into figuring out how you will get to your final destination if you indeed miss your connection. Use the time to search for other flights or look into alternatives, such as a rental car for the next leg of your trip. Or a hotel if you'll need an overnight stay. Action puts you in control and melts away anxiety.

Another common example is not speaking up for yourself. You might know you need to ask someone for a favor or for help but are anxious about it—you worry what if you're turned down?—so you procrastinate. But putting off something you know you need to do only makes it harder and more difficult.

Anxiety may be irrationally scaring you into inaction, when you rationally know that you need to speak up for a situation to improve. Using anxiety as a tool for motivation, rather than avoidance, is a key way to use it to your advantage.

Simply rebranding anxiety's signals can give you the upper hand, too. For instance, if your heart beats fast at the thought of go-ing on a blind date, don't focus on the fear of potential rejection. Instead focus on the opportunity to meet somebody new and your excitement about it.

Stomach tied up in knots over the thought of saying "I'm sorry" to someone? Look at your worry as a sign that you care about the person who needs to hear your apology.

Important: As with any new habit, the more you practice using anxiety as a tool, the better you'll get at it.

You Can Overcome Your Fear of Flying

Martin N. Seif, PhD, ABPP, is a clinical psychologist who has spent the last 30 years developing treatments for anxiety disorders. He has a private practice in Greenwich, Connecticut, and New York City, is associate director of The Anxiety and Phobia Treatment Center at White Plains Hospital Medical Center in New York and is a founding board member of the Anxiety and Depression Association of America. He is also co-author of *What Every Therapist Needs to Know About Anxiety Disorders* and *Overcoming Unwanted Intrusive Thoughts*. Using techniques that he developed, Dr. Seif overcame his own crippling fear of flying. DrMartinSeif.com

---

If you have a "fear of flying," you know how debilitating it can be. Is there any way you can possibly get over it?

A flying phobia is more than an inconvenience. (A phobia is an intense fear that is out of proportion to the actual danger posed by the situation or object.) Most people who are afraid to fly recognize that flying is safe, yet they find air travel very frightening.

If you have a flying phobia, you're not alone. About 20% of the population has a fear of flying that interferes with their work and social lives.

The Causes

Fear of flying is caused by a variety of underlying fears and phobias, which have complex genetic, developmental and environmental causes. In my experience, about 70% of those who have a fear of flying are triggered primarily by feeling trapped on a plane. Others have a fear of heights, crashing, terrorism, being far from home, physical harm such as a heart attack or stroke or even a fear of panic or losing control. Another aspect of this phobia is anticipatory anxiety—anxiety experienced in anticipation of doing something fearful in the future.

Most people with a fear of flying have experienced an unexpected episode of panic while flying. Symptoms of panic can include extreme dread, sweating, breathing difficulties, dizziness and more. This typically first occurs between the ages of 17 to 34, but it can happen later in life or as early as age 11 or 12. It often occurs during a time of significant change, good or bad, which can include a birth or death…a marriage or divorce…a new job or getting fired. Very few of these fears originate with an actual technical problem during the flight.

As a result of this panic episode and possible additional episodes, the individual becomes sensitized to these feelings…and to flying. He/she may start to fear that the scary symptoms will return and begin to avoid getting on a plane, which only stokes the fear.

Getting Over the Fear

Overcoming a fear of flying takes work and commitment but is entirely possible. Identifying the triggers that produce your anxiety with the help of a qualified therapist is the first step. Exposure to feared triggers while armed with the right tools is the key for overcoming the problem.

Types of therapy: Cognitive behavioral therapy (CBT)—a form of psychotherapy that helps you recognize unhealthy or unreasonable thoughts and behaviors and replace them with healthy strategies—can be tailored to fear of flying. And group therapy programs that meet at airports, available in a few areas of the country, sometimes culminate with a flight guided by the therapist. Virtual reality programs that expose patients to flight simulations can be helpful as well.

No matter what type of therapy is chosen, techniques for managing anxiety will typically be taught, such as helping patients to avoid fighting feelings of anxiety, which can make them worse. Anxiety thrives on ignorance and feeds on "what if" thinking. Learning the facts about flying including how a plane flies, the meaning of various sounds, what actually causes turbulence, etc., can also help with anxiety management.

Medications that treat anxiety and depression such as selective serotonin reuptake inhibitors (SSRIs) and serotonin-norepinephrine reuptake inhibitors (SRNIs) can be helpful to some people, particularly for those who have additional anxieties, but these drugs must be taken every day for a long period of time and they do have side effects. Short-acting antianxiety drugs, such as *lorazepam* (Ativan) or *diazepam* (Valium), can also provide relief for some—especially for the anticipatory anxiety—but they have side effects as well and don't allow patients to work on underlying triggers and develop coping tools.

To find a therapist and other programs that treat fear of flying, go to the website of the Anxiety and Depression Association of America at ADAA.org and click on "Find Help" and/

Hypnosis Helps Your Stomach Distress

Hypnosis improves irritable bowel syndrome (IBS) and other stomach issues, according to Megan Riehl, PsyD. The brain and gut exchange chemical messages with each other, so when people are under hypnosis, targeted suggestions about abdominal and bowel discomfort help them develop coping mechanisms that reduce pain and improve quality of life. Cognitive behavioral therapy also helps, and both methods are recommended by the American Gastroenterological Association.

Megan Riehl, PsyD, is a gastrointestinal health psychologist and assistant professor of medicine at University of Michigan, Ann Arbor.

or type "Fear of Flying" in the search box to get more information on the topic.

Use Self-Hypnosis to Stop Bad Habits

Grace Smith, a master hypnotherapist certified by the International Association of Counselors and Therapists, National Guild of Hypnotists and others, who is based in Vero Beach, Florida. She is author of *Close Your Eyes, Get Free: Use Self-Hypnosis to Reduce Stress, Quit Bad Habits, and Achieve Greater Relaxation and Focus* and founder of Grace Space Hypnosis (GSHypnosis.com) and Grace Space Hypnotherapy School.

If you've got a bad habit that you can't break, you may assume that you're just not leveraging enough willpower or using your logical thinking skills the right way. But that's not true.

The fact is, the thought processes that drive willpower and logic reside in the conscious mind. But lasting behavioral change starts in the subconscious—where beliefs, emotions, values, habits, intuition and imagination reside.

A Window to the Subconscious

Self-hypnosis is widely recognized as one of the most effective ways to access the subconscious. My self-hypnosis techniques use a combination of a slow countdown and some mental-imagery practices to relax your body and mind so deeply that you enter the theta brain wave state.

Once your mind is producing theta brain waves (as opposed to beta, alpha or delta waves), you feel ultrarelaxed, and you experience an increase in problem-solving abilities, as well as enhanced creativity. By comparison, the beta brain wave is wide awake and engaged…alpha is reflective…and delta is the brain wave we enter when we're asleep.

The theta state is the key to self-hypnosis because it allows you to make new connections in the brain very quickly and thoroughly. In other words, you become open to suggestion—but only the suggestions you want to absorb. Once you are in the theta state, you repeat the suggestions, or hypno-affirmations, thereby increasing the likelihood that these thoughts will become reality.

The Do-It-Yourself Approach

Self-hypnosis is a good choice for many people because it can be done anytime, anywhere—except while driving or performing some other activity that requires your full attention.

It's free and powerful enough that short, focused sessions, ranging from one to five minutes, are all you need. About three months (or 90 days) of daily practice is sufficient to retrain your subconscious completely and leave bad habits in the past, without any assistance from a hypnotherapist or a recording. Aim for three to five sessions a day.

6 Simple Steps

To jump-start your self-hypnosis practice, use the following general, 60-second script. After reading it a few times, you'll start memorizing it, at which point you can close your eyes while practicing. Once you've mastered that, you can tailor it to tackle the specific habits you wish to transform by changing the hypno-affirmations in Step 4 and the visualizations in Step 5.

First, begin by ranking your stress level on a scale of zero (completely relaxed) to 10 (panic attack). *Then…*

STEP 1: **While sitting in a comfortable chair** with your hands in your lap and both feet on the floor, take four slow, deep breaths. Inhale through the nose for four counts, exhale through the nose for eight.

STEP 2: **Imagine a color you love flowing in through the top of your head,** down through your entire body, out the bottoms of your feet and down into the ground. This color is washing away any stress.

STEP 3: **With your eyes still closed, count down from 10 to one,** repeating, silently or aloud, I am going deeper and deeper after each number. For example, Ten, I am going deeper and deeper. Nine, I am going deeper and deeper, etc...

STEP 4: Next, repeat the following hypno-affirmation 10 times, silently or aloud—I am safe. I am calm. I choose to be here.

STEP 5: Take a few deep breaths as you see, feel and experience yourself feeling happy and calm for the rest of the day.

STEP 6: Open your eyes and notice your new, lower stress level on the scale (again, zero is no stress), and congratulate yourself on how quickly you improved your state.

About half of all adults will relax by 50% or more during their first self-hypnosis session. Those who relax by less than 50% during their first session simply need a bit more conditioning and will learn to relax that deeply over the course of a week or so with repeated practice. There is no one who can't be hypnotized—all that varies from person to person is the amount of conditioning that's needed.

To Tackle Bad Habits

After you've run through the process described above a few times, incorporate the following hypno-affirmations to initiate powerful changes in your life. *For example...*

• **To go to bed earlier.** Proper rest is critical for cognitive functioning, mood and memory. Practice this hypnosis ritual two hours before your preferred bedtime for maximum efficacy.

Sample hypno-affirmation: During Step 4, repeat, I easily and effortlessly go to bed at X pm. When I go to sleep early, I enjoy my life even more. During Step 5, imagine yourself getting into your comfortable bed at your chosen time, sleeping soundly through the night and then waking up refreshed, ready for a productive and rewarding day.

• **To lose weight.** Steady, long-lasting weight loss requires meaningful behavior changes rather than short-term deprivation.

Sample hypno-affirmation: During Step 4, repeat, I choose to nourish my body with healthy foods. Every day in every way, I am losing weight and feeling great. During Step 5, imagine having already lost the weight

you wish to lose. See, feel and experience yourself feeling strong, happy and healthy.

• **To reduce anxiety.** Lots of people feel anxious before giving a speech or going on a job interview. But if you wrestle with these feelings on a regular basis, you know how exhausting and painful they can be.

Sample hypno-affirmation: During Step 4, repeat, I am safe. I am calm. I choose to feel relaxed. I have more than enough time. I am safe. During Step 5, visualize yourself remaining calm throughout your entire day, especially during situations that used to cause anxiety. See, feel and experience yourself feeling safe, calm and relaxed throughout the entire experience.

Important: With self-hypnosis, it is better to tackle one area at a time than to simultaneously work on, say, weight loss and procrastination. Pick one self-hypnosis topic, practice for 90 days (or until you experience the results you desire), and then move on to the next topic.

DIY Anxiety Relief with Acupressure

Kathleen Lumiere, DAOM, LAc, associate professor and DAOM program director, department of acupuncture and East Asian medicine, Bastyr University, Seattle.

If "anxious" feels like your default emotion, you don't have to just accept that. While relaxation techniques such as meditation, counseling and even medication can help, there's another very effective, quick-and-easy way to "get a handle" on your anxiety—literally. We're talking about pressing acupressure points on your body to turn off the angst. *Here's how to do it...*

Acupuncture is commonly used to treat anxiety and the symptoms associated with it. Acupressure works on the same principles and uses the same pressure points but without the needles. It's also easy to do yourself on your own body, so it's a great remedy that you always have with you.

Like acupuncture, acupressure is based on a theory that energy flows through a system of lines or meridians that crisscross the body. This energy flow can become blocked at pressure points located at the edges of muscles, and anxiety is one of the problems that can result. Stimulating the pressure points opens the flow of energy and relieves the anxiety. Acupressure can relieve not only physical symptoms such as headache, nausea, sweating and heart palpitations…it also can relieve emotional symptoms such as excessive fear, worry, apprehension and irritability.

The seven pressure points below are especially good at relieving anxiety and associated symptoms. When you're working on a particular pressure point, you can either apply steady pressure or gently massage it for a few minutes, whichever works better for you. Repeat as often as you like—acupressure is perfectly safe. You can further enhance the effectiveness by taking slow, deep breaths and/or closing your eyes while you're pressing or massaging. It doesn't matter which points you try, how many of them, in what order or whether you apply pressure to a particular point on one or both sides of the body. Focus on the points (and the side of the body) that work for you.

Seven points to try…

• **Pericardium 6 (PC 6).** PC 6 is a very well-researched acupressure (and acupuncture) point. In fact, it's the pressure point stimulated by motion sickness wristbands to reduce nausea. (Wearing one of these bands also helps relieve anxiety!) Find it at the center 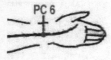 of your inner wrist, about an inch above the crease. PC 6 not only reduces the nausea caused by anxiety, it also can reduce palpitations.

• **Heart 7 (HT 7).** Find HT 7 on the outside of your inner wrist (the side opposite your thumb), just above the palm of your hand in the crease area. Pressure here may relieve nervousness, fear and palpitations.

• **Yintang.** YinTang is located right between your eyebrows, an area sometimes called the third eye. It is an especially powerful pressure point for relieving anxiety and calming the whole body. Yintang also is useful for reducing anxiety headaches and insomnia.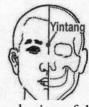

• **Jianjing or Gallbladder 21 (GB 21).** This point is located at the top of your shoulder about halfway between your shoulder and neck and in line with your nipple. Since trying to reach your shoulder with the hand on the same side is awkward, you will need to cross your arms to reach each shoulder with the opposite hand (or let 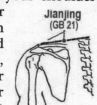 someone press this pressure point for you). Pressing GB 21 is wonderful for relieving the neck pain and tension that can accompany anxiety. It also can lower blood pressure.

• **Liver 3 (LR 3).** Locate L 3 by finding the web between your big toe and the next toe (you'll need to take off your shoes and socks), then follow that space up about two inches toward your ankle. Pressure on LR 3 can relieve feelings of tension, irritability and stress.

• **Stomach 36 (ST 36).** Find this point about two inches below your knee just on the outside of your shinbone. Pressure here can relieve anxiety-associated nausea and indigestion.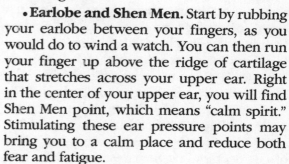

• **Earlobe and Shen Men.** Start by rubbing your earlobe between your fingers, as you would do to wind a watch. You can then run your finger up above the ridge of cartilage that stretches across your upper ear. Right in the center of your upper ear, you will find Shen Men point, which means "calm spirit." Stimulating these ear pressure points may bring you to a calm place and reduce both fear and fatigue.

What else helps: Eating anxiety-reducing foods such as cooked vegetables, leafy greens and mushrooms…avoiding foods that promote anxiety, namely processed, deep-fried and spicy foods as well as sweets (which can relieve anxiety temporarily but then make it worse)…getting regular exercise.…and getting enough sleep also help keep anxiety at bay.

Finally, if all these steps don't help or don't help enough, discuss with your doctor what other steps you might need to take. You should also let your doctor know that you have heart palpitations, especially with shortness of breath or dizziness, even if you think they're caused by anxiety, as they could be a sign of a more serious health problem.

Feeling Lonely? Getting More Sleep May Fix That

Study titled "Sleep loss causes social withdrawal and loneliness," by Eti Ben-Simon, PhD, Matthew P. Walker, PhD, both University of California, Berkeley, published in *Nature Communications*.

If you often feel lonely, you're likely to ponder how you might increase your social opportunities. Join a club? Sign up for a class? Volunteer with a youth sports league? All worthy ideas—but there's something else you probably wouldn't think about to fix your loneliness: Get more sleep. But that's exactly what new research suggests you should do.

The Sleep-Loneliness Connection

How could a lack of sleep make you lonely? It's all about how you behave when you're sleepy…and how others perceive you. It's been known for a while that people tend to withdraw from others when they're sleepy. So psychologists at University of California at Berkeley decided to investigate whether lack of sleep could actually lead to loneliness.

The first part of their study involved 18 healthy adults and took place in a lab. After one full night of sleep and after one night of not sleeping, participants were given two "social distancing" tests…

Test #1: Participants were asked to say "stop" when another person walking toward

them reached the point that felt uncomfortably close.

Test #2: Participants were hooked up to MRI machines that scanned the parts of the brain that respond to threat, then they watched a person come closer on a computer screen. Afterward, they answered questions about their moods and feelings while taking the test.

Results: In both the real-life and the computer-generated social-distancing tests, participants preferred significantly more distance from other people after not sleeping. And their brain scans confirmed that threat-sensitive areas of the brain were stimulated by an approaching person after a sleepless night—but not after a night of full sleep.

For the next part of the study, about 100 participants kept journals in which they rated each night's sleep quality and the degree of loneliness they felt on the following day. Again, there was a clear pattern of more loneliness after nights of poor sleep.

Finally, recorded videos of the first part of the study were "judged" by about 1,000 other participants. Not only were the "judges" able to identify the people who were feeling lonely—but the loneliness was "contagious." The participants who were watching the videos said that watching videos of lonely people made them feel lonely. In fact, the lonelier the person on the video was, the lonelier the watcher felt. The watchers also said that in social situations, they would be inclined to avoid such lonely-seeming people.

Sleep deprivation is a serious public health problem in America, according to the Centers for Disease Control and Prevention. So is loneliness and social isolation. If you're one of the four out of 10 adults getting less than seven hours of sleep a night, now is a good time to change that. For instance, trade staying up late to watch television for an earlier bedtime—so you can wake up feeling refreshed enough to be sociable and make others want to be sociable with you.

Chapter 6

FOOD AND FITNESS

Let Yourself Love Your Body

I'll do that when I lose 10 (or 20 or 30) pounds…

If you've ever said that (or something similar) to yourself, you're not alone. So many of us postpone things we want to do—from buying a new pair of pants to going on a beach vacation—all because we're dissatisfied with our bodies.

The trap: Because the overwhelming majority of dieters eventually gain back the weight they lose, it's becoming increasingly clear that dieting is not the answer. Instead, research now shows that you are more likely to maintain a healthy body weight and eating habits when you focus your efforts on "befriending" your body instead of constantly striving to make it "just right."

For a fresh perspective and real-world advice on how to achieve this, we spoke with Heidi Schauster, MS, RDN, CEDRD-S, a nutrition therapist and leading authority on overcoming dieting cycles and poor eating habits.

Why do so many people focus so intently on the ideal body? Ironically, we can learn something about this from toddlers. Obviously, they aren't worried about their appearance. If you watch young children before they have any ideas imposed on them about what they should or shouldn't eat, they'll have just a bite of a cookie and won't eat any more if there is something else more entertaining to do. Most adults, however, have a hard time not finishing a treat.

Research shows that if we offer children a variety of foods, they'll intuitively choose a well-balanced diet over time even if they focus on one type of food at a given meal. This just goes to show that the focus on an ideal body and an ideal way to eat is culturally imposed.

When people don't like their bodies, doesn't that mean they have body dysmorphia? Not necessarily. Body dysmorphic disorder (BDD) is a mental illness in which a person has a distorted perception of his/her own body. It could be related to an eating disorder, such as anorexia, in which you're not seeing your body size accurately, or you may believe that there's something wrong

Heidi Schauster, MS, RDN, CEDRD-S, founder of Nourishing Words Nutrition Therapy in Somerville, Massachusetts. Schauster is a certified eating-disorders registered dietitian. She is author of *Nourish: How to Heal Your Relationship with Food, Body and Self* and an adjunct faculty member at Plymouth State University's graduate-level Eating Disorders Institute. ANourishingWord.com with some part of your body—your nose is too big or your shoulders are crooked—and everyone else notices. When people have BDD, they struggle deeply in their work life and relationships because of these intrusive thoughts about their bodies.

Far more people simply go about their daily lives without fully accepting their bodies. As a result, they put parts of their lives on hold by denying themselves the opportunity to fully enjoy themselves—to go swimming, get dressed up for special occasions or even have sex. This lack of acceptance and self-denial, too, can be a huge burden.

So why doesn't dieting work for adults? As anyone who's ever dieted knows all too well, avoiding entire food groups or severely limiting food intake creates a deprivation mindset. When we feel deprived, we become more anxious and are less likely to make choices from a feeling of being in charge. It's also an innate survival mechanism to resist starvation of any type. Our bodies are wired so that our metabolism naturally slows down when we're not eating enough in order to keep us from starving.

It takes a conscious effort—and practice—to get back to a self-connected way of eating that most toddlers do instinctively. It involves slowing down and paying close attention to your body and what it's asking for. It involves listening closely for cues of hunger and fullness and choosing to respond to them appropriately. Sometimes it also requires asking, "What's eating me?" and getting to the feelings underneath.

It also helps to be sure that meals and snacks contain carbohydrates, proteins and fats so that we feel satisfied and are able to make it to the next eating episode without significant cravings.

What other factors affect our weight aside from our diet and activity levels? A well-known study from the Netherlands looked at infants born to women during a famine. Ironically, as those infants grew up, they struggled more with being "overweight" than their siblings did. Scientists theorize that because the moms were starving when the ba-bies were in utero, something activated their genes to make them more likely to store energy as fat.

Hormones also play a role in our body size. For example, women who have gone through menopause are more likely to store body fat on their abdomens, while younger women with more circulating estrogen are more likely to store fat on their hips, thighs and buttocks. Poor sleep increases cortisol levels, and this can increase appetite and, therefore, body weight.

We need to stop blaming ourselves for our body size. Not only is it unfair, but when we don't feel good about our bodies, we often don't take care of them, either.

Even if people accept their bodies, shouldn't they lose weight if they are clearly overweight? According to many studies, weight loss itself does not bring good health—but certain habits do. Those habits center around eating fruits and vegetables and exercising regularly. This supports the thinking that a focus on healthy lifestyle habits is more productive than a singular focus on an ideal body weight.

To help you accept your body and improve your relationship with food…

• **Toss the scale.** The only time you need to step on a scale is at the doctor's office. The number itself is unimportant, and reinforcing it every day can be destructive. Is that how you want to frame your identity every morning?

• **Keep a journal.** A "food and feelings" journal can move you toward crucial awareness. Don't obsess about portion, amounts or calories. Instead, rank your hunger level from zero to 10 before and after a meal. Finish each day's entry by noting your physical activity levels, self-care practices (including good sleep and downtime) and what you felt good about. Even after just a few days of this, take notice of your food and exercise habits and your relationship with food. Do you skip meals only to be ravenous and overeat? Do you crave food when you feel bored, lonely or tired?

• **Eat your meals mindfully.** Pay close attention to your hunger and fullness levels (see above) and then respond to these cues. They are far better guides to your eating than habitual times of day, emotions or other external signals that often prompt us to eat.

• **Clarify your goals.** When you know what you really want to accomplish in life, whether personally or professionally, you begin to understand what really fills you up. Create a values checklist of traits that are important to you, such as being adventurous, authenticity, curiosity, forgiveness, humility, persistence or spirituality. Food tends to fall into place when you connect with what really matters and spend less time obsessing about changing your body.

• **See yourself through others' eyes.** Ask yourself why your family and friends like being around you—is it your sense of humor, your quiet determination or your zany fashion sense that they admire? Recognizing your innate qualities will help you shift your focus away from an idealized body.

For Better Breast Health, Eat This Way

The study "Consumption of Mediterranean versus Western Diet Leads to Distinct Mammary Gland Microbiome Populations," led by researchers at Wake Forest Baptist Medical Center in Winston-Salem, North Carolina, and published in *Cell Reports*.

The so-called gut "microbiome" has gotten a lot of attention for its effect on one's digestive health and its impact on chronic diseases. But researchers have now discovered that microorganisms that comprise the microbiome also live in breast tissue…and the implications could be significant when it comes to breast cancer risk.

Study details: As a stand-in for human subjects, researchers studied 38 female monkeys—half of whom were fed a typical American diet (high in unhealthy fats and refined carbohydrates)…with the other half receiving a plant-focused Mediterranean diet.

Results: After two and a half years (the equivalent of about eight human years), the groups had significantly different bacteria in their breast tissue. Compared with the standard diet group, the Mediterranean-diet monkeys had more bile acid metabolites and about 10 times as much Lactobacillus in their breasts—both of which have been shown to reduce breast cancer risk.

Why it matters: While the microbes that live in the human digestive tract have been well-researched, this is the first time that the breast gland has been found to have a microbiome and that it, like the gut microbiome, can be affected by diet. An imbalance in the gut microbiome has previously been linked to inflammatory bowel disease, irritable bowel syndrome, obesity and even type 2 diabetes.

"We were surprised that diet directly influenced microbiome outside of the intestinal tract in sites such as the mammary gland," explained Katherine Cook, PhD, assistant professor of surgery, hypertension and cancer biology at the Medical Center, a part of Wake Forest Baptist Medical Center. "However, we are just at the early stages of understanding how dietary effects on the microbiome might be used to protect women from breast cancer."

Researchers are digging deeper: More studies are under way to determine whether supplements such as fish oil and probiotics can affect the breast microbiome. Results from those studies may be a few years away.

Takeaway: Even though this research is preliminary, you don't have to wait to eat a Mediterranean diet, including plenty of fruits and vegetables, whole grains, legumes, nuts, olive oil and more fish than red meat. In addition to its potential to improve your breast flora, this diet has been shown to lower levels of LDL "bad" cholesterol, reducing heart disease risk.

The New Frontier in Healthy Eating

Laurie Steelsmith, ND, LAc, licensed naturopathic physician and acupuncturist in private practice in Honolulu. She writes Bottom Line's "Natural Healing Secrets for Women" blog and is coauthor of three books—the best-selling *Natural Choices for Women's Health*, the critically acclaimed *Great Sex, Naturally* and her latest, *Growing Younger Every Day.* DrSteel smith.com

At this very moment, trillions of microbes are making themselves quite at home in your intestines. That's a good thing, because that community of microbes—your microbiome—is key to good health. And the most important factor for a healthy microbiome is what you eat.

Here's how it works: A well-balanced microbiome is chock-full of bacteria that produce certain short-chain fatty acids that positively influence health. These include acetate, propionate and, especially, butyrate—highly biologically active compounds that support gut health, blood sugar regulation, optimal blood fat levels, appetite control and immunity. They also cross the blood-brain barrier and so influence your mood. A healthy microbiome protects against obesity, diabetes, heart disease, certain autoimmune diseases and depression.

Those good-for-you bugs need nourishment, primarily fiber that stays undigested until it reaches the intestines. But the typical Western diet—high in animal protein and fat while low in fiber—effectively starves the microbiome. The solution isn't to just eat more fiber or even more fruits and vegetables— certain foods promote a healthy microbiome in powerful, specific ways. They work in different ways, so eating a bountiful variety is best. *Start by saying "yes" to these foods…*

Walnuts

People who eat walnuts have more favorable cholesterol levels, as well as less diabetes, than people who rarely eat them. Why?

One key reason: Eating a handful of walnuts each day—about one-third cup, or 16 walnut halves (about 215 calories)—can change the microbiome in a good way by increasing the bacteria species that generate butyrate. Other nuts that support a healthy microbiome include almonds, cashews, pistachios, hazelnuts and pecans.

Ghee

Ghee is a type of clarified butter, originally from India, that is simmered and allowed to caramelize before the milk solids are removed. What's left is flavorful and aromatic butter fat without dairy proteins but with high levels of short-chain fatty acids—including butyrate. The flavor is concentrated, so a little goes a long way. One tablespoon a day (about 110 calories) is fine. Ghee is used in cooking and as a condiment.

FOS Foods

Fructooligosaccharides (FOS) are complex sugars that generally pass undigested through your digestive system until intestinal microbes break them down. FOS are the perfect diet for certain butyrate-producing bacteria. In animal studies, just two weeks on a high-FOS diet significantly increased butyrate production. FOS are found in many everyday foods including bananas, onions, leeks, garlic, asparagus, jicama and Jerusalem artichoke.

Caveat: For some people, FOS-rich foods are hard to digest and can cause gastrointestinal trouble. See "When Gut-Friendly Foods Are Bad for You" on the next page.

Polyphenol-Rich Food and Drink

The powerful antioxidants called polyphenols found in tea, coffee, berries, grapes, cocoa and certain vegetables (including artichokes, olives and asparagus) are strongly associated with the prevention of diabetes and heart disease. Credit the microbiome, at least in part—90% or more of polyphenols are metabolized by microbes, and they increase levels of the protective bacteria Bifidobacteria and Lactobacillus. *Examples*…

• **Olive oil.** In studies, the microbiomes of animals fed olive oil had higher levels of four bacteria that are known to reduce insulin levels (associated with diabetes prevention) and increase levels of leptin, a hormone that helps control appetite.

• **Cocoa.** Dark chocolate and cocoa powder are rich in flavanols, a type of antioxidant. In a study at University of Reading in the UK, adults who followed a diet rich in cocoa flavanols had an increase in healthful Bifidobacteria and Lactobacilli populations.

My recommendation: Add two or three tablespoons of raw cacao powder to a smoothie a few times a week…or bake with it.

• **Fermented foods.** Yogurt is made when friendly bacteria, usually Lactobacillus bulgaricus and Streptococcus thermophilus, are added to milk. Sauerkraut and kimchi (a salty Korean side dish) are made by allowing beneficial bacteria to digest the natural sugars in cabbage leaves. Other gut-friendly fermented foods include sourdough bread, certain natural cheeses (see below), olives, soy sauce, miso and tempeh. Fermented foods not only contain very high numbers of healthful microbes, but these good-for-you bacteria are particularly likely to survive the passage through the digestive tract—where they can thrive.

Tip: You already know that yogurt has health benefits, but don't neglect cheese. In one study at University of Copenhagen in Denmark, healthy volunteers produced more butyrate when they included cheese in their diets.

Best cheeses for your gut bacteria: Fresh mozzarella, aged Parmigiano, Camembert and raw-milk cheeses.

Foods to Avoid

Eating good-for-your-gut foods isn't enough. Certain eating patterns, as well as common additives used by the food industry, can throw a monkey wrench into your microbiome. *Be wary of…*

• **Emulsifiers.** Animal studies show that the microbiomes of mice fed diets with relatively low levels of emulsifiers—chemicals added to stabilize processed foods—were less robust than microbiomes of mice that weren't fed emulsifiers.

Even more concerning: Certain common emulsifiers have been found to chip away at the colon's mucous membrane, which is nature's way of keeping microbes inside the gut so they don't enter the bloodstream where they can do harm.

Avoid: Carboxymethylcellulose (aka cellulose gum, or CMC) and polysorbate-80. You also may want to avoid foods that contain the common emulsifier carrageenan, which can irritate the intestinal wall.

• **Artificial sweeteners.** Sucralose, aspartame and saccharin all have been shown to disrupt the balance and diversity of gut microbiomes.

Example: Mice fed sucralose for six months had higher levels of bacteria that promote inflammation. It's also wise to avoid sugar alcohols such as xylitol, which can cause stomach distress in many people.

Fine to use: Monkfruit sweetener or stevia.

Bottom line: The changes to the microbiome from what you eat may occur quickly, within 24 hours, but they don't last long. Making good diet choices each day is your best strategy to keep your microbiome—and you—healthy.

When Gut-Friendly Foods Are Bad for You

Here's a dilemma—some foods that promote a healthy microbiome can cause gastrointestinal distress for certain people.

Solution: Heal the gut first, then slowly introduce these foods to see if they can be tolerated.

Example: FODMAP is an acronym for "fermentable oligosaccharides, disaccharides, monosaccharides and polyols." Many people have trouble digesting these complex molecules—especially if they have irritable bowel syndrome—and restricting them often leads to symptom relief. But fructooligosaccharides

(FOS) in particular help feed a healthy microbiome. Cutting out FODMAPs can reduce Bifidobacterium and other beneficial species.

Solution: If you need a low-FODMAP diet, work with a health professional such as a naturopathic physician on an elimination diet. But as your symptoms improve, gradually reintroduce some foods. Adding them in slowly allows the gut flora to get used to them. You may need to stop eating onions permanently, for example—but bananas might be just fine.

A gluten-free diet poses a similar dilemma. People with celiac disease, as well as those with gluten intolerance, need to avoid wheat and other grains that contain gluten. But skipping wheat often means missing out on fiber that your microbiome needs. People on gluten-free diets have been found to have reduced levels of healthy Bifidobacterium and Lactobacillus and higher levels of unhealthful E. coli and Enterobacteriaceae bacteria.

Solution: If you are avoiding gluten, be sure to eat plenty of high-fiber foods, including whole grains such as oats (be sure they are certified as non-cross-contaminated with gluten), brown rice and millet. You may want to add in psyllium powder to boost your fiber intake, too. As with low-FODMAP diets, people who start out gluten intolerant can sometimes improve their gut health enough that they can reintroduce gluten-containing grains such as whole wheat.

Omega-3s for Vegetarians

Sharon Palmer, RDN, a registered dietitian nutritionist and author of *The Plant-Powered Diet*. She also holds an MSFS degree, a master's of science in sustainable food systems. Read her blog at "The Plant-Powered Dietitian" at SharonPalmer.com.

For people who don't eat fish, marine algae can be a great way to add healthful, plant-based omega-3s to their diets. This option could appeal not only to vegetarians, who eschew animal products and may or may not consume dairy products, but also to vegans, who eat no animal products (including fish) or animal-derived products. Even people who simply don't like the taste of fish may want to consider marine algae as a good source of omega-3s.

Though you may not realize it, the omega-3s found in fish oil mainly come from the marine algae that the fish consume—or from eating krill and other fish that feed on algae. So essentially the primary source of omega-3s is marine algae.

Marine algae can be consumed in food sources, too, including nori seaweed (typically found in sheets that are used in rolling sushi or as a crunchy, salty snack that can be added to rice bowls and soups) and kelp (available in sprinkles that can be used as a topping for salads and/or a substitute for salt). However, it can be difficult to get an appreciable amount of the long-chain omega-3s EPA and DHA from these food-based sources.

Bonus: Chlorophyll, the green plant pigment found in algae, also has potential health benefits, such as helping to boost immunity and reduce inflammation. The powdered supplements chlorella and spirulina are rich in chlorophyll and can be added to smoothies or juice.

In addition, marine algae are now grown in controlled environments and can be extracted and concentrated into supplements. Studies have found that the EPA and DHA in marine algae supplements have a similar ability to lower levels of blood lipids, including triglycerides, as fish oil supplements. It's important to note, however, that marine algae supplements may have variable levels of EPA and DHA compared with fish oil supplements.

Most healthy people should consider taking a supplement that contains 250 mg of EPA and DHA per day (roughly the equivalent of eating fish twice per week). If you have a known heart condition, your doctor may want you to have higher levels of EPA and DHA. To ensure that you are choosing a quality supplement, look for "third-party tested" or some other third-party certification on the label.

Best Bread for Digestion

The best bread for digestion is the old-fashioned slow-rising kind—especially for people with irritable bowel syndrome (IBS). When bread dough is allowed to rise twice, for at least four hours total, nearly all the hard-to-digest sugars known as FODMAPs are eliminated. These often are responsible for abdominal pain, diarrhea or constipation that some IBS sufferers experience when they eat bread. Bake your own or find artisanal bakers who allow breads to rise for four hours or longer.

William D. Chey, MD, is director of the Digestive Disorders Nutrition and Lifestyle Program at Michigan Medicine, Ann Arbor.

Keep a Food Diary: The Secret to Eating Healthier

Lisa R. Young, PhD, RDN, a nutritionist in private practice and an adjunct professor in the department of nutrition, food studies and public health at New York University in New York City. She is author of Finally Full, Finally Slim: 30 Days to Permanent Weight Loss One Portion at a Time.

Every few years, another dietary fad sweeps the country. If you do this one big thing—say, eat fewer carbohydrates or fill up on protein—you'll be healthier and thinner.

But in real life, healthful eating depends on the dozens (if not hundreds) of small decisions that you make every day…assuming that you even make decisions. Most people eat without thinking, nibbling at leftovers as you store them after dinner…grabbing a snack when rushing out the door…or taking a few quick swigs of a soft drink.

How many healthy (or unhealthy) foods do you actually consume? You probably don't have a clue. The only way to know for sure is to write down everything you eat.

Compelling research: People who keep a food journal lose weight at twice the rate as those who don't keep track, according to a study published in *American Journal of Preventive Medicine.*

In addition to raising your awareness to what and how much you're eating, a food diary makes you aware of your habits—which can ultimately help you change your behavior and make healthier food choices so that you eat less of the wrong foods and more of the right foods.

Find Your Eating Style

It might seem like a hassle to keep a food diary. But you don't have to do it forever…a month is usually long enough. And it's an extremely powerful tool for changing behavior. In fact, it's the best way to identify your eating patterns. Nutritionists have discovered a few main patterns that define an individual's eating style. *For example…*

• **"See food" eaters** might cook healthy, well-balanced meals but still consume hundreds of unnecessary (or unhealthy) calories by eating whatever appears in front of them—doughnuts at the office…sugar next to the coffee maker…soda in the refrigerator, etc.

• **Emotional eaters** turn to food whenever they feel extra-stressed.

• **Mindless eaters** grab food on the run because they're often too busy or harried to enjoy leisurely meals.

You can easily consume 1,000 extra calories a day without even thinking about it. Some people are aware of their eating patterns, but many never realize where the bulk of their calories comes from.

A food diary—including a "cheat" diary (see next page) to account for the dozens of quick, mindless bites that you probably take every day—will help you identify your eating patterns…where your calories are coming from…and the quality of your diet. Are you getting enough antioxidants and fiber? Are you overloading on sugar? Writing it down is the only way to really know.

Keep It Simple

One month is the recommended length of time to keep a food diary because that's about how long it takes people to change their habits. One of my clients, a busy hedge-fund manager, soon realized that she would munch mindlessly on junk food. After recording all of these "cheats" for six days, she realized that she needed to think before snacking. (She went on to lose 20 pounds over the next two months.)

The four pillars: A food journal only needs to include four basic pieces of information—what you ate…how much…the food group (fruits…grains…vegetables…meats and alternatives…and dairy)…and how you prepared it. The details are important because people tend to engage in what's known as "perception deception." You may see yourself as an active, healthy person and discount aspects of your behavior that don't align with your self-image.

Example: You may think that you're eating a healthful diet because you include a whole grain with every meal, but what if you only take a bite or two of brown rice and a double-helping of steak…or the broccoli that you sauté is swimming in butter? Details matter!

Just a Few Minutes a Day

I advise clients to make diary notes every time they eat, if possible. You'll forget things if you wait until the end of the day…and jotting down an entire day's notes can make it feel like too much work.

If you're comfortable with computers/phone apps (MyFitnessPal is a popular app), there are dozens of programs for tracking calories, food groups and portion sizes. But it's just as easy to carry a pen and a notebook…send yourself a simple text or an e-mail. After you've done it for a few days, it almost becomes automatic.

A pre-diary is good for those who are really committed to improving their diets…and for planners who prefer not to do things on the fly. Every day, write down what you plan to eat—the food groups, the portion sizes, preparation methods, etc. You can use the same diary (using a different-colored pen) to write down what you actually ate.

A cheat diary is one of the most helpful tools. The calories and unhealthful ingredients from foods that you mindlessly pop into your mouth can add up fast. Especially for people who are too busy to keep a more detailed diary, a cheat diary is a good way to become aware of the unhealthy food choices.

Focus on portions. Research has shown that people underestimate how much they eat and drink. They often don't realize that today's supersized portions have far more calories than they imagine.

Example: When I asked students in an introductory nutrition class how many calories were in an eight-ounce serving of a popular soda compared with the calories in a 64-ounce "double gulp," 70% underestimated the proportional increase. (An eight-ounce serving has 100 calories, and a 64-ounce soda contains 800…but most students estimated that the larger beverage only had 300 calories!)

Larger portion sizes may have started in restaurants/packaged foods, but now they're also a problem at home. You need to know how much you're eating—not how much you think you're eating. I advise everyone to buy stackable measuring cups and spoons. You can also buy dishware that marks off serving sizes and even wineglasses with fill lines (the standard serving size is five ounces).

Weigh your foods. A kitchen scale (like the EatSmart Precision Pro Digital Kitchen Scale, among many others) is a great way to know exactly how much, say, a four-ounce serving really is. After using a scale for a while, most people learn to "eyeball" portions with decent accuracy.

Ketogenic Diet: More Than a Weight-Loss Fad

Tanya J. W. McDonald, MD, PhD, a practicing epileptologist and assistant professor of neurology in the department of neurology at the Johns Hopkins University School of Medicine in Baltimore. She is lead author of "The Expanding Role of Ketogenic Diets in Adult Neurological Disorders," a review article published in *Brain Sciences*.

The ketogenic diet has shaped up as the biggest weight-loss trend of the last few years.

What's not being talked about: Even though there are positive anecdotal reports on using this high-fat, very-low-carbohydrate diet for weight loss—and research is promising (see next page)—few people know about its current and potential uses for neurological conditions and other chronic diseases…

Neurological Conditions

• **Epilepsy.** Diet therapy was a common epilepsy treatment until the development of antiseizure drugs in the 1930s. Now researchers are taking a second look at the ketogenic diet because some patients with epilepsy are drug-resistant—that is, they have failed to respond to two different medications…and have less than a 5% chance of becoming seizure-free with the use of additional drugs.

Scientific evidence: Research has confirmed that 40% to 50% of adults with epilepsy will improve on the diet with the most benefits seen in patients who stick with it.

Among the many possible mechanisms, the diet is thought to dampen the brain-cell "excitability" that's associated with seizures. It also improves the balance of intestinal bacteria, which appears to provide seizure protection.

The ketogenic diet doesn't replace anti-epilepsy drugs—most patients will continue to take medication, although many will require fewer drugs and/or a lower dose. I advise a variety of epilepsy patients to try the diet for at least three months. If it's effective,

they stick with it. If not, they slowly resume their consumption of carbohydrates, under the supervision of a medical professional or nutritionist.

• **Brain cancer.** Glioblastoma, a type of malignant glioma, is the most frequently diagnosed primary brain tumor. Early research suggests that a ketogenic diet could help patients with this type of cancer, particularly when combined with radiation and/or other treatments.

In laboratory studies, animals given a ketogenic-like diet showed improved survival times of 20% to 30%. Small studies—many of them case reports (descriptions of individual patients)—have shown improvements in disease progression and survival.

The diet may help because the cells that fuel cancer depend on glucose as an energy source. When you take away glucose with a ketogenic diet, cancer cells may lose the ability to proliferate.

My advice: If you or a loved one has been diagnosed with this type of cancer, ask your doctor if a ketogenic diet might help—and if he/she recommends participating in one of the clinical trials listed at ClinicalTrials.gov. (There are also trials that focus on the use of this diet for other types of cancer.)

• **Alzheimer's disease.** Like the cancer cells described above, the amyloid deposits that are the hallmark of Alzheimer's may depend on high levels of glucose in the blood.

In laboratory studies, animals given extracts that put their bodies into a ketosis-like state (see next page) showed improved learning and memory. Studies involving Alzheimer's patients or those with mild cognitive impairment have shown that people given similar extracts had improvements in working memory and visual attention.

My advice: Because the research is too preliminary to conclude that the diet is—or isn't—effective for this purpose, I wouldn't advise Alzheimer's patients to try the diet without close medical supervision. But if you've been diagnosed with Alzheimer's—or have a high risk of developing it—you might want to discuss it with your doctor.

Other Uses

• **Weight loss.** The ketogenic diet is a far cry from the plant-rich diets that most experts recommend for weight loss. In its most restrictive form, it limits many vegetables, fruits, beans and grains—all of the foods that can help you lose weight.

Yet people who switch to a ketogenic diet (the plans for weight loss are somewhat less restrictive than those used for some of the conditions described above) do lose weight—and they lose it quickly.

Caveats: Most experts agree that people who follow the diet can lose weight. But it doesn't appear to be any more effective than other, more conventional diets, and the dropout rate is probably much higher.

• **Diabetes.** People with diabetes are usually advised to eat less fat because weight loss and a lower-fat diet have been thought to go hand in hand. But experts are taking another look at the ketogenic diet for diabetes control.

Reasons: Not only can the diet promote weight loss, but there's some evidence that it improves insulin sensitivity and lowers blood sugar.

Caution: People with diabetes who follow a ketogenic diet have an increased risk for diabetic ketoacidosis, a life-threatening condition due to elevated blood sugar and blood acids (ketones).

More from Dr. McDonald...

How the Diet Works

The term "ketogenic" has become a catchall phrase for any high-fat, low-carbohydrate diet. But in the medical community, the diet calls for a severe restriction of carbohydrates and high amounts of fat. The requirements are so rigorous that the diet should be attempted only with the supervision of a doctor, as with any medical therapy.

How it works: Normally, blood sugar (glucose) from carbohydrates is your main source of energy. But when glucose is restricted, your body starts breaking down fat, a process that releases ketone bodies into the bloodstream. Cells use ketone bodies as an alternative fuel source until you start eating carbohydrates again.

If you stay on the diet long enough, the body enters ketosis. (You experience a mild form of ketosis when you've gone all night without food.) Ketosis mimics a starvation state—it triggers metabolic changes, including those that promote weight loss and improve insulin sensitivity.

The diet emphasizes foods high in fat, moderate in protein and low in carbohydrates (eggs, cheese, avocados, butter, olive oil, cream, bacon, steak, salmon, sardines, nuts, seeds, etc.).

Easier Than a Diet... and Great for Health

Tina Marinaccio, RDN, integrative registered dietitian nutritionist and adjunct professor in clinical nutrition and food studies at Montclair State University in New Jersey. She leads the nutrition element of Dr. Dean Ornish's Program for Reversing Heart Disease. TinaMarinaccio.com

---

I am the first to admit that fasting sounds even worse than dieting. But some kinds of fasting can be easier than dieting—and have benefits that go well beyond weight loss. In fact, even people who are not overweight can get amazing benefits from fasting, including healthier hearts, stronger muscles and clearer thinking.

The technical term for what I'm talking about is "intermittent fasting," which means fasting for short periods—sometimes, just 12 hours—on a regular basis. Most intermittent-fast techniques are not daily, and many allow for some calories even on "fast" days. This is definitely not a hunger strike! Some researchers believe that these intermittent fasts are easier to maintain than daily "caloric restriction"—aka traditional dieting, which basically requires that you eat less than you want every single day forever. Intrigued?

Here's more on the benefits of intermittent fasting and how you could easily try it…

Why Intermittent Fasting Is So Healthy

Studies have shown that intermittent fasting can help people lose weight without losing muscle. Maintaining muscle is key to keeping weight off and healthy aging. People on intermittent fasts find it easier to control their appetite even on nonfasting days.

One reason: They are producing less insulin, a key "hunger hormone."

But there are many more benefits. These kinds of fasts have been shown to reduce blood pressure…reduce blood glucose levels and improve insulin sensitivity…reduce levels of triglycerides (blood fats) and improve the cholesterol profile…reduce inflammation…enhance muscle endurance…and even improve learning and memory. In animal studies, intermittent fasting can reverse type 2 diabetes, slow the progression of cardiovascular disease and prolong life.

Why is this kind of fasting so good for the body? One hypothesis is that our gut biome—the mix of gastrointestinal bacteria that's key to health—needs a rest to function optimally. In addition, fasting has been shown to help the body get rid of damaged cells and regenerate healthy new ones. Humans likely evolved eating this way—food was scarce, and we couldn't spend every day eating and snacking every few hours like we can now. Periodic fasting respects—maybe even resets—our internal body clocks.

Choosing a Way to Fast

The best fast is the one that fits into your lifestyle. *Here are three options supported by scientific evidence…*

• **Time-restricted eating.** This is the easiest fast to pull off. Every day, you simply restrict eating to a specific stretch of the day. You'll get the most benefits by limiting yourself to eating during just an eight-hour stretch—say, 10 am to 6 pm. But time-restricted eating is something you can ease into—for example,

by restricting your eating to 12 hours…and then gradually scaling back to eight hours.

Eating at night, in particular, interferes with the body's natural day-night cycle, disrupting hormones in a way that favors weight gain. And there's psychology—choosing an endpoint to the day's eating helps eliminate nighttime eating.

Let's face it: No one is sitting in front of the TV at night eating carrot sticks. It's more likely to be ice cream or chips.

Tip: Get most of your calories early in the day, meaning you eat a big breakfast and a smaller lunch and dinner. It's fine to eat breakfast several hours after you wake up—that's healthy as long as it's not paired with late-night eating.

• **Periodic fasting.** On two consecutive days, you cut way back on calories—by 75%. The rest of the week, you eat in a normal fashion. The popular 5:2 Diet is an example of this approach.

• **Alternate-day fasting.** In this approach, you alternate days when you restrict calories—to perhaps 500 calories for the day—with days when you eat a normal, healthy diet. This way of fasting is one day on, one day off. It's effective, but some people find that they are too hungry on fasting days to sustain it.

Tip for periodic or alternate-day fasting: To meet your calorie goal and assure good nutrition on partial-fast days, make protein shakes with fruit and some form of healthy fat, such as ground flax or a no-sugar-added nut butter. A low-sugar plant-protein powder serves as the base. Two brands I like are Vega and Kashi GoLean (I'm fond of the Vanilla Vinyasa flavor).

Caution: Before you start any fast, discuss it with your health-care provider. That's especially important if you have a medical condition. For example, although fasting may help improve diabetes, people who take blood sugar–lowering agents need to be especially careful about low blood sugar. Plus, some medications need to be taken with food.

More tips for successful intermittent fasting…

• **See a registered dietitian (RD).** An RD can help you determine which of the eating patterns—if any—makes sense for you and help you put a plan into place. He/she can help you choose the most nutritious foods (especially important on days when you don't eat as much as you normally do)…and, if you need them, recommend nutritional supplements.

• **Be extra wary when you eat out on partial-fasting days.** Restaurants use more fat and sugar than you would at home, and portions are huge. It's easier to eat at home so that you know what you're taking in.

• **Consider professional metabolic testing.** How can you know what to eat to cut calories by, say, 75%? You start by calculating the calories you burn at rest—your resting metabolic rate, aka RMR—and then add everyday activities plus physical exercise. Online RMR calculators are notably inaccurate.

Better: An FDA-approved calorimeter, which measures your RMR when you breathe into it. These instruments are too expensive to make it worth buying one for home use, but many RDs have them in their offices.

• **"Cheat" with nonstarchy vegetables.** If you find yourself extra-hungry on a fasting day, don't suffer too much. The best way to "cheat" is with low-glycemic vegetables, many of which have lots of filling fiber and all of which have very little effect on blood sugar or insulin levels.

Examples: Salad greens, cruciferous vegetables (broccoli, cabbage, cauliflower, etc.), radishes, zucchini, summer squash, eggplant, tomatoes and mushrooms.

Bonus: These types of vegetables are especially good at feeding beneficial gut bacteria.

One caution, though: Don't pile on potatoes, winter squashes, corn, peas and the like—these are starchy vegetables that you shouldn't cheat with.

Carb Cutting and Fat Boosting Burns Calories

People who have slimmed down may be able to lose another 15 to 20 pounds without further limiting calories.

Recent finding: For each 10% decrease in calories from dietary carbohydrates and 10% increase in fat, people burned an average of 50 more calories a day. The results need further study, but meanwhile, consuming more oil and less bread won't hurt.

David Ludwig, MD, PhD, is codirector of New Balance Foundation Obesity Prevention Center at Boston's Children's Hospital, and coauthor of a study published in *The BMJ.*

Can Organic Food Prevent Cancer?

The studies "Association of Frequency of Organic Food Consumption with Cancer Risk" by a team of researchers at the Sorbonne and other French institutions and published in *JAMA Internal Medicine* and "Organic Food Consumption and the Incidence of Cancer in a Large Prospective Study of Women in the United Kingdom" by researchers at the University of Oxford and published in *British Journal of Cancer.* Sharon Palmer, RD, author of *The Plant-Powered Diet.* SharonPalmer.com

Exercising, applying sunscreen, getting health screenings—you know the drill to help prevent cancer. Now a French study suggests adding another step to the list—eating organic.

The study: Researchers from respected institutions across France followed nearly 70,000 adults, mostly women with the average age of 44, for five years. Participants filled out questionnaires detailing how often—"never," "occasionally" or "most of the time"—they chose organic versions of 16 categories of foods, from fruits and veggies to dairy, meat, fish, eggs, coffee, tea, wine, chocolate and sugar. They also provided yearly health updates, including any cancer diagnoses, but were not asked about any other behaviors that could raise or lower cancer risk.

The results: Participants whose diet included the highest proportion of organic foods had 25% fewer cases of cancer compared with those who never ate organic foods. The most significant reductions were seen with lymphoma (76% overall and 86% for non-Hodgkin lymphoma) and postmenopausal breast cancer (34%).

The limitations: The study didn't pinpoint which foods in particular offered the most cancer protection. (Chances are it wasn't the sugar!) The theory is that cancer reduction comes from an overall reduction in pesticide ingestion. After all, three such chemicals—glyphosate (the notorious ingredient in the weed killer RoundUp), malathion and diazinon—have been rated "probably carcinogenic to humans" by the International Agency for Research on Cancer.

This is the second study to find a link between eating organic and a reduced risk for non-Hodgkin lymphoma. However, the first one, done four years earlier in the UK and involving 623,000 middle-aged women, showed little or no decrease for any other types of cancer.

How might you put these findings into action? *Here's advice from registered dietitian Sharon Palmer…*

• **Prioritize your produce.** We already know that eating lots of fruits and veggies in general is a big part of a cancer-prevention diet. If you can't afford to buy all organic produce, buy organic versions of foods known to have high levels of pesticide residues, notably strawberries, spinach, nectarines, cherries, apples, tomatoes, peppers and potatoes. Each year, the nonprofit Environmental Working Group puts out the "Dirty Dozen," a list of produce with the highest levels of pesticides, and the "Clean 15" with the lowest levels of pesticides. Use these lists as shopping guides. Where can you skip organic? In general, foods that have a tough or thick outer peeling such as melons, avocado, pineapple and citrus fruits have lower pesticide residues—but do wash them well before you cut them to avoid contaminating the fruit inside. Cruciferous vegetables such as cabbage, broccoli and cauliflower often require less pesticide so can also be bought "conventionally grown."

• **Shop farmer's markets.** Ask local growers how they cultivate their crops. Although they may not be certified organic, they could be forgoing synthetic pesticides and farming in a way that's more protective of the soil and local ecosystem and more cost-effective for you.

• **Grow your own food.** This is the least costly way to eat organic. If you grow your own tomatoes and lettuce and herbs and other crops without spraying them with pesticides or using synthetic fertilizers, these are essentially home-grown "organic."

• **Reallocate dollars within your overall food budget.** Move the dollars you spend on sugary, nutrient-poor foods to the organic foods column. Consider other expensive items you can cut back on, such as meat, and spend that money on organic grains (including flours), beans, fruits, vegetables and eggs.

Beyond Peanut Butter

Sharon Palmer, RDN, a Los Angeles–based registered dietitian nutritionist and author of *The Plant-Powered Diet* and *Plant-Powered for Life.* Palmer also is editor of the newsletter *Environmental Nutrition* and nutrition editor for *Today's Dietitian.* SharonPalmer.com

What can compete with—or even beat—the classic jar of peanut butter for nutrition, taste and all-around versatility? Actually, a lot these days, thanks to the growing number of nut and seed butters popping up in most supermarkets and natural-food stores.

You can even find hand-churned versions at many farmer's markets. Or make your own! Nut and seed butters are poised to be the next big thing in tasty and convenient high-nutrition foods.

A Nutritional Powerhouse

No matter what nut or seed butter strikes your fancy, they are all nutritional heavy-weights—especially when it comes to heart health. Tree nuts, including almonds, walnuts, pistachios, hazelnuts, cashews, Brazil nuts, macadamias, pine nuts and pecans, can reduce LDL "bad" cholesterol and help curb chronic inflammation, which is a root cause of heart disease.

Peanuts, which are technically a legume, are not only rich in protein, vitamin E, niacin, folate, magnesium, phosphorus and manganese, but they also have a hefty amount of arginine (an amino acid that can help improve blood flow in your arteries) and resveratrol (the same antioxidant compound found in red wine).

But I'm not the only one heaping on the praise. The FDA has given nut and peanut butter manufacturers the green light to claim on product labels that eating 1.5 ounces per day of most nuts as part of a healthy diet may reduce the risk for heart disease.

So what's so great about tree nuts and peanuts? They are filled with unsaturated fats, as well as vitamins, minerals, fiber and phytochemicals (plant compounds with antioxidant and anti-inflammatory activities).

Seeds, such as flax, sesame, sunflower, pumpkin, hemp and chia, may not have garnered quite the recognition for their health benefits at this time, but these tiny kernels possess similar nutritional powers as nuts.

Worth noting: Even though nut and seed butters are rich in the healthful variety of fat, they are still concentrated in calories. Most nut butters provide about 180 to 190 calories per serving (two tablespoons)—so a little goes a long way. That's why sitting down with a spoon and an open jar isn't the best way to enjoy these butters.

Instead, spread them on your favorite whole-grain breads…use as a dip with vegetable sticks or apple slices…add to smoothies…mix into your breakfast cereal…use them as a healthful fat source (instead of butter or margarine) in baking…and stir them into sauces and vinaigrettes.

Bonus: Nut and seed butters are a great plant-based protein option for vegetarians and people who want to cut back on their consumption of red meat—high amounts of which have been linked to increased risk for diabetes, heart disease and certain cancers. It's also a good idea to read the labels of nut and seed butters to avoid unwanted added ingredients, such as sugars and hydrogenated oils.

Nut and Seed Butters Worth Trying

- **Almond.**

How to enjoy it: With its mildly nutty, sweet taste, almond butter is delicious when it's spread on avocado and tomato sandwiches. It also makes a terrific dip for fruit and veggies.

For a yummy, healthful surprise: Try adding almond butter to baked goods, such as oatmeal cookies and banana bread.

Special quality: Almond butter is a good source of calcium, providing about 8% of the Daily Value per serving (two tablespoons).

Nutritional value: In addition to being a reliable source of protein (5 g per serving), almond butter contains riboflavin, vitamin E, magnesium, phosphorus and manganese.

- **Walnut.**

How to enjoy it: Try walnut butter in sauces to accent savory foods, such as seafood or lentil patties, as well as in wraps and on toasted whole-grain raisin bread.

Special quality: Walnuts have something unrivaled in the nut world—they have omega-3 fatty acids…and a lot of them. That's a big part of the reason why walnuts are good not only for the heart but also for the brain.

Nutritional value: Walnut butter has 5 g of protein per serving and is rich in magnesium, phosphorus, copper and manganese. With their nutty and mildly astringent taste, walnuts also offer a high level of healthful phytochemical compounds.

- **Pistachio.**

How to enjoy it: To incorporate pistachio butter into your diet, add it to vinaigrettes for grain salads, biscotti dough and muffins.

Special quality: Pistachio butter is one-of-a-kind because of its color—a lovely shade of green! The green hue comes from lutein, a carotenoid that has antioxidant action, helping to lower blood pressure and fight chronic conditions such as heart disease and stroke, as well as protect eye health as we age.

Nutritional value: Pistachio butter is creamy and rich in protein (6 g per serving), fiber, thiamine, vitamin B-6, phosphorus, copper and manganese.

●**Sunflower seed.**

How to enjoy it: Spread sunflower seed butter on banana sandwiches, fill dates with it and stir it into butternut squash soup.

Special quality: This sweet, golden butter is a great alternative for people who might be allergic to tree nuts or peanuts. Sunflower seed butter is also a superstar for its impressive levels of vitamin E (it has 37% of the Daily Value in one serving). Research has linked this powerful antioxidant to improved immunity.

Nutritional value: It's packed with protein (6 g per serving), fiber, vitamin B-6, niacin, folate, pantothenic acid, phosphorus, zinc, copper, manganese and selenium.

●**Sesame seed (tahini).**

How to enjoy it: Sesame seed butter (tahini) is what gives hummus that earthy, nutty taste. But it's also delicious and nutritious in its own right. Try using tahini as a dip for falafels, as a spread in pita sandwiches, as a pasta sauce with noodles and as an addition when baking soft cookies.

Special quality: Tahini is a good source of plant-based calcium (providing 12% of the Daily Value). It also has cholesterol- and blood pressure–lowering effects.

Nutritional value: Pale in color, tahini is bold in nutrition, packing in protein (5 g per serving), fiber, thiamine, calcium, iron, magnesium, phosphorus, zinc, copper and manganese.

Foods That Fight Disease

Eggs may help reduce risk factors associated with diabetes in overweight and obese people. Eating about 1.5 ounces of pecans daily cuts risk for both heart disease and diabetes in overweight adults age 45 and older. Yogurt protects against colorectal cancer. Vegetables and berries reduce risk for Parkinsonism (a group of neurological movement-problem disorders similar to those seen with Parkinson's disease) and slow its progression. Drinking three or more cups of coffee a day reduces the risk for liver disease.

Overview of multiple research projects recently presented at a meeting of the American Society for Nutrition.

Lentils: The Healthiest Food You Don't Eat— But Should

Dil Thavarajah, PhD, associate professor in the departments of plant and environmental science at Clemson University, a research scholar at its School of Health, and coauthor of the studies "Can lentil reduce the risk of obesity?" published in *Journal of Functional Foods* and "The impact of processing and cooking on prebiotic carbohydrates and lentil" published in *Journal of Food Composition and Analysis.*

Dan Ramdath, PhD, research scientist at Guelph Research and Development Centre of Agriculture and Agri-Food Canada in Guelph, Ontario, Canada and coauthor of "Carbohydrate replacement of rice or potato with lentils reduces the postprandial glycemic response in healthy adults in an acute, randomized, crossover trial" published in *Journal of Nutrition.*

When was the last time you cooked with lentils? If you're like most Americans, it wasn't too recently—if you ever have. What a shame! Lentils are often called the "poor man's meat" because they have lots protein. But there's nothing poor about what they can do for your health (they can help you feel great), and there's an unlimited number of delicious ways you can prepare them.

To help you get great health benefits and enjoyment from lentils, we went to someone who grew up in Sri Lanka eating them three times a day—and who now happens to be one of the world's leading lentil biofortification scientists: Dil Thavarajah, PhD, a plant physiologist at Clemson University. *Here are her top reasons to dig into lentils…*

Lentils Deliver on Nutrients

Lentils provide a wide array of micronutrients, including iron, zinc, selenium and potassium. These nutrients help enhance red blood cell formation, thyroid function, eye health and wound healing and help prevent birth defects, among other benefits. Lentils are also a great source of fiber as well as polyphenols, which are bioactive compounds credited with promoting health and helping prevent diseases ranging from heart disease to cancer. In terms of protein, one cup of cooked lentils has 24 grams, close to the protein content of three ounces of chicken.

Lentils Keep Your Gut Happy

Eating lentils improves your gut microbiome, or healthful gut bacteria, thanks to their high level of prebiotic carbohydrates. You can even double their prebiotic content by cooking lentils, cooling them in the fridge and then reheating them at meal time. (You'll still get some of the prebiotic boost if you decide to have them cold in a salad, though not as much as if you reheat them.)

Having more "good bacteria" in your gut is key to losing weight or maintaining a healthy weight, improving insulin sensitivity and reducing cholesterol and triglyceride concentrations, Thavarajah said.

The dietary fiber in lentils also keeps your digestive system happy and humming along. One cup of cooked lentils has on average 15 to 20 g of fiber, half the daily requirement.

Lentils Reduce Blood Sugar

According to a new study done at Agriculture and Agri Food Canada's Guelph Research and Development Centre, simply replacing half a serving of rice with lentils lowered the rise in blood sugar caused by rice alone by about 20%, and replacing half a potato portion with lentils lowered the blood sugar rise caused by potatoes alone by 35%. This is important if you're trying to manage—or prevent—diabetes or prediabetes. Study author Dan Ramdath, PhD, explained that lentil consumption is followed by a slow rise in blood sugar, possibly due to the combined effects of starch that is resistant to digestion (called resistant starch) and starch that is rapidly digested starch.

Note: The researchers replaced only half the servings of potatoes and rice for the study because people typically eat lentils in combination with other starches as part of a larger meal—but feel free to replace 100% of your rice or potatoes or even pasta with great-for-you lentils.

Fast Facts

The lentils used in the Guelph study were ordinary varieties found at most markets. Even though some recipes call for a particular color of lentil—brown, green, French green, red or black—all varieties are nutritious. The color of some lentils can change dramatically with cooking. For instance, red lentils, which are actually a salmon color in the package, will turn yellow.

Unlike beans, the dried lentils you buy don't need to be pre-soaked before cooking, making them very convenient to use. They're a key ingredient in Indian, Middle Eastern and Southern US cooking, so you can explore many cuisines and never get bored.

Give Cheesy "Nooch" a Try

Janet Bond Brill, PhD, RDN, FAND, is a registered dietitian nutritionist, a fellow of the Academy of Nutrition and Dietetics and a nationally recognized nutrition, health and fitness expert who specializes in cardiovascular disease prevention. Based in Allentown, Pennsylvania, Dr. Brill is author of *Blood Pressure DOWN, Cholesterol DOWN* and *Prevent a Second Heart Attack*. DrJanet.com

It may not sound appetizing, but hold on and give this hugely popular vegan food additive a second look. Nutritional yeast—referred to affectionately by many people as "nooch"—is a nonactive, cultured strain of the single-celled organism *Saccharomyces cerevisiae* (technically classified as a fungus). Saccharomyces cerevisiae is grown on molasses and then harvested, washed and dried with heat to kill or "deactivate" it. Because it's inactive, it is not like regular yeast, meaning it doesn't froth or grow like baking yeast does, so it has no leavening ability.

Note: If you have a known sensitivity to eating mold/yeast, try a small amount of this product. If you have a reaction, don't add it to your diet. Nooch is sold either as a yellow powder or flakes (larger grocery stores might have the Bob's Red Mill brand or Bragg brand in the natural-food section).

Why eat it? There are two simple reasons: Taste and nutrition. Nutritional yeast is added to foods to create a savory, nutty flavor that really does taste a lot like cheese. Nooch is a nourishing nondairy substitute for those who can't or choose not to eat dairy. But even if you're not vegan, nooch offers a load of nutrients with few calories and little saturated fat. It also has less sodium than real cheese.

Nutritional yeast is rich in B vitamins, folic acid, selenium, zinc, fiber and protein (a complete protein at that). It's gluten-free and contains no added sugars or preservatives. Most, but not all, commercially sold nutritional yeast has been fortified with B-12. Vitamin B-12 is found in animal foods, so prudent vegans must supplement their diets with a reliable source of B-12. Most healthy adults require 2.4 micrograms (mcg) of vitamin B-12 each day. Bob's Red Mill Nutritional Yeast, for example, contains 3.5 mcg of the vitamin in a two-tablespoon serving.

Best ways to enjoy nooch: Use it much like you would Parmesan cheese—sprinkle it on popcorn or roasted vegetables...add it to pasta sauce or salads...or mix into yogurt-based dressings and flours.

These 4 "Super Spices" Have Hidden Benefits

Joshua Levitt, ND, a naturopathic physician and medical director at Whole Health Natural Family Medicine in Hamden, Connecticut. Dr. Levitt is a clinical preceptor for Yale School of Medicine and collaborates with the Integrative Medicine Center at Yale New Haven Hospital. He is author of *The Honey Phenomenon* and numerous other books and articles. WholeHealthCT.com

When it comes to "superfoods," fruits and veggies aren't the only heavy hitters. A handful of popular spices also have gained a rightful place on this list because of their own research-supported therapeutic effects.

Examples of the best known: Cinnamon for diabetes. Garlic for high cholesterol. Ginger for nausea. Cayenne for pain relief.

What you may not realize: Those same spices have even more benefits—little-known but powerful—that are also backed by scientific evidence. *How to use these spices for even greater preventive and curative effect...*

Cinnamon

A small daily dose of cinnamon has been proven in many studies to lower and help regulate blood sugar—crucial for those trying to prevent or manage type 2 diabetes.

Little-known benefit: Cinnamon also can lower high blood pressure.

Scientific evidence: In a recent study published in *Lipids in Health and Disease*, people who ingested 3 g (about two-thirds of a teaspoon) of cinnamon daily had a significant drop in blood pressure after four months—from averages of 136/88 to 122/80.

How to get more: Because cinnamon is so tasty, it's easy to include more in your diet. As a heavy cinnamon user, I buy organic Ceylon cinnamon (the highest quality) by the pound.

Note: Supermarket cinnamon is usually cassia (or Vietnamese), which contains a compound called coumarin that may damage the liver at high doses in susceptible individuals.

Cinnamon is great on roasted sweet potatoes and squash and adds delightful sweetness to pancakes and waffles. Plus, because it's such a powerful antioxidant, a sprinkle of cinnamon stops apple slices from turning brown—making the treat more delicious and more appetizing.

Garlic

This potent spice—a rich source of many healing compounds—is proven to lower cholesterol, reducing your risk for heart disease.

Little-known benefit: Eating garlic regularly also may help reduce your risk for colorectal cancer.

Scientific evidence: When Italian researchers analyzed seven case-control studies on garlic consumption and colorectal cancer, they found that people who ate the most garlic reduced their risk for the disease by 37% compared with people who ate the least. These studies measured garlic intake in various ways, so there is no optimal intake. To be fair, there is also research showing no correlation between garlic and colorectal cancer risk, but even the potential benefit makes garlic a smart addition to one's diet.

How to get more: Lightly sautéed fresh cloves are likely the healthiest way to consume garlic, but you also can use garlic flakes or powder. I use garlic (usually combined with lemon) in nearly every cooking liquid, sauce and marinade that I make in my kitchen.

Ginger

Dozens of studies have proven ginger's usefulness in easing nausea and vomiting due to everything from chemotherapy to motion sickness to morning sickness.

Little-known benefit: Ginger also inhibits the COX-1 and COX-2 enzymes that play a role in the production of inflammation-causing compounds in the body. This means it works the same way as pain-relieving drugs such as *ibuprofen* (Motrin) and aspirin.

Scientific evidence: A study published in *Phytotherapy Research* found that ginger supplements are comparable to aspirin, ibuprofen, *naproxen* (Aleve) and other over-the-counter painkillers in easing muscle pain caused by exercise and other types of strenuous activity.

Research also has shown that ginger is just as effective as the migraine drug *sumatriptan* (Imitrex).

How to get more: For a therapeutic, pain-relieving dose of ginger, take a 1,000-mg supplement, twice daily. For migraine, I recommend up to 1,000 mg at the onset of a migraine. If you want to use ginger to help prevent migraine, add fresh ginger to your daily diet or take a ginger supplement (250 mg to 500 mg daily).*

In the kitchen, add fresh ginger—finely diced or crushed—to sauces and marinades. Used three or more times a week, ginger in doses commonly consumed in the diet can have a mild pain-relieving and anti-inflammatory effect. Ginger is also great in smoothies.

Cayenne

Cayenne is a powder made from dried, red chili peppers, and it's very hot when used to spice food. But the natural intensity of cayenne and its active ingredient capsaicin affect more than your taste buds.

It's the only natural compound that—when applied topically—can degrade substance P, a neurotransmitter that tells the brain to trans-

---

*If you take blood thinners such as *warfarin* (Coumadin) or if you have gallstone disease, talk to your doctor before using ginger supplements.

mit pain signals. With less substance P, there's less pain—which is why capsaicin is a common ingredient in many creams, ointments and salves for pain problems such as arthritis, nerve pain, foot pain and back pain.

Little-known benefit: Cayenne can also help you lose weight. Capsaicin and other compounds in cayenne work because they have several effects that help you shed pounds—they suppress appetite…increase calorie-burning ("basal metabolic rate")…and burn up ("oxidize") body fat.

In a recent meta-analysis of nine studies on capsaicin and weight loss, published in *Critical Reviews in Food Science and Nutrition*, researchers concluded that the spice "could be a new therapeutic approach in obesity."

How to get more: For patients who want to lose weight, I usually recommend adding cayenne to the diet or using low-dose (2 mg) capsaicin supplements daily. (High-dose supplements can irritate the gastrointestinal tract.)

As a weight-loss aid, I recommend drinking one or more cups a day of warm water with a pinch of cayenne, juice from half a lemon, a teaspoon of honey and ground ginger (using a chunk of fresh ginger the size of half your thumb, from knuckle to tip). Cayenne is also excellent in marinades for fish and poultry and sprinkled on eggs. Plus, it adds a kick to salad dressings.

Have Some Cardamom with Your Coffee…

The phenolic compounds in this spice have been shown to aid in digestion, protect the heart and fight depression.

Good news: Research has found that these healthful compounds survive the brewing process when cardamom is added to coffee, a beverage already packed with disease-fighting antioxidants.

What to do: Add cardamom seeds to your coffee beans before grinding or cardamom powder to ground coffee. The highly fra-

grant spice, which tastes similar to nutmeg, also can be added to tea and mulled wine.

Urszula Gawlik-Dziki, DSc, professor of food technology, University of Life Sciences, Lublin, Poland.

Cold Brew Myth

A better brew? *New finding*: Hot-brewed coffee has more antioxidants than cold-brewed versions…and despite marketing claims, the pH (a measure of acidity) of cold-brewed coffee isn't any lower.

Scientific Reports.

The Healthiest Roast for Your Coffee

Study titled, "Cellular Antioxidant and Anti-Inflammatory Effects of Coffee Extracts with Different Roasting Levels" by researchers at Ewha Womans University, Seoul, Republic of Korea, and colleagues, published in *Journal of Medicinal Food*.

If you're reading this, there's a better than even chance that you've had or will have coffee today. According to the latest stats, 62% of American adults drink some form of java daily. It's a healthy habit, statistically linked to a reduced risk for heart disease, diabetes, certain cancers, dementia and depression.

But there's a way to make it even healthier.

Lighter Coffee Makes You Stronger

Coffee, according to the latest dietary survey, is actually the number one source of antioxidants in the US diet. Coffee's primary antioxidant—making up as much as 10% of green coffee beans by weight—is chlorogenic acids (CGA). It is also a powerful anti-inflammatory compound. CGA makes cells more responsive to insulin, which helps explain how coffee fights diabetes. CGA also protects DNA from damage, which helps explain the link to reduced risk for certain cancers.

It's good news, but there's a way to make your coffee work harder for your health—buy beans that are roasted "light" rather than "medium" or "dark." Roasting means exposing coffee beans to air and high temperatures. The more intense and long-lasting the roasting process, the more chlorogenic acid breaks down into other compounds that don't have the same health benefits.

Korean researchers recently compared coffees of several different roasting levels, analyzing their levels of chlorogenic acid and how they affect human cells. They exposed extract of different darknesses of roasted coffee to human cell cultures to test their antioxidant and anti-inflammatory properties.

Result: Not only did light-roast extracts have higher CGA levels, but they were also better able to protect human cells against oxidation (cell damage) and inflammation. Medium-roast coffee, not surprisingly, was not as anti-inflammatory as light roast but better than dark roast. The research was published in the *Journal of Medicinal Food*.

So the next time you choose a brew, consider the lighter side of things. If you love the darker side of java, rest assured that you'll still get some antioxidant and anti-inflammatory benefits—just not as much as you could get with a lighter- or medium-roast brew.

Yummy Dairy

Whole-fat dairy in moderation is not harmful, as once believed, and it may even be healthful. In a large international study, people who consumed, on average, two to three servings per day of full-fat dairy had lower risk for heart disease and stroke when compared with people who ate less than one-half serving of whole-fat dairy per day. One serving could be one cup of yogurt, one slice of cheese or a glass of milk.

Mahshid Dehghan, PhD, is a nutritional epidemiologist at Population Health Research Institute at McMaster University, Ontario, Canada, and lead author of the study published in *The Lancet*.

What Sorghum Can Do for Your Health

Andrea Thompson, RDN, LDN, nutritionist and dietitian with expertise in gluten-free diets, Penn State Health St. Joseph Hospital, Reading, Pennsylvania.

If you read food labels, you've probably been seeing a lot of sorghum listed, especially in gluten-free baked goods such as pretzels and crackers. You may have wondered what it is—just another starchy filler that happens to be gluten-free?...or maybe something with actual nutritional value?

Happy to say, it's the latter—sorghum is an age-old grain that's a staple food in parts of Africa and Asia. It's gluten-free, highly nutritious (as long as you're eating the whole grain), and happens to be getting trendy. In fact, including sorghum among the whole grains in your diet is healthy. Sorghum is a good source of protein, iron and fiber. Studies suggest that sorghum may have a nutritional edge over other whole grains. *For instance, research shows that sorghum…*

• **Is better than other grains at regulating blood glucose and insulin response,** important not just for people with diabetes but for everyone. (University of Arkansas)

• **Has more antioxidant phytochemicals than other grains.** In fact, the antioxidant properties of sorghum are similar to those of fruits. *Note for weight watchers*: Sorghum's antioxidant tannins help inhibit weight gain. (Texas A&M University)

• **Promotes heart health.** The waxy outer layer of sorghum contains policosanols, compounds that are present in other grains but in much smaller amounts. Policosanols reduce total cholesterol and LDL "bad" cholesterol while increasing HDL "good" cholesterol. In fact, research suggests that policosanols may be more effective than statin drugs.

Want to add more sorghum to your diet? Many processed foods that are purposely made gluten-free, such as cereals, pretzels and crackers, are made with it. But while the nutrient-rich outer hull of sorghum grains is edible and is not always removed for processing, processed food is still processed food—typically loaded with added salt and sugar. So if you really want to incorporate the goodness of sorghum into meals, opt for whole grain. It's best to stick with regular whole grain sorghum rather than "pearled" sorghum, which has the bran (outer layer) and some of the germ removed. Pearled sorghum cooks faster and is softer when cooked, but you won't be getting all of sorghum's nutritional benefits.

Sorghum has a mild earthy taste that can be somewhat sweet. Cook whole sorghum the same way you'd cook rice…and use it the same way you'd use rice as a side dish and in salads, casseroles, soups and stir-fries. Whole-grain sorghum can also be popped like popcorn—just heat in a little oil on your stovetop. The popped kernels are smaller and softer than popcorn, but they taste nearly the same. Substitute whole-grain sorghum flour for other flours in recipes for breads, pancakes, muffins and cakes. And if you're a beer drinker, try sorghum beer—it's made with sorghum in place of wheat and/or barley and is gluten-free. Tasty varieties include Bard's Beer and Dogfish Head Tweason'ale.

However, even if they contain sorghum, you won't improve your health by going on a diet of beer and pretzels. Sorry!

Very Common Drugs That Rob Your Body of Nutrients

Hyla Cass, MD, integrative physician in private practice in Los Angeles. She is author of several books, including *8 Weeks to Vibrant Health* and *Supplement Your Prescription: What Your Doctor Doesn't Know About Nutrition*. CassMD.com

If you're taking a prescription medication every day, it may be interfering with your nutrition—and your doctor may not know it. This problem is so common that I wrote the book *Supplement Your Prescription: What Your Doctor Doesn't Know About Nutrition*.

Fortunately, you can protect yourself. When I treat patients who are taking prescription medications, I almost always prescribe specific nutritional supplements to head off deficiencies that the drugs can cause.

Important: These are the minimum doses for my standard nutritional prescriptions. You may benefit from higher doses, which you should discuss with your health-care provider.

If you take *metformin (Glucophage, Glumetza, Fortamet):* This diabetes drug can deplete vitamin B-12. Metformin also may deplete the body of the antioxidant and cardiovascular protector coenzyme Q10 (CoQ10). A study published in *Archives of Internal Medicine* showed that people with diabetes taking metformin had B-12 levels that were, on average, less than half the levels of people not taking the medication. Metformin also depletes folate (vitamin B-9). You most often will see this vitamin supplied as folic acid, which is then metabolized in the body to folate. (It also can be supplied as methylfolate for poor metabolizers of folic acid.)

Daily supplements needed…

- **Vitamin B-12 (1,000 mcg)**
- **Folic acid or methylfolate (400 mcg)**
- **CoQ10 (100 mg)**

If you take a corticosteroid such as *prednisone, prednisolone, betamethasone, budesonide, triamcinolone, cortisone or methylprednisolone:* While these anti-inflammatory drugs often are prescribed for short-term use to manage conditions such as allergic rashes, people with certain autoimmune conditions such as rheumatoid arthritis, Crohn's disease, ulcerative colitis and lupus often take them indefinitely. The nutrients they can deplete include calcium, folate, magnesium, potassium, selenium, vitamin D and zinc.

Daily supplements needed…

- **Calcium (600 mg)**. *Note*: Most of your calcium should come from food.
- **Folate (400 mcg)**
- **Magnesium (400 mg)**
- **Potassium (99 mg)**
- **Selenium (100 mcg)**

- **Vitamin D (1,000 IU)**
- **Zinc (25 mg)**

If you take an ACE inhibitor blood pressure drug such as *benazepril* (Lotensin), *enalapril* (Vasotec), *lisinopril* (Prinivil) or *ramipril* (Altace): These medications can deplete zinc.

Daily supplement needed: Zinc (25 mg).

If you take a calcium channel blocker for high blood pressure such as *amlodipine* (Norvasc), *diltiazem* (Cardizem), *felodipine* (Plendil), *isradipine* (DynaCirc), *nicardipine* (Cardene), *nisoldipine* (Sular) or *verapamil* (Calan, Covera-HS, Isoptin, Verelan): These medications deplete potassium.

Daily supplement needed: Potassium—the average daily requirement is 4.7 grams (4,700 mg), best obtained through eating potassium-rich foods including bananas, cooked spinach and many other fruits and vegetables. Supplements top out at 99 mg (found in your multi), while pharmaceutical supplements are higher but also contain a lot of unneeded chemicals. Have your potassium blood level checked, and go by your health practitioner's recommendation.

If you take a beta-blocker for high blood pressure and/or heart disease: It can deplete CoQ10.

Daily supplement needed: CoQ10 (100 mg).

If you take a statin to reduce cholesterol: It can deplete the body of CoQ10, which is vital for heart health.

Daily supplement needed: CoQ10 (100 mg).

If you take an antibiotic even for a short time: It can deplete the nutrients biotin, inositol, vitamins B-1 (thiamine), B-2 (riboflavin), B-3 (niacin), B-5 (pantothenic acid), B-6 (pyridoxine), B-12 (cyanocobalamin) and vitamin K—and interfere with the beneficial bacteria in your gut.

Also: Fluoroquinolones (any antibiotic that has a generic name that ends with the suffix "-floxacin," including the well-known ciprofloxacin, aka Cipro), can deplete calcium and iron. Tetracyclines (ending with the suffix "-cycline") can deplete calcium and magnesium. Trimethoprim-containing antibiotics (Trimpex, Proloprim, Primsol) can deplete folic acid. Penicillins (ending with the suffix "-cillin") can deplete potassium.

Daily supplements needed...
You needn't worry about how to find and take all those nutrients! The doses of magnesium, calcium and other nutrients contained in a good multivitamin/mineral supplement should cover your needs for these nutrients during a course of antibiotic therapy.

- **Additionally, find a high-potency B-complex supplement that contains close to these ingredients and doses.** B-1 (25 mg), B-2 (25 mg), B-3 (50 mg), B-6 (50 mg), folic acid (400 mcg to 800 mcg), B-12 (10 mcg), biotin (50 mg) and B-5 (50 mg). A "B-50" formula generally will provide these levels.
- **B-12 (1,000 mcg), taken in sublingual tablets for better absorption.**
- **Vitamin K (30 mcg to 100 mcg)**
- **After a course of antibiotics, take a probiotic supplement** to restore the beneficial bacteria in your gut. Choose one that contains at least one billion live organisms per daily dose and includes both *Lactobacillus acidophilus* (L. acidophilus) and *Bifidobacterium bifidum* (B. bifidum).

The Best Diet You're Not Following

Alan Lee Hinderliter, MD, associate professor of medicine, University of North Carolina School of Medicine, Chapel Hill, and lead author of the study "Lifestyle Interventions Reduce the Need for Guideline-Directed Antihypertensive Medication," presented at the American Heart Association's Joint Hypertension 2018 Scientific Sessions with coauthors Patrick Smith, PhD, Andrew Sherwood, PhD, and James Blumenthal, PhD, from Duke University, Durham, North Carolina.

The DASH diet has an image problem—it's just not sexy, no crazy foods, no extreme requirements, no stories to amuse your friends with...just a healthy way of eating that can steadily reduce your blood pressure and risk for heart disease and stroke. It can even allow some people to stop taking blood pressure drugs. All of that is why it's recommended by health organizations ranging from the American Heart Association and the Academy of Nutrition and Dietetics to the National Kidney Foundation. And although it wasn't initially created as a weight-loss diet, it gets high marks for that as well if you limit calories while following the DASH food group guidelines.

So why the ho-hum reaction to DASH—short for Dietary Approaches to Stop Hypertension? One reason is that people may not give it enough time to work. Or they might not make calorie and exercise adjustments that can maximize results. But a new study has found exactly what it takes to be successful on this powerhouse plan.

Researchers from the University of North Carolina and Duke University divided 129 overweight men and women with high blood pressure (but not yet on any hypertension medication) into three groups. One group followed DASH only, another followed an enhanced DASH with an exercise plan and diet tweaks for weight loss, and the third—the control group—didn't change anything about their lifestyle.

After 16 weeks, the researchers compared their results. The DASH-only patients reduced systolic (the top number) blood pressure by 11 mmHg and diastolic blood pressure by 8 mmHg, and the number of people in this group who might need blood pressure medication dropped from 51% to 23%. But the results were even more impressive in the DASH diet and exercise group—those participants reduced their systolic blood pressure by 16 mmHg and their diastolic blood pressure by 10 mmHg, and only 15% remained candidates for needing medication. What's more, they also each lost, on average, 19 pounds. Not surprisingly, numbers barely budged for the control group.

Whether you want to reduce high blood pressure, lose weight or both, here's how to make the enhanced DASH plan work for you...

• **The diet itself.** The standard DASH diet does not make you feel deprived. It allows eight to 10 servings of fruits and vegetables, six to eight servings of whole grains, two to three servings of low-fat or nonfat dairy, two to three servings of healthy fats such as olive oil and up to six ounces of lean meat, poultry or fish every day. It also allows four to five servings a week of beans and/or nuts and even allows sweets as long as you limit them to a few servings a week. The DASH diet is a healthy eating plan for just about anyone, but because it was developed with a focus on blood pressure, it includes a daily sodium limit: 2,300 mg.

• **Calorie cutting.** If you're at a healthy weight, eating about 2,000 calories a day for a man or 1,600 for a woman (depending on your metabolism and activity level) on DASH will help you reduce blood pressure while maintaining your weight. But if you want to lose weight (and most people with high blood pressure should), cut your total daily DASH calories to about 1,200 if you're a woman or 1,500 if you're a man.

Note: If you haven't yet cut out sweets, do so now to lose weight. If you already have, cut the food group limits proportionally from the plan described above.

• **Exercise.** The enhanced-DASH group walked on a treadmill for 30 minutes three times a week at a moderate intensity, meaning they worked hard enough that they could talk but not sing during the exercise. Though this is below the 150-minutes-per-week fitness guideline recommended by the CDC, it's a good starting point for people new to exercise and gives you a solid foundation to add to.

• **A support system.** The enhanced-DASH group had weekly small group sessions led by a dietitian. Having a shared goal is a powerful motivator and, as anyone who has ever tried dieting alone knows, it's hard to do on your own. Consider joining an in-person or online diet group and/or ask whether your health insurance covers sessions with a weight-loss counselor.

• **Patience.** Study participants committed to the program for four months. You might start seeing results sooner, but also keep in mind that DASH is designed as a lifelong program and that results will continue to build over time. Stay on DASH long enough, and you'll be rewarded with good results every time your blood pressure is taken or you step on a scale.

When You Eat Matters

Michael F. Roizen, MD, chief wellness officer at Cleveland Clinic and chief of its Wellness Institute. Board-certified in internal medicine and anesthesiology, he is coauthor, with Michael Crupain, MD, MPH, of *What to Eat When: A Strategic Plan to Improve Your Health & Life Through Food.*

In the never-ending diet debates, people focus almost exclusively on what to eat. But when you eat may be nearly as important.

Your body's circadian rhythms—the daily cycles that dictate when you awaken, when you're alert, etc.—don't just influence your behaviors like sleepiness. The time-specific, daily release of hormones determines when you get hungry and how much you eat…as well as your body's metabolism—how efficiently you utilize fats, carbohydrates and other nutrients.

What scientists are now discovering: Chrononutrition—the concept that food habits should align with circadian rhythms for optimal health—can have a dramatic impact on your chances of developing a variety of serious conditions. *What you need to know…*

Why Timing Matters

Suppose that you eat the same carbohydrate-rich meal twice a day—once in the morning and again in the evening. Both meals will trigger a rise in your blood sugar (glucose) levels, but the rise will be higher after the evening meal.

The "master clock" that controls circadian rhythms in humans and other mammals is located in a tiny brain area called the suprachiasmatic nucleus. The clock constantly sends out chemical messages that control key functions in your body. The effects can be profound.

In a study published in *Proceedings of the National Academy of Sciences*, nurses who changed their schedules to night shifts burned about 250 fewer calories a day, even though their jobs were the same. When researchers examined the findings of 17 studies on the effects of shift work, their analysis concluded that night-shift workers were 40% more likely than other workers to develop cardiovascular disease—possibly because their work hours were in opposition to their natural circadian rhythms.

Benefits of Early Eating

Most people get hungriest at night. But to realize the health-promoting effects of chrononutrition, the best time to eat most of your daily calories is before 2 pm.

Here's why: The body's cells respond more readily to insulin early in the day—important for food metabolism and healthy weight maintenance, as well as preventing diabetes.

Research has shown that insulin sensitivity is higher during the hours when you're most active. This makes sense because you need energy from your glucose reserve (which depends on insulin) when your muscles are moving. At night, when most people's energy needs are lower, you need less glucose.

The "Three-Quarter" Challenge

What happens when you eat earlier in the day? It's well-established that people who consume most of their calories during the daytime are less likely to be obese. That's why I recommend consuming three-quarters of your daily calories at breakfast and lunch.

Of course, changing your eating schedule isn't easy. People are naturally primed to eat more at night, probably because our ancient ancestors needed to store more calories to survive…and because they didn't live long enough to suffer the effects of harmful conditions such as arthritis, dementia and diabetes.

To get started: Try to get most of your daily calories between about 8 am and 2 pm for at least three days a week—more often if you can. As you become more accustomed to eating mainly during these hours, you can transition into this schedule seven days a week.

If you get hungry at night, have a healthy snack, like raw, crunchy vegetables (or roasted veggies if you prefer).

Improve Your Blood Sugar

As mentioned earlier, insulin resistance (the reduced ability of insulin to transport glucose into cells) is higher at night than during the daylight hours. Insulin resistance is a serious health problem because it increases the risk for diabetes, obesity—and even heart disease, cancer and dementia.

Animals given high-fat meals at night are more likely to consume more calories, gain more weight and have more insulin resistance than those that are given the same meals earlier in the day.

Similar changes occur in humans. The weight-management program at Cleveland Clinic encourages not only eating 75% of daily calories before 2 pm but also increased walking and a reduction of simple carbohydrates (such as chips, white bread and other processed foods). People with diabetes who follow the program for as little as two months often improve so much that they're able to discontinue one or two diabetes medications.

Boost Your Heart Health

A consistent finding is that daytime eating lowers high blood pressure, a leading cause of heart disease. The reduction is significant enough, in many cases, that it equals the effects of taking a blood pressure–reducing drug.

When you improve the metabolic state of the body by eating earlier (and healthier) meals, you also reduce the whole-body inflammation that can cause a gradual impair-

ment of kidney function. Reduced kidney function can impair the renin-angiotensin system, a group of hormones that helps regulate blood pressure.

Other benefits: Daytime eating causes a decrease in triglycerides and LDL "bad" cholesterol…an increase in beneficial HDL cholesterol…and a lower risk of developing metabolic syndrome, a life-threatening constellation of symptoms that includes high blood pressure, high blood sugar and elevated triglycerides.

We interviewed Michael F. Roizen, MD, chief wellness officer at Cleveland Clinic and chief of its Wellness Institute. Board-certified in internal medicine and anesthesiology, he has authored 175 peer-reviewed publications and served 16 years on FDA advisory committees. He is coauthor, with Michael Crupain, MD, MPH, of *What to Eat When: A Strategic Plan to Improve Your Health & Life Through Food*.

A Healthier Eating Plan

An optimal eating schedule can't overcome the effects of a poor diet. Everyone should avoid most processed foods and simple sugars (such as white flour) and eat more "whole" foods, including whole grains, beans, veggies, etc. *Also…*

• **Eat your breakfast!** There are surprisingly few randomized trials on the health benefits of eating breakfast, but research has shown that people who skip this meal are more likely to have higher LDL "bad" cholesterol levels. Those with diabetes often have higher blood sugar levels later in the day when they skip breakfast.

Make breakfast either the largest or the second-largest meal of the day. People who aren't normally breakfast eaters should at least practice "less-late" eating and get most of their calories at lunch.

• **Get some protein at breakfast.** A bit of protein reduces food intake later in the day.

Examples: Greek yogurt (with no added sugar), salmon, steel-cut oats and nuts or seeds. Aim to get about 25 g of protein at breakfast each day.

•**Skip the big suppers.** Get no more than about 25% of your total daily calories from snacks/supper combined. If you do eat at the regular supper hour (around 6 pm or 7 pm), have something like a small salad, accompanied by a small portion of a protein-rich food.

Whey for Muscles

Whey protein rebuilds muscle after inactivity. Adults who consumed whey supplements were able to regain more muscle mass that had been lost during a period of inactivity, such as a hospitalization or an illness, compared with people who consumed collagen supplements. Total protein intake was twice the recommended daily allowance. Whey also is beneficial for healthy adults who are involved in strength training.

Sara Oikawa, MSc, is a PhD candidate in the department of kinesiology at McMaster University, Ontario, Canada, and coauthor of a study published in *American Journal of Clinical Nutrition*.

The Surprising Way to Get More from Your Exercise

Paul A. Estabrooks, PhD, behavioral scientist, professor and Harold M. Maurer Distinguished Chair of the department of health promotions at University of Nebraska Medical Center in Omaha. He is an author of "Group-Based Physical Activity for Older Adults Randomized Controlled Trial," recently published in *Health Psychology*.

If you're skeptical that group workouts could offer more than an intense solitary jog on your treadmill, there's a body of research that gives some convincing reasons why going solo may not be the best approach. *Compared with solo exercise, group workouts are linked to…*

•**Less pain.** When adults exercised for 45 minutes on rowing machines, those who had rowed in groups demonstrated a higher pain tolerance versus solitary rowers, according to research published in *International Journal of Sport and Exercise Psychology*. Researchers theorize that physically syncing up with others stimulates a release of feel-good endorphins.

•**Greater motivation to push harder.** A phenomenon called the Köhler effect motivates people to strive harder when working in a group. Research conducted at Kansas State University found that this phenomenon really kicks into high gear when you exercise with people you perceive as stronger than yourself, inspiring exercisers to work out nearly 200% longer and harder than when working out alone.

Caveat: Simply being in a room with other people isn't enough to reap all of these great benefits. The key is finding what researchers call a "true group class."

The Magic of a True Group Class

A true group class is one in which the instructor takes steps to promote bonding among participants and a collective goal. For example, your instructor might start class by saying, "Over the next 45 minutes, we are going to collectively walk the equivalent of three laps around the Parthenon."

Important: Typically, group-based fitness classes are more effective than solo workouts only when they use these types of group dynamic strategies. In a meta-analysis published in *Sport & Exercise Psychology Review*, researchers compared the benefits of home workouts, standard exercise classes and true group classes.

Result: True group classes were deemed the most beneficial—mainly because people stick with exercise longer when they are working out in these groups. Solo exercise at home ranked last.

The special ingredient seems to be the bonding that takes place in these classes.

Feeling like you belong to a group is a very basic human need...one that research has linked with improved health and longevity—especially as one ages.

What to Look For

To find a class with this dynamic...

- **Find an instructor you love.**
- **Exercise with people your age.** Look for a class with members who are within about five years of your own age.
- **Look for a class with competition built in.** Boot camps and boutique fitness classes encourage friendly competition by allowing participants to compare their performance results.
- **Experiment with virtual group classes.** No class available? You can still reap the benefits of a collective workout with a virtual group class, such as those offered by Peloton, which provides cycling workouts you can do while streaming live and on-demand fitness classes with instructors and fellow participants.

Note: While on-demand classes offer the benefit of friendly competition, they do not provide the positive effects associated with bonding.

Get Up and Go

Calorie-burning varies with time of day. People burn 10% more calories when at rest in the late afternoon and early evening than when they are at rest in the early morning. The exact reason is not known, but it appears to be tied to the body's natural circadian rhythm. This may help explain why people with irregular eating and sleep schedules are more likely to gain weight than ones with regular schedules.

Study by researchers at Brigham and Women's Hospital and Harvard Medical School, both in Boston, published in *Current Biology*.

See What's Missing from Your Workout...

Tom Holland, MS, CPT, an exercise physiologist, certified sports nutritionist and certified strength and conditioning coach. He is founder and president of Team Holland, a fitness-consulting company in Darien, Connecticut, and author of four fitness books, including *Beat the Gym: Personal Trainer Secrets—Without the Personal Trainer Price Tag.* Team Holland.com

---

First things first: If you exercise regularly, pat yourself on the back. But if you're like most people and do just one exercise over and over again, listen up.

By simply varying your exercise routine, you can greatly improve the health benefits of your workout...overcome any boredom that might creep in...and even reduce your risk for injury.

The good news is, you don't need a lot of fancy equipment to vary your workout. *Here's how to mix it up if your favorite exercise is...*

Walking

If you are a walker, add high-intensity interval training (HIIT). Whether you frequent your local outdoor track or use a treadmill, walking is arguably one of the best forms of exercise there is.

But to maximize the benefits, you need to ramp up your speed (and/or perhaps incline or resistance if you're using a treadmill). The best way to do this is to up the ante on your workout with some HIIT, which intersperses short bursts of increased intensity.

While your regular walking routine may feel like a five on a scale of one to 10, during HIIT intervals, you should feel like you're exercising at a seven or an eight. The variety makes a low-intensity, steady exercise like walking more interesting and fun, and people who have fun when they exercise are more apt to stick with it.

If you're trying to lose weight: HIIT burns extra calories both during and after the workout.

To try it: Walk or use a treadmill at a comfortable warm-up pace for three minutes, then alternate 60 seconds at a normal pace with 60 seconds at a faster pace or higher incline for the remainder of the workout. (Pumping your arms helps—use the safety cord if you're on a treadmill.) Be sure to do a three-minute cooldown at a slower pace. Try adding HIIT to your walking routine one to three times per week. (For more information on HIIT, see page 141).

Tennis

If you love tennis, add some foam rolling. Pulled muscles and strains are ubiquitous among tennis players in their 50s, 60s and beyond, thanks to the quick, sudden movements and direction changes. But just a few minutes of pre-tennis self-massage with a foam roller could be enough to keep you on the court.

Why foam rolling? Because this technique, which involves moving a foam roller back and forth along different parts of the body, enhances blood flow to different muscles, performing it preworkout can improve flexibility and range of motion, reducing one's risk for injury, according to research published in *International Journal of Sports Physical Therapy.*

Also: Foam rolling lower-body muscles prior to exercise alters perception of fatigue, so you won't tire as quickly.

To start rolling: Target your calves, quadriceps and iliotibial bands, the thick connective tissue running down the outside of each hip to just below the knee.

For calves, sit on the floor and place the roller perpendicular underneath your outstretched legs. While supporting most of your weight with your hands, lift your hips and slowly move the roller up and down your calves for 10 to 30 seconds.

Flip over to roll out your quads…and turn on your side for the iliotibial bands—roll these areas for 10 to 30 seconds each. Try this rolling routine before tennis matches and a few times per week.

Yoga

If yoga is your thing, add cardio exercise. Yoga offers balance, flexibility, strength and stress relief. But unless you're practicing a fast-paced vinyasa yoga that has your heart working hard enough to make conversation difficult, it's probably not counting toward the standard recommendation of at least 150 minutes weekly of moderate cardiovascular exercise.

Mix things up with jogging or fast walking, biking, swimming or fast-paced aerobics classes. Just make sure that you're spending most of your time at your target heart rate for 30 minutes a day, five days a week. It's fine to do three 10-minute sessions to reach your goal.

Your target heart rate: Aim for 50% to 85% of your maximum heart rate, which is 220 minus your age. So if you're 55, your maximum heart rate is 165, and your target heart rate 83 to 140 beats per minute.

Exciting recent finding: Heart disease patients practicing yoga in addition to aerobic exercise had twice the reduction in blood pressure, cholesterol levels and body mass index compared with those who did either exercise alone.

Also: For all types of exercise, do strength training two days a week for a well-rounded regimen.

How to Exercise Despite Pain

Marilyn Moffat, PT, DPT, PhD, a practicing physical therapist and professor of physical therapy at New York University, New York City. She is author of two books for the lay audience and four professional books in the field. Steinhardt.nyu.edu/faculty/Marilyn_Moffat

Exercise is the magic elixir. It protects the heart, strengthens bones, lifts mood, increases energy, improves memory, boosts metabolism and prevents disease. But how can you get these benefits if your body hurts?

That is the problem for millions of Americans with chronic pain, especially knee pain or back pain. You want to exercise, but getting over that "pain hump" while you exercise is just too tough.

The irony is that pain not only makes regular exercise tougher—it also makes it more important. Why? It's a path toward less pain and a greater ability to do everyday tasks.

To learn how to get exercise when jogging or even walking is painful, we spoke with physical therapist Marilyn Moffat, PT, DPT, PhD. She homed in on two of the biggest obstacles that keep most people away from pain-relieving exercise—knee pain and back pain. *Her recommendations…*

Finding Your Own Path

I'll provide exercises below that almost everyone can do. But no single exercise is perfect for everybody, and your unique limitations and physical condition will dictate your ideal activity. Many people with chronic joint or back pain benefit from a detailed individual plan developed with a physical therapist. Ask your health-care provider for a recommendation or go to the website of the American Physical Therapy Association (MoveForwardPT.com), and click on "Find a PT" at the top of the page. It's always a good idea to check with your doctor before beginning a new exercise program.

When trying these exercises, start slowly, be cautious and pay attention to doing them correctly.

Important: Many people may need to build up to the "hold" times. For example, if an exercise calls for you to hold a pose for 30 seconds and that's too hard, try doing it for 10 seconds. If even that's too hard, just hold it as long as you can. You'll get stronger over time.

Stop immediately if any particular movement causes sharp pain, especially in a joint area. On the other hand, muscle fatigue (even

burn) should be expected, especially with strengthening exercises. It's a good thing!

Let's get moving…

If You Have Knee Pain

The best way to reduce knee pain is to increase the strength and flexibility in the muscles that support your knee. The key is to find exercises that permit pain-free range of motion. That means taking the load off the joint as much as possible. Walking in waist-deep water is a great way to do this—but not everyone has regular access to a pool. *Alternatives…*

•**Seated straight-leg raises** build up the quadriceps, which help support the knees.

What to do: Sit on the floor with your back against a wall. With one knee bent and the other leg straight out in front of you, wrap your hands around your bent leg, then slowly raise the straight leg up, keeping the knee as straight as possible—hold for 30 seconds. Then slowly lower the straight leg back to the floor. Do the exercise two or three times on each side.

•**Bridges** strengthen the hamstrings and quadriceps (key knee muscles), as well as the glutes and both the front and back of your body's core.

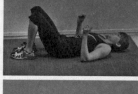
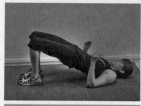
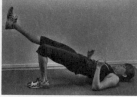

What to do: Lie on your back with your knees bent, and your feet and upper arms on the floor. Bend your elbows to a 90-degree angle, with your fingers pointing to the ceiling. Lift your glutes (butt muscles) off the floor, then straighten one leg out in the air at the level of the opposite knee and hold for 30 seconds. Bend the knee down, put your foot back on the floor and lower your butt. Alternate legs. Do this exercise two or three times per leg.

If You Have Back Pain

People with spinal stenosis (narrowing of the spaces within the spine) or other degenerative changes in the low back have a hard time with many exercises. Even walking can be difficult with spinal stenosis because each step slightly extends the spine, which narrows the spinal canal, exacerbating the pain.

What helps: Increasing flexibility and core strength. Yoga planks with the spine straight or slightly rounded are especially beneficial—they strengthen the core muscles that support the back as well as the arm and leg muscles. Pay attention to good form.

•**Basic front plank.** Start on your hands and knees with your hands directly under your shoulders and your knees directly under 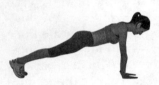 your hips. Straighten one leg all the way back, then the other leg, and you should be in perfect position. (If weight bearing on straight arms is too difficult, do a plank on your forearms.) Tuck your chin in so that your neck is straight and you are looking at the floor. Your spine should be in a straight line and not arched. Maintain as straight a line as is comfortable from your head through to your ankles. Hold for 30 seconds. Do two or three times.

•**Side plank also strengthens the core muscles and the arms and legs.** Start by lying on your right side and with your right hand directly under your right shoulder. Ideally your feet should be stacked one on 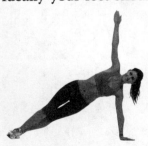 top of the other, but it's fine to start with the bottom knee bent. Lift your hips off the floor, and keep a straight line from your head through your shoulder, hips and feet. As you lift your hips, push your right hand into the floor. (Again, if weight bearing on a straight arm is too difficult, do the side plank on your forearm.) Hold for 30 seconds. Alternate sides. Do two or three times on each side.

Aerobic Fitness for Anyone with Pain

Whether you have pain in your knees or back (or hips or somewhere else), getting aerobic activity to improve your circulation and protect your heart can be challenging. But it's vital! *Here are ways to do it…*

•**Recumbent exercise bikes** (the kind where you are seated against a backrest) and seated stepper machines allow you to build your aerobic capacity. Being seated while doing aerobic exercise usually is easier for your back and reduces the forces on your knees that would occur if you were using a treadmill. The seated stepper, which resembles a recumbent elliptical machine, engages your arms as well as your legs. Many gyms have these machines.

What about walking? It's great if you can do it comfortably.

Tip: To absorb impact, wear sneakers that have good cushioned bottoms, add gel inserts into the sneakers and wear padded socks.

•**When walking on a treadmill,** use the handrails for support and to off-load some of the force of the body weight on your back and knees.

•**When walking outside,** choose school tracks or nature paths if possible—they're a little easier than paved sidewalks and roads—and you might consider walking poles. They help to absorb some impact, engage your upper body, help intensify your workout and improve stability. They are available at sporting-goods stores and online. Be sure to use two poles for the best balance and posture.

The Easy Way to Do HIIT

Robert Zembroski, DC, DACNB, a functional medicine physician, board-certified chiropractic neurologist, clinical nutritionist and director of the Darien Center for Functional Medicine in Connecticut. He is author of *Rebuild: Five Proven Steps to Move from Diagnosis to Recovery and Be Healthier Than Before.*

High-intensity interval training (HIIT) is one of the most exciting trends in fitness, but the word "intensity" can scare away all but the most committed. Exercise is already hard, you may be thinking, and now experts want to make it harder?

Actually, it's the opposite. Most people find HIIT easier than traditional cardio workouts, such as jogging, swimming or even shoveling snow. Compared with cardio training, HIIT more effectively improves your metabolic rate (for burning calories)...and improves your VO2 max—a parameter associated with cardiovascular health—according to research. In addition, it strengthens the immune system.

What most people don't realize: Even though HIIT alternates periods of all-out exertion with periods of lower-intensity exercise, the intense segments of the workout don't have to be too grueling. *Facts you need to know to get started with HIIT...*

The Magic of HIIT

With HIIT, you exercise as hard as you can for 30 seconds to a minute. (The actual exertion level and duration of the "burst" will vary from person to person.) Then you slow down to a lower intensity for a minute or two...then repeat the hard-easy sequence a few more times. The total length of the workout depends on your fitness level and physical abilities.

It's the "explosive" part of the workout that creates what can only be called "magic." People who engage in HIIT have better cardiovascular health—including improved cholesterol profiles and less insulin resistance—than those who do conventional endurance workouts, according to research published in *Experimental Gerontology.*

Ease into HIIT

HIIT is a safe form of exercise, which poses no more risk for sprain/strain injuries than any other exercise regimen. As with any new workout, however, it's a good idea to get the go-ahead from your doctor before starting HIIT.

I tell people who are elderly or have physical limitations—or are merely new to exercise—to start with a low-intensity version of HIIT.

Example: If you're a 65-year-old who has mainly been sedentary, you might start out with a slow walk (the easy part of the exercise at up to 3 mph), then pick up your speed—walking at around 4 mph to 5 mph while swinging your arms for the hard part. After 30 seconds or a minute of fast-walking/arm-swinging, you'd drop back to a stroll for a minute or two, then maintain the cycle for four to five rounds. *To get started...*

• **Choose your sport.** With HIIT, it doesn't matter which activity you choose. You can do the exercise/rest cycles in a swimming pool or on a treadmill or an exercise bike—or using your own two feet. All that matters is that the activity allows you to go all-out for a brief period of time...drop down to a slower level...then go all-out once again. For most people, four of these intervals are enough to get an excellent workout.

• **Don't exercise on an empty stomach.** If you don't have enough blood sugar when you exercise, your body will pull sugar from the muscles first. That's the opposite of what you want to happen. To improve body composition, you want to preserve muscle and burn fat. The best way to do this is to exercise within one to three hours after having a small meal.

Good pre-workout meal choices: A couple of scrambled eggs with a few slivers of avocado and a side of veggies. Or a healthful protein bar such as RXBAR, Oatmega or SimplyProtein Whey Bar.

141

•**Work with your limitations.** Many of my patients have some physical limitations. They might be overweight…out of shape…or deal with arthritis, leg pain or other minor (or not so minor) disabilities. You can still engage in HIIT—you just have to find what works for you. A personal trainer can offer advice.

•**Go low and slow.** To start, I recommend doing an HIIT workout three days a week, for about 10 minutes each time. You'll slowly increase the total time—by increasing the number of intervals and/or the duration of the exertion/rest components—as you get stronger. Aim to work up to 20 to 30 minutes for each session.

•**Don't forget the warm-up and cooldown.** When you start your workout, whether it's biking, jogging or using a Stair-Master, slowly go through these movements for the first few minutes…and shift into low intensity of the same exercise for a few minutes of cooldown at the end of the workout.

Each week, you'll find that you can gradually increase the duration and intensity of the workouts.

Chapter 7

GET THE BEST MEDICAL CARE

Is That Symptom Serious or Not?

Google is not your friend when you're investigating a mysterious new symptom. Do you rush to the doctor...or try to wait it out?

What doctors know: The vast majority of symptoms that bring people to doctors' offices turn out to be minor—or at least manageable. But unless you've had years of medical training, you won't know what's serious and what's not. Some seemingly "minor" symptoms really do need to be checked out...others can be ignored...and some should send you racing to the ER. *Common symptoms—and what to do...*

Light-Headedness

It usually means that your brain isn't getting enough blood. That sounds scary, and it can be—but not always.

Relax if you sometimes feel light-headed when you get out of bed or stand up from a seated position, particularly when the sensation lasts a few seconds or less and isn't so severe that you feel like you're going to pass out. All it means is that your change of position is forcing blood to move against gravity—there's a slight lag before your blood pressure compensates and the brain gets enough blood and oxygen.

Exception: Light-headedness that occurs every time you stand up...lasts more than a minute...or forces you to sit/lie down could be due to orthostatic hypotension, a large drop in blood pressure that's often caused by dehydration...side effects from certain medications (such as beta-blockers and diuretics)...or bleeding (from an ulcer, for example) that may or may not have been detected. You'll want to see a doctor the same or next day.

Note: If you're bleeding and feel light-headed, go to the ER.

Make an appointment if you have worsening light-headedness during exercise. I worry most when a patient is age 50 or older and gets light-headed during mild exertion. This could indicate that the heart isn't supplying enough blood to the muscles—which can occur because of aortic stenosis, a stiffening of

Christopher Kelly, MD, a physician at Columbia University Medical Center in New York City. His research has been published in *The New England Journal of Medicine* and other professional journals. He is coauthor, with Marc Eisenberg, MD, of *Am I Dying?!: A Complete Guide to Your Symptoms—and What to Do Next.*

the main valve that separates the heart from the aorta, the large vessel that conveys oxygen-rich blood to your entire body—or weakening of the heart muscle from blockages in the arteries (atherosclerosis). Your doctor will probably recommend an ultrasound and possibly a stress test or other tests to assess the health of your cardiovascular system.

Call an ambulance if you feel light-headed and your heart is racing out of control. You could be experiencing a rapid and irregular heart rhythm, such as atrial fibrillation or ventricular tachycardia, that can be deadly without quick treatment. After you call 911, lie down while you're waiting for an ambulance and elevate your feet.

Headaches

They're among the most common symptoms that bring people to doctors' offices and ERs. They're painful but usually not serious—with some exceptions.

Relax when headaches feel like a band of pain around your skull…improve with rest and medication, such as acetaminophen (Tylenol) or *ibuprofen* (Advil)…and tend to occur at high-stress moments in your life. They're probably just tension headaches, thought to be caused in part by muscle spasms in the scalp. They rarely last long and aren't a problem for most people.

Make an appointment if your scalp hurts when you brush your hair, your jaw tires quickly while chewing and you're age 50 or older. It could be temporal arteritis, an uncommon autoimmune disease that affects the temporal arteries that carry blood to the head. It can eventually cause severe pain and/or vision loss.

Temporal arteritis can usually be diagnosed with blood/imaging tests, although a biopsy of the affected artery may be needed.

Treatment: Oral steroids (such as prednisone) taken for a few months to a year or more. High-dose intravenous steroids may be given at the time of diagnosis. The condition can't be cured, but drugs will stop the pain and reduce the risk for complications.

Call an ambulance if the headache pain is sudden and among the worst you've ever had—like an ice pick stabbing into your head. It could be a subarachnoid hemorrhage, a ruptured blood vessel in the head. It may be accompanied by neck pain, nausea or vomiting. About one in eight people don't live long enough to get to a hospital. Get help immediately!

Fatigue

The causes of fatigue run the gamut. But if you feel constantly run-down—even when you get enough sleep (see below)—there's probably something wrong.

Relax if you've started a new medication. Fatigue is a common drug side effect, even among drugs that people don't associate with sedation.

Common offenders: Blood pressure medications—such as *atenolol* (Tenormin), *metoprolol* (Lopressor) and other beta-blockers—along with pain relievers, antihistamines and many antidepressants.

My advice: Talk to your doctor if you notice fatigue after starting any new drug. In most cases, all you'll have to do is switch to a different drug or take a lower dose. Also, remember that there are numerous causes of fatigue, including stress.

Make an appointment if you're also suffering from constipation…have gained weight…and often feel cold. These are symptoms of hypothyroidism, an underactive thyroid gland. It's easily diagnosed with simple blood tests. Most people will get back to normal when they start a thyroid-replacement medication, such as *levothyroxine* (Synthroid).

Other possibilities: Sleep apnea, in which breathing intermittently stops and starts during sleep—and prevents you from getting a good night's rest. People with sleep apnea usually aren't aware of it, but their partners often complain about loud snoring and/or gasping. It's clinically diagnosed with a sleep test.

Progressively worsening fatigue combined with weight loss can be a red flag for cancer. This, too, warrants a visit to your doctor.

Call an ambulance if you suddenly experience bone-deep fatigue that's accompanied by any degree of mental confusion. There are multiple life-threatening conditions that can cause sudden, severe fatigue/confusion, including a brain infection, stroke or sepsis.

Is It Time to Get Your Hormone Levels Checked?

James B. LaValle, RPh, CCN, a clinical pharmacist and board-certified clinical nutritionist based in Foothill Ranch, California. He is author of four books, including *Your Blood Never Lies: How to Read a Blood Test for a Longer, Healthier Life* and *Cracking the Metabolic Code: 9 Ways to Optimal Health.* JimLaValle.com

We've all had routine blood tests—to check our cholesterol levels, blood glucose, thyroid hormone and other important health indicators. But there's a lot that you could be missing.

To get a fuller picture: Talk to your doctor about blood tests that check levels of hormones that are often overlooked. As chemical messengers that affect virtually every function in your body, these hormones play a crucial role in everything from your immune system and brain health to your sex drive, mood and energy levels.

The problem is, such hormone levels are usually tested only when a problem is suspected. But many integrative-health experts now recommend annual testing (or a schedule recommended by your practitioner) of specific hormone levels for adults over age 30, especially to learn more about...*

•**Cortisol is the King Kong of hormones**—levels of all other hormones can be affected, in one way or another, by one's cortisol levels.

Commonly known as the "stress hormone," cortisol is released from the adrenal

*Normal ranges for these hormones vary depending on a person's age, sex and the laboratory where the blood samples were tested.

glands in response to psychological and/or physical stress. Constant worrying and rushing through life can raise your cortisol levels. Physical stressors, such as pain and overexercising, also can elevate cortisol.

Over time, high cortisol levels can result in increased blood sugar, decreased or imbalanced immune function, decreased bone formation and impaired memory.

Worse: If cortisol levels remain too high for too long, levels can then drop too low. Symptoms of low cortisol include extreme fatigue, muscle weakness and depression.

•**Testosterone plays a critical role in male sexual development and function,** but it also promotes brain function and increases muscle mass and energy levels...and it boosts libido in both sexes.

As we age, testosterone naturally drops in men and women. But low testosterone also can be due to such factors as chronic stress and obesity...and the use of certain drugs, including opioid painkillers and corticosteroids (such as prednisone).

Important: Get testosterone levels tested before using a testosterone replacement.

In women, low testosterone can lower mood and libido and reduce muscle mass, bone density and energy.

Note: When practitioners test testosterone levels, they should also test levels of another type of testosterone called dihydrotestosterone (DHT). When elevated, DHT can cause "male-pattern" baldness in women.

•**Estrogen influences sexual development and reproductive and sexual health in both women and men.** In women, overly high levels of estrogen may cause estrogen-related cancers, such as endometrial and breast cancers.

Especially among women after menopause, low estrogen is very common. It might also be seen in women with very low body fat or certain medical disorders. Over time, low estrogen in women can lead to osteoporosis, heart disease and/or stroke. Symptoms include decreased libido, hot flashes, night sweats, depression, anxiety, memory problems, headaches and fatigue.

• **Progesterone is the companion hormone to estrogen.** It's also needed to counterbalance the effects of estrogen. Low progesterone can result from chronic stress, lack of exercise and/or poor diet. Over time, it can contribute to increased risk for heart disease in men and women…and increased risk for uterine fibroids, endometriosis and breast and ovarian cancers in women.

In addition, low progesterone is thought to be related to premenstrual syndrome (PMS) symptoms in women, including painful menstrual cramps. It also may be related to an increased risk for infertility and miscarriage.

Symptoms of low progesterone include anxiety, depression, insomnia, fatigue, loss of libido and mood swings.

• **DHEA (dehydroepiandrosterone)** is produced mostly in the adrenal glands and is a building block material that can be used to create estrogen and testosterone. DHEA is important for the immune system, and it plays a role in insulin sensitivity and fat metabolism—both key factors in diabetes.

DHEA levels can fall due to aging or chronic stress. Symptoms include fatigue, muscle and joint pain, weight gain, trouble sleeping, low libido, poor memory and depression.

What Next?

Testing for these hormones is one of the best preventive measures people can take, in my opinion, because it can identify the impact that stress may be having on you.

If any of your hormone levels falls outside the "normal" range, talk to your doctor about next steps. Lifestyle changes—especially including stress-management techniques (such as meditation, yoga and/or deep-breathing exercises)…sufficient sleep…and appropriate levels of exercise, which help relieve stress and improve testosterone levels—support hormone health.

Note: Excessive exercise often leaves you feeling very tired, and you may get sick more often.

In some cases, however, medical treatment (such as hormone replacement therapy) may be needed. In addition, there are supplements (see below) that can be used to support better hormone balance and levels. To ensure that your health-care provider is knowledgeable about optimizing your hormone profile, consider seeing a naturopathic physician. To find one near you, check The American Association of Naturopathic Physicians, Naturopathic.org.

Supplements That Help

Even though lifestyle measures, such as those described earlier, are useful, some people may need certain over-the-counter (OTC) supplements that can help support and rebalance hormones.

Before beginning self-treatment, consult your doctor on dosing and to make sure that a supplement you are considering will not interact with a medication or another supplement you may be taking. *Supplements that can be useful for…*

• **Cortisol and DHEA—Relora.** Helps lower cortisol. And as cortisol decreases, DHEA will start to be restored. It also reduces stress-related carbohydrate cravings.

• **Ashwagandha.** Restores balance in cortisol, whether high or low, as well as supports DHEA and thyroid hormone balance.

Caution: It may increase the effects of hypnotics and sedatives (such as barbiturates). Use only with physician approval if you have a thyroid disorder or if you take a blood thinner or antiplatelet drug.

• **Testosterone—Eurycoma longifolia.** Also known as tongkat ali and Malaysian ginseng, this herb helps improve the testosterone-to-cortisol ratio.

• **Estrogen—Rhapontic rhubarb.** Used for hot flashes and other menopausal symptoms.

• **Progesterone—Chasteberry.** Good for symptoms associated with low progesterone, such as PMS.

Caution: Do not use if you are pregnant or breast-feeding, or if you have a hormone-sensitive condition, such as breast cancer or uterine fibroids.

Doctor vs. Nurse Practitioner

Trisha Torrey, founder of EveryPatientsAdvocate. com, Leesburg, Florida.

Have you ever made an appointment with your doctor, only to be seen instead by a nurse practitioner? Is that legal? There's nothing illegal about a medical practice changing your provider from a doctor to a nurse practitioner (NP) or physician's assistant (PA), but you should be told in advance.

Why this may have happened: Maybe the doctor was sick that day, was overbooked or had an emergency, among other reasons.

What to do: When you make an appointment, tell the scheduler who you want to see and confirm that he/she will be available. Also ask the scheduler to let you know ahead of time if a change needs to be made.

Note: The quality of care provided by an NP or a PA has been shown to be equal to (or sometimes better than) what you'd get from a medical doctor if it's a routine visit or it's a basic and acute problem such as the flu or a rash. And many people actually prefer to see an NP or a PA due to better availability, extra time for questions and perhaps lower costs. However, it's best to see your doctor if you're having unusual symptoms or you have a chronic condition that needs constant monitoring and you're not being seen by a specialist.

Sail Through Surgery: An Anesthesiologist's Guide

Jill Zafar, MD, assistant professor of anesthesiology at Yale University and medical director of presurgical evaluation at Yale New Haven Hospital in Connecticut.

It's official, you need surgery. You understand its importance for your health, but there's no denying that your nerves are on edge. First, take a deep breath to take any panic out of the equation. Then start to prepare for it, just as you would any goal you want to accomplish. To show you how, we turned to Jill Zafar, MD, medical director of presurgical evaluation at Yale New Haven Hospital in Connecticut.

Why an anesthesiologist? Often an unsung hero in the operating room, this is the doctor who not only maps out your anesthesia plan but also keeps you comfortable and safe during surgery and helps with pain control afterward. Dr. Zafar's insider view on surgery-suite prep will help you get through your procedure with flying colors.

Before Surgery

"Train" the way you would for a fitness event: You wouldn't think of running a 5K race without preparing for it, says Dr. Zafar, who suggests you look at surgery the same way. In fact, an operation can stress your body as much as running that race would. If you have the luxury of time before your procedure, go into it in the best shape possible through exercise and a nutritious diet…with guidelines from your doctor or surgeon that take into account your general health. Doing so may make your recovery quicker and more comfortable. Make sure you eat enough protein, take any regular medications and continue to exercise. Cut back on alcohol.

SURPRISING TIP: **Some hospitals have formal surgery wellness programs** designed to help patients sail into surgery in the best shape possible. Ask whether your hospital or surgery center has such a program, and get on board if it does.

Stop smoking: If you still haven't kicked the habit, let surgery provide the impetus to finally quit. Dr. Zafar says that's the case for a good number of people. Take advantage! Your lungs and heart don't work as well when you smoke, and this may make you more likely to develop breathing problems during or after surgery. You're also at higher risk of getting pneumonia. Smoking slows down blood flow, so your incision may heal more slowly or become infected.

SURPRISING TIP: **You should quit smoking now, of course.** But even quitting the day before your procedure can reduce your risk for complications.

Get the most out of your pre-op appointment: Although you may have met your surgeon already, you'll likely have a specific pre-op meeting (and possibly one with your anesthesiologist) in the days or weeks leading up to the procedure. Together, you'll review all your medical conditions and make sure that you're healthy enough for the procedure. Use this time to go over any medications, herbs and supplements you take. If you take any daily, ask which ones you're able to take on the morning of your surgery. Some drugs may need to be stopped a week or so before surgery—certain ones interact with anesthesia and can trigger low blood pressure, while others can cause bleeding complications. If you'll be spending at least one night in the hospital, confirm that your surgeon will give a list of your meds to the hospital so that you'll be given those drugs during your stay.

Expect your doctor to ask about lifestyle habits that could interfere with anesthesia such as drinking alcohol and using recreational drugs as well as smoking. And be honest about everything—your doctors are not there to judge you but to protect you.

Important: Don't forget to mention if you have or think you have sleep apnea. Anesthesia is riskier for people with this breathing problem, so special precautions are necessary.

You might need certain tests if you haven't had them recently…

• **A chest X-ray to assess your lung function.**

• **An electrocardiogram to check your heart.**

• **Blood or urine tests.**

Depending on your unique health profile and any chronic conditions you have, you may need other tests or need to see other specialists.

Most people won't meet their anesthesiologists until the day of surgery. So early on, ask your surgeon about what kind of anesthesia is most commonly used for your procedure.

There are four main types…

• **General anesthesia.** You're fully unconscious. Drugs are delivered through an IV or a breathing mask.

• **Sedation analgesia.** You may have heard this called twilight sleep. The anesthesiologist can sedate you minimally, moderately or deeply depending on what procedure you're having done. The lightest form means you're awake but relaxed and can answer questions. If you get the deepest kind, you'll sleep through the whole operation and probably won't remember anything. Sedation analgesia often causes fewer side effects than general anesthesia.

• **Regional anesthesia.** This blocks pain in a large area, but you remain fully conscious.

• **Local anesthesia.** Just a small part of your body is numbed—think Novocain used at the dentist's office.

You may get a sedative along with local or regional anesthesia to make you more comfortable.

Share your concerns: If you've ever had a bad reaction to anesthesia, tell your surgeon or reach out directly to the anesthesia department in advance of your procedure to discuss it. Based on this history, your anesthesiologist might alter your anesthesia plan or add a medication such as something to prevent vomiting if that's the problem you had.

Something more serious: It's rare, but some people have a severe reaction under anesthesia called malignant hyperthermia (MH). It causes high fever and other problems and can be life-threatening. You're more susceptible to having such a reaction if you have a certain genetic mutation passed down to you by a parent. If you know that someone in your family developed MH during surgery, your anesthesiologist will likely treat you as if you have it, too, as a precaution. There is a blood test that can look for the gene mutations most commonly associated with MH, but the only way to truly confirm or rule out susceptibility is with a muscle biopsy, a test done at only certain centers around the country. You can find out more at MHAUS.org.

Don't be afraid of anesthesia: Some people, even those who have had anesthesia with no problems in the past, fear going under more than the surgery itself. You may even be worried about waking up from general anesthesia during surgery. That can happen in high-risk procedures such as open heart or emergency surgery if the anesthesiologist has to err on the side of keeping you alive versus giving you enough anesthesia to keep you fully unconscious. But it's very rare, and even if you have some awareness, it's unlikely you'll feel pain.

The Day of Surgery

Follow pre-op instructions: Typically, you won't be able to eat past midnight the day before surgery. That's because if there's anything in your stomach, you could regurgitate it, inhale it into your lungs and end up with pneumonia. So follow the eating and drinking directions you're given to the letter.

SURPRISING TIP: Studies have found that a carbohydrate pre-op drink (think of a liquid version of the carbo-loading that marathon runners do the night before their race) can lead to better outcomes. A prolonged starvation period can itself produce stress and dehydration, explains Dr. Zafar. It turns out that the carb drink can lead to more stable blood sugar when you're in recovery. Do not do this on your own, however, because it may not be safe for everyone. Ask your doctor whether this drink is an option for you and, if so, where to get it and when exactly to drink it.

What happens when you get to the hospital: The surgery center or clinic is a lot like the airport—there's a lot to do before you get where you're going. Pack your patience—it takes time to safely prepare you for your surgery. *During this busy time...*

• **Your surgeon will stop by to discuss the operation again,** answer your last-minute questions and possibly mark the surgical site with a pen.

• **Your anesthesiologist will review your medical records,** explain exactly what kind of anesthesia you'll receive and get your written consent. Ask about how much pain to expect after surgery and how it will be controlled. Mention your good or bad experiences with specific pain medications in the past.

• **Nurses will take your vital signs,** likely start IV fluids and give you light sedation.

• **If you're anxious, share your specific concerns with the anesthesia team.** This talk may calm your fears so that you're less stressed heading into the operating room.

If you're having general anesthesia, the anesthesiologist may place a breathing tube in your throat to keep your airway open after you're unconscious. If it's needed, it will likely be removed before you wake up.

During surgery, the anesthesiologist will continually monitor your anesthesia levels and your vital body functions to make sure that you're handling the surgery well.

After Surgery

In the recovery room, you'll probably feel groggy and maybe briefly confused. You may have side effects such as nausea or vomiting or, if you had a breathing tube, a sore throat. If you had local or regional anesthesia, the injection site may be sore.

You'll be in some pain: The amount will depend on the surgery you had. The anesthesia team can give you pain medications or a nerve block to make you more comfortable.

The majority of surgeries today take place at outpatient facilities. *If you're going home the same day of your operation...*

Have someone there to take you home: You won't be able to drive yourself home, but don't attempt to take a bus or even a cab if you can help it. You need someone not only to help you in and out of the car but also to stay with you and see to your needs for at least a few hours as the anesthesia works its way out of your system.

Make sure that you understand post-op instructions: Your medical staff will give you instructions specific to your surgery.

You'll also learn about the signs of risky post-op complications and what to do if any develop. Ask the person who will drive or accompany you home to listen to any verbal instructions and take notes because you still may be a little fuzzy from the anesthesia.

Take these precautions: For 24 hours after surgery, even if your surgery doesn't limit your activities, respect the fact that you had anesthesia and don't drink alcohol, make any important decisions or use potentially dangerous machinery—many people scoff at this last one, but the advice isn't limited to forklifts or bandsaws. Snowblowers and lawn mowers fall into this category, too. Your body needs time to recover its strength even if your head feels clear.

Take your pain medication as prescribed: Most people are sent home with opioid pain medications after surgery. The opioid abuse crisis has made some people afraid of taking them, but if you're in so much pain that you can't move around, you could develop complications such as pneumonia or blood clots. Your doctor may also prescribe ibuprofen or acetaminophen-based pills to cut back on the need for opioids, but in some cases, opioids are simply the most effective option.

If you're concerned about them, talk to your doctor about exactly how to safely take them before you leave the hospital, and don't hesitate to call your surgeon's office about this or any other aspect of aftercare as you recover.

When "Simple" Surgeries Turn Deadly

Frank Overdyk, MD, a patient-safety advocate and anesthesiologist in Charleston, South Carolina. Dr. Overdyk is a member of the board of advisors of the Physician-Patient Alliance for Health & Safety, PPAHS.org. He received the 2018 AAMI (Association for the Advancement of Medical Instrumentation) & Becton Dickinson Patient Safety Award.

Some surgeries and procedures are considered "minor" when compared with lengthy, invasive operations such as heart or brain surgery…or a hip or knee replacement.

The so-called simple procedures—performed about 40 million times each year in the US—often take place in ambulatory surgery centers (ASCs), where you're sent home in a few hours. But what happens when simple surgeries go wrong—or even turn deadly?

Not so simple after all.

Since their introduction in the US in the 1970s, ASCs have been a valuable resource, helping patients avoid hospital-acquired infections and speeding recovery at home in more comfortable surroundings.

However, the risks are real. Deaths resulting from treatment at ASCs are not officially tracked, but according to a recent investigative report published by USA Today Network and Kaiser Health News, more than 260 ASC patients died from surgical complications (such as internal bleeding and cardiac arrest) over the last five years. *Some key risks—and how to protect yourself…*

•**Cosmetic surgery (such as a face-lift).** *What can go wrong:* Particularly during any type of cosmetic surgery, in which a surgeon is operating near the mouth, nose, vocal cords or neck, general anesthesia (the use of a drug to make the patient unresponsive and unconscious) or "deep sedation" (similar to general anesthesia but often does not involve a breathing tube) can interfere with a patient's ability to breathe.

To protect yourself: If your surgeon plans to use deep sedation, ask whether a dedicated sedation provider will be involved (by law, general anesthesia requires an anesthesiologist, nurse-anesthetist and/or anesthesiologist assistant). Or ask whether the surgeon can use local anesthesia or a nerve block instead. With a nerve block, local anesthetic is injected near nerves and specific body parts that will be affected by the surgery. Nerve blocks have different risks from general anesthesia and deep sedation but usually don't impede your ability to breathe or your level of consciousness.

• **Tonsillectomy.** Nearly 300,000 tonsil-removal surgeries are performed each year in adults—often prompted by frequent sore throats. But chronically swollen tonsils also contribute to sleep apnea, which raises risks for serious conditions, such as heart attack and stroke.

What can go wrong: Tonsillectomy involves the airway and blood vessels. Persistent bleeding in the airway after tonsillectomy is an infrequent but serious complication that requires immediate attention and can arise hours after the procedure…long after the ASC closes.

To protect yourself: Ask to be the first case of the day. This is the best time to schedule any procedure—but especially this one. Scheduling early in the day gives the most time for any complication to be addressed on-site.

• **Bunionectomy.** *What can go wrong:* Recovery from bunion removal can be very painful, and opioid pain relievers often are prescribed for the immediate post-op period and beyond. This can be dangerous, especially for patients with sleep apnea, obesity or advanced age. In addition to depressed breathing, opioids can trigger a variety of side effects, including nausea/vomiting and urinary dysfunction.

To protect yourself: Before your procedure, discuss the plan for post-op pain management. Ask your doctor how you can limit opioid use by instead relying on alternatives, including nonsteroidal anti-inflammatory drugs (NSAIDs) and the COX-2 inhibitor *celecoxib* (Celebrex). These drugs target enzymes responsible for inflammation and pain without such a high risk for side effects.

• **Endoscopy.** *What can go wrong:* With endoscopy, which involves the use of deep sedation, both the doctor performing the procedure and the anesthesia provider are working inside your airway. This means that contents from your stomach could get into your lungs (aspiration).

To protect yourself: Make sure you are a suitable candidate and without an acute illness (see below).

Are You an ASC Candidate?

If you're elderly and/or have chronic health problems that increase your risk for complications during or after your surgery—such as moderate-to-severe sleep apnea, morbid obesity or chronic obstructive pulmonary disease (COPD), discuss with your primary care doctor and the doctor performing the procedure whether you're a suitable candidate for outpatient surgery at an ASC.

Also, if you have a cold, the flu or a fever, call to notify your outpatient facility—you may be asked to reschedule the procedure to a time when you are well. Similarly, if your blood sugar or blood pressure is high or unstable…or you have shortness of breath from asthma or heart failure, notify the doctor performing the procedure and get advice on the best plan of action.

Other Safeguards You Need

Before undergoing treatment at an ASC, also make sure that…

• **The facility only rarely needs to transfer a patient to a hospital** for more advanced care. The hospital also should be relatively close.

• **There will be electronic monitors and "crash carts" on-site.**

• **A dedicated anesthesiologist,** nurse-anesthetist or anesthesiologist assistant will be on hand during the procedure. This is crucial if you will be receiving general anesthesia or deep sedation. Deep sedation carries greater risks than "conscious sedation," during which the patient is able to respond to verbal prompts and commands.

Note: If you are comfortable with taking oral medication for anxiety and prefer not to take the additional risks associated with deep sedation, ask for conscious sedation, and make sure your consent form indicates this.

• **Your oxygen saturation and exhaled carbon dioxide ("capnography")** will be continuously monitored by the dedicated provider mentioned above during all procedures requiring deep sedation or general anesthesia. Oxygen saturation also should be monitored continuously during recovery from deep sedation or general anesthesia. The recovery area should be staffed by a qualified professional trained in basic and advanced cardio life support.

• **The doctor performing the procedure has board certification** by a board that is a member of the American Board of Medical Specialties, ABMS.org. This credential is highly recommended and offers an added layer of safety.

Know the Warning Signs of Post-Op Problems

Alana Elise Sigmund, MD, FHM, medical director for arthroplasty at Hospital for Special Surgery, New York City, where she oversees the medical care of postoperative patients. Her research into preoperative stress testing and postoperative management of arthroplasty patients has appeared in *JAMA Internal Medicine, The Journal of Arthroplasty* and most recently in *Mayo Clinic Proceedings*. She is also a member of the Society of Hospital Medicine Research Committee.

You're back home and feeling relieved that your surgery—major or minor—was a success. As the last vestiges of anesthesia or IV pain medication wear off, you realize that you were fairly woozy when you left the hospital or at least distracted by the tumult of the discharge process. And now that you're propped up on your familiar sofa and feel an unexpected twinge of pain, you realize that you don't really remember all that information about "complications" the nurse warned you about when you were discharged. And that piece of paper with a list of reasons to call the surgeon's office? Suddenly the descriptions all seem very vague.

Are you in trouble?

It's important to know what's most likely normal and what could be a sign of trouble when you're recovering at home, especially when you're an outpatient and are healing away from the watchful eye of nurses and doctors. Of course, any complications or side effects will depend on the specific type of surgery you had. But Alana Elise Sigmund, MD, internist and perioperative medicine specialist at Hospital for Special Surgery in New York City, has some guidelines.

Suggestion No. 1: After an outpatient procedure, you may still feel groggy when you're discharged, so ask the person picking you up to take notes. That way you'll know what your surgeon recommended.

Then use this surgery side effect checklist to quickly recognize a variety of roadblocks on your path to recovery…

• **Side Effect: Drainage.**

Normal: What's a reasonable amount of drainage—fluid that leaks from the incision after surgery—depends on the type of surgery, and your surgeon should give you a time frame for when yours should slow down and then stop.

Not normal: If you notice drainage increasing, call your doctor. Generally, the fluid should be clear or light pink. If it turns yellow or another color, this could be a sign of infection. If the fluid develops an odor, pick up the phone.

• **Side Effect: Redness and Swelling.**

Normal: Some redness and swelling around an incision is a normal part of healing. You should see it decrease as you heal.

Not normal: If redness and/or swelling gets darker or starts to spread, you could have cellulitis, an infection in the deep layers of skin and the tissue beneath it, or a surgical site infection that needs to be treated with antibiotics.

Smart tip: If you're concerned or are just unsure, snap a picture of the area with your phone and see if you can send it to the doctor.

• **Side Effect—Pain.**

Normal: It's almost impossible not to have any pain after surgery and, depending on the type of surgery you had, it could be worse on the second day. But you should start to feel a little better every day after that. If you need pain medication, make sure you take no more than directed.

Not normal: If you feel a sudden and big uptick in pain, that's a red flag, and your doctor needs to know right away. Another reason to give a call is if you just don't feel that your pain is fading over time.

●**Side Effect—Fever.**

Normal: People often run slight fevers for about two days post-op. If you suspect you have a fever, take your temperature. If it's less than 101.4°F, check again about four hours later to make sure it's going down.

Not normal: If your temperature reaches 101.4°F or higher and occurs two days or more after surgery, there's a greater chance that the fever is due to an infection, especially if you have other symptoms like painful urination or a bad cough. Call your doctor.

●**Side Effect: Lower Leg Pain**

Normal: Post-op leg cramps—when the muscle seizes up—are common and often are caused by abnormalities in electrolytes, the various minerals in your body fluids, and you should certainly tell your doctor about leg cramps. You might need nothing more than food and water. If that's not working, reach out to your physician's office.

Not normal: There's another reason you might have leg pain after an operation—and it's a more immediate concern. Pain in your lower leg or calf could be a sign of deep vein thrombosis (DVT), a dangerous type of blood clot that can break free and block an artery in your lung—a potentially fatal condition called a pulmonary embolism (PE). Surgery can raise your risk for DVT. If you have calf pain postoperatively, call your care team. Your doctor may order an imaging test, such as ultrasound, to diagnose a DVT and, if one is found, will then treat you, typically with a blood thinner to dissolve the clot.

Always Cause for Concern

There's no "normal" for some post-op reactions. *Here are symptoms that definitely require prompt action...*

●**Trouble Breathing.** If you feel short of breath but can still speak in full sentences, alert your care team by phone. The problem may be related to your surgery or another condition you have, like asthma or allergies. But if it's so bad that you can't get out a sentence, call 911. Sudden trouble breathing can be a sign that a DVT has broken free and that you're experiencing a PE.

●**Bleeding.** Normal post-op bleeding can happen after some operations such as sinus surgery. Your doctor should have told you if you're likely to bleed after your procedure and, if so, how much bleeding to expect and when it should stop. If bleeding wasn't mentioned or if it seems different than what was explained to you, contact your doctor. If bleeding is profuse, of course, call 911.

●**Shock.** Shock in medical terms is when the body doesn't have enough blood flowing to its organs. Severe blood loss is a major cause of shock, itself a life-threatening emergency. *Symptoms of shock can include...*

●Rapid heartbeat and rapid breathing.

●Pale skin and sweating.

●Confusion.

●Weak pulse.

●Unusually cool hands and feet.

●Chest pain.

●Call 911 if you think you could be in shock!

Surgery can stress every system of the body, including the heart. The risk of heart problems after most types of surgery is low for most people, but you're at greater risk if you had major surgery and already have heart disease. In the days after surgery, if you feel pain or any strange sensation in your chest, one or both arms, your jaw or even your stomach that isn't obviously a normal result of the surgery, call 911. You could be having a heart attack.

Special note for women: Women often hurt in other places like the arms, jaw or even the nose.

It's not uncommon for patients to develop an irregular heart beat rhythm called atrial fibrillation (AF) a day or two after an operation. It's often related to the amount of intravenous fluids you're given to support your blood pressure during surgery, and some people may be especially susceptible to AF. If you develop AF, you might notice that your heart is racing or you might feel short of breath. Call your doctor, because AF raises your risk for stroke. Your doctor will let you know whether it's best to go to the office…or to the ER to determine whether you are experiencing AF.

Older Surgeons Have Lower Patient Death Rates

Among 892,187 Medicare patients who had one of 20 types of emergency surgery (such as hysterectomy or a heart valve procedure), those performed by surgeons who were age 50 and older had lower death rates during a four-year study period than procedures done by younger surgeons.

Yusuke Tsugawa, MD, PhD, assistant professor, David Geffen School of Medicine, UCLA, Los Angeles.

Urgent-Care Centers Overprescribe Antibiotics

Nearly half of patients with respiratory infections that don't require antibiotics receive prescriptions in urgent-care facilities. That's roughly double the proportion of inappropriate antibiotic prescriptions given in emergency departments and medical offices.

Caution: Unnecessary antibiotics lead to antibiotic resistance and other adverse side effects.

Katherine E. Fleming-Dutra, MD, is medical epidemiologist with the Office of Antibiotic Stewardship at Centers for Disease Control and Prevention, Atlanta, and corresponding author of the research, published in *JAMA Internal Medicine*.

If You've Got Cancer, Stay Out of the ER!

Nathan Handley, MD, MBA, an oncologist specializing in genitourinary cancers and assistant professor of medical oncology at Thomas Jefferson University in Philadelphia. He is lead author of "Best Practices for Reducing Unplanned Acute Care for Patients with Cancer," published in *Journal of Oncology Practice*.

Picture this scenario: A 62-year-old widow—let's call her "Mrs. Gand"—has recently been diagnosed with cancer. Two days after her first chemotherapy session, she's at home resting when she is overcome with nausea. It's 9 pm, and she can't get her doctor on the phone. Not knowing what to do, she drives herself to the local hospital ER. After sitting in a cramped waiting room for three hours, the ER doctor admits her to the hospital, where she remains for two days.

What most people don't know: For many cancer patients, a trip to the ER is not only unnecessary, it's time-consuming, costly—and possibly dangerous. For one thing, ER doctors are less familiar with the side effects of cancer treatments—especially newer ones like immunotherapy, which can cause unusual symptoms such as rashes and thyroid abnormalities. A non-cancer specialist may decide that it's safer and easier to admit the patient and wait for more specialized help.

Another important reason to steer clear: After arriving, you'll likely be stuck in a waiting room while more life-threatening cases, such as car accident victims, are seen. Hospitals are notorious sources of hospital-acquired infections. Because cancer patients usually have weaker immune systems due to chemotherapy, they are more susceptible to such infections than people who are healthy.

How to Avoid the Hospital

Cancer patients have alternatives to the ER… but usually don't know about them. To address this problem, researchers at University of Pennsylvania reviewed the medical literature to identify the best ways for cancer patients to avoid unnecessary visits to the ER and hospitalizations. *The smartest strategies…*

STRATEGY #1: **Plan ahead.** Many conditions that send cancer patients to the ER can be treated with prescription medications available at the pharmacy. With proper planning, someone like Mrs. Gand would have known that IV antinausea drugs given during chemotherapy usually wear off in 48 hours or less.

She and her oncologist could have then developed a plan to manage potential symptoms, including possibly using a prescription medication, such as *ondansetron* (Zofran) or *prochlorperazine* (Compazine), at home.

Helpful: If a cancer patient can't keep fluids down, IV fluids can sometimes be administered at the clinic where chemo is given so that an ER visit can be avoided.

What to do: Prior to chemo or any cancer treatment, ask your doctor to review any possible side effects—and what to do if any occur.

Important: White blood cell counts drop to their lowest point seven to 14 days after chemo, increasing susceptibility to infection. Knowing this ahead of time allows a cancer patient to take steps, including some of the tactics outlined in this article, to avoid a trip to a germ-laden ER during this crucial window.

Not all infections or fevers warrant hospitalization. If a cancer patient develops symptoms of an infection while at home, such as fever and/or chills, his/her oncologist may be able to see him the same day…or perhaps a colleague can squeeze him in. If you are ever unsure, you should always call your oncologist!

Exceptions: If fever, diarrhea or vomiting is accompanied by shortness of breath, racing heartbeat, stiff neck, new pain or altered mental status, call your doctor—you may have a potentially life-threatening infection known as sepsis. If your doctor is unavailable, head to the ER. When you arrive, say, "I have cancer and am concerned about infection and sepsis" to boost your odds of being seen more quickly.

STRATEGY #2: **Check out local urgent care.** More oncology practices and hospitals are opening urgent-care clinics specifically for cancer patients, often with same-day appointments and extended hours.

What to do: Before starting treatment, ask your oncologist about alternative places to seek care so you're not scrambling for help should a problem arise. Ask if your oncology clinic offers same-day appointments for symptom management…or if it has an affiliated urgent-care center. Even if the oncology clinic can't accommodate you, some practices are affiliated with specific ERs, allowing for smoother exchange of medical information.

STRATEGY #3: **Stay connected.** Simply relaying your symptoms to your doctor could keep you out of the ER and the hospital.

New study: Outpatient chemotherapy patients who got weekly e-mails encouraging them to report 12 common symptoms between appointments at Memorial Sloan Kettering Cancer Center in New York City fared better physically, mentally and emotionally than those who didn't get the messages. The patients also lived five months longer, on average.

Why did the e-mails help? They encouraged patients to proactively report side effects, which promotes faster treatment…and relief.

What to do: If your oncologist's office doesn't offer weekly e-mail or text check-ins or other telehealth options, craft a plan with your doctor where you agree to touch base with any unpleasant symptoms, perhaps via a secure online portal. You can also ask if there's a nurse available for such check-ins.

STRATEGY #4: **Ask about palliative care.** Early palliative care, which focuses on relief from the symptoms and stress of a serious illness, enhances quality and duration of life for patients with chronic or end-stage cancer. Meeting with a palliative care physician early on—soon after diagnosis, ideally—can help ease pain, depression and more.

These specialists are usually covered by insurance and collaborate with you and your oncologist to keep you comfortable and out of the ER. A specialist isn't always necessary, though—most oncologists have some training in palliative care, too.

Important: Palliative care is not hospice. Hospice focuses on a person's final six months, when curative treatment is no longer possible. Palliative care can help nonterminal patients and is used in conjunction with treatment.

Getting to Know Your Behind-the-Scenes Doctor: The Pathologist

Michael J. Misialek, MD, associate chair of pathology at Newton-Wellesley Hospital and medical director of the Vernon Cancer Center, both in Newton, Massachusetts, where he directs the Chemistry Laboratory and Point of Care Testing. A clinical assistant professor of pathology at Tufts University School of Medicine in Boston, he is also active with the College of American Pathologists and compiles the Path Report website, PathReport.org.

Here's something to ponder: Chances are, you have never seen the doctor who is at the front lines of determining virtually all of the key decisions about your health care.

Your pathologist is the behind-the-scenes player who handles laboratory testing that drives nearly 80% of all medical diagnoses and treatments. But this doctor is hardly ever mentioned—much less someone you're likely to meet.

How could that be? On TV shows like CSI, pathologists examine corpses and investigate suspicious deaths. In real life, their work is much more far-reaching. Pathologists are commonly recognized for their role in diagnosing cancer when a biopsy is performed. But these medical doctors also analyze laboratory tests—checking for everything from elevated cholesterol levels and infections to kidney disease and the cause of skin growths.

You can think of it this way—anything that is biopsied, scraped off, drawn from your veins, coughed up or excreted will pass under the microscope of a pathologist, who looks at physical specimens for signs of risk and disease.

Integral for Cancer Care

If you've been diagnosed with cancer, your initial diagnosis and the subsequent treatment plans always start with a pathologist.

Example: Your doctor might suspect that you have breast cancer—based on a mammogram, physical findings (like a breast lump), symptoms, etc.—but the actual diagnosis will depend on what's discovered from a tissue sample that's examined in a laboratory.

The cancer diagnosis is just the beginning. The pathologist will use microscopic criteria to "grade" tumors according to their severity...identify hormone receptors (such as those for estrogen or progesterone) that predict how tumors are likely to behave...and determine what treatments are most likely to be effective.

Will you do better if you have surgery first, followed by radiation or chemotherapy? Or will your cancer respond more readily to preoperative chemotherapy and/or radiation? The treatments that your doctor ultimately chooses, including the order of treatments, are largely guided by pathology findings.

Recent development: "Liquid biopsy," which is based on a blood draw rather than a tissue sample, is an emerging technology that is transforming not just cancer care but virtually every disease process. To ensure accuracy and precision, pathologists are often involved in the design, validation and oversight of these tests.

Smart idea: If you're diagnosed with cancer or any other serious condition, ask to see the pathologist's report. Pay particular attention to the "diagnosis" section to learn the pathologist's conclusion and the "comments" section, which gives additional information on any subtleties of your case.

Tracking Disease

Many diseases (such as diabetes) and risk factors (including elevated cholesterol) can be diagnosed only by laboratory findings. But about 20% of pathology tests are requested after a diagnosis to determine how well a treatment is working.

An oncologist, for example, might order additional biopsies and/or other tests to track a tumor's response to radiation or chemotherapy…and still more tests to fine-tune the treatments by adding or subtracting drugs, changing doses, etc.

Another example: You'll need laboratory tests to determine if (or how well) medication to treat thyroid disease is working. The same goes for drugs such as insulin, blood thinners and cholesterol-lowering statins.

An Imperfect Science

Most pathologists will come to the same conclusions when they look at tissue samples—but not always. Doctors are only human. They have different opinions and biases…and they sometimes make mistakes.

Example: In a Johns Hopkins study published in *Cancer*, researchers reviewed biopsy slides from more than 6,000 patients and found that 86 patients were given wrong diagnoses that could have led to unnecessary or inappropriate treatments.

Research published in *JAMA*, looking at biopsies for breast cancer, found that 13% of cases of ductal carcinoma in situ (abnormal cells that are found within milk ducts) were not universally agreed upon by pathologists. This doesn't always mean that the pathologists made mistakes—there's disagreement among experts about how to diagnose this condition or interpret laboratory findings. But the study suggests that patients and doctors should view pathology reports with some healthy skepticism.

My advice: Don't hesitate to get a second pathology opinion, particularly if you're dealing with a rare disease…when the treatment for a disease (often the case with cancer) largely depends on pathology findings…or when a pathology report doesn't completely line up with your doctor's best judgment.

Important: A second pathology opinion will not require an additional biopsy—another pathologist is simply asked to review the slides from the first tissue sample.

These second opinions might be covered by insurance, but not always. Check with your insurance company before making the decision. Also, don't assume that you must use a pathologist who practices in your area for a second opinion. Biopsy slides can be shipped anywhere. Your doctor can often coordinate a second pathology opinion. Just be sure that the pathologist is board-certified and that the work is being performed in a laboratory credentialed by the College of American Pathologists.

Meet Face-to-Face

Most patients never meet the pathologist(s) involved in their medical care, but they should. I urge patients to come forward with questions, particularly when they're dealing with a rare or complicated disease…or when they have questions about the diagnosis that their primary doctor cannot fully answer.

Personal story: I received a call from a breast cancer patient who felt overwhelmed by information. I was familiar with her case because I had made the initial diagnosis. I explained what her diagnosis meant and what the biopsy showed (in terms that a layperson could understand). Just as important, I was able to give reassurance that her treatment plan was appropriate.

It's not yet routine for patients to consult with pathologists. But where I work, breast cancer patients are always given the chance to meet with a pathologist, just as they meet with oncologists and other members of their care team. While this practice is not widespread, it is gaining acceptance throughout the medical community.

My advice: Ask whether your hospital offers the opportunity to meet the pathologist, how to schedule the meeting and whether there is any cost associated with the visit—most of the time there is not.

More From Dr. Misialek

Pathologists Also Can Diagnose Drug Abuse

More than 115 Americans die every day from opioid overdoses—not just from heroin and other illegal drugs but also from prescription painkillers such as fentanyl, according to recent statistics. Primary care doctors are the first-line responders in this crisis, but many aren't sure how to interpret the tests that determine if patients are misusing their medications—or not taking them at all.

Example: A patient who is given oxycodone (a powerful narcotic) for chronic pain. The patient's doctor might order a basic urine drug test to ensure that the drug is being used correctly, but the results are inconclusive. If the doctor suspects (but isn't sure) that the patient is misusing drugs, he/she might call me for advice. In such a case, I may recommend that the doctor order a urine test that looks for metabolites of oxycodone. The test will show conclusively if a drug is being used correctly.

Stop Fibbing to Your Doctor

Danielle Ofri, MD, PhD, associate professor of medicine at NYU Medical Center in New York City and editor in chief of the *Bellevue Literary Review.* She is author of *What Patients Say, What Doctors Hear.* DanielleOfri.com

You know the drill. Your doctor asks, "How are you?" and that's your cue to explain that new pain you're wrestling with or that weird rash you've recently noticed. But be honest—do you bare all the facts when talking to your doctor? If you're like most people, probably not.

Shocking research: When more than 4,500 adults were surveyed, 60% to 80% admitted to omissions, distortions and outright lies when talking to their doctors about topics such as how often they exercise, whether they take dietary supplements and how much alcohol they drink, according to research published in *JAMA Network Open.*

Why the cover-up? There are a variety of reasons why patients aren't completely honest with their doctors. *Among the most common…*

• **Shame** (such as not wanting to reveal things they may consider socially unacceptable)…embarrassment (including a reluctance to admit they didn't take their medications because they couldn't afford them)…a desire to be liked (wanting to appear to be a "good patient," they may say they've given up smoking, for example, and replaced KFC with kale when that's not true)…and fear of bad news (failing to mention worrisome symptoms because they are afraid the information might point to a serious illness).

A Bigger Problem

There also can be larger communication issues at play that may interfere with honest dialogue—even if that is the patient's goal—due to today's strained health-care system with shorter doctor visits, electronic record-keeping and overburdened medical personnel.

For one thing, doctors generally dominate the conversation. Even when patients are invited to voice their concerns, research shows that doctors interrupt them within 11 seconds. This isn't simple rudeness—doctors are trained to zero in on diagnosis.

If you start by complaining of a pain in your shoulder, for example, your doctor wants to quickly figure out the source of the pain. But if you wanted to bring something else to your doctor's attention, this may be left unsaid.

Sobering finding: In a recent study published in *Journal of General Internal Medicine,* patients' agendas—what mattered to them—got sufficient attention during only one-third of doctor visits.

Listening also can be a problem in which both doctors and patients fall short. Nervous, rushed and upset by a troubling diagnosis or news about your condition, you may miss much of what you are told. Meanwhile, omissions in your story may occur if your doctor is distracted by the computer on which he/she is entering notes…or is preoccupied with unraveling an earlier symptom.

Truth or Consequences

With all these inherent traps in doctor-patient communications, the likely result is overlooked symptoms, misdiagnoses and missed opportunities for the most effective medical intervention.

To avoid such consequences…

•**Make good communication your top priority.** It's the part of your doctor visit that deserves the most time and energy. If this happens, all the other pieces, such as the physical exam, blood tests and X-rays, will fall into place.

•**Bring a list of all your questions and concerns.** But don't expect your doctor to address a dozen symptoms. Instead, show the doctor your list and ask him to pick out what's most important.

Helpful: If there's an item that's especially important to you, let the doctor know by saying, "I want to be sure we get to X."

•**Don't censor yourself.** Don't be ashamed to bring up whatever matters to you—even if you're not sure whether it's medically important.

•**Ask a family member or close friend to be a second listener and take notes.** If you're alone at the appointment and can't take notes, ask your doctor if it's OK to record the conversation on your smartphone.

•**Be sure the doctor is listening.** If he's not, say, tactfully, "Could you please stop looking at the computer for a minute while I get my story out? I'll be brief."

•**Confirm how to stay in touch.** Whether it's a patient portal, e-mail or number to call, find out how to ask additional questions or request clarifications on anything you don't understand.

•**Don't stick with a doctor with whom you're unable to speak freely.** If you don't feel able to get your story heard, think seriously about changing doctors.

Also: You'll be less likely to lie, fudge or skip over things with a doctor you trust and feel comfortable with.

How Safe Is Your Drug Plan?

Charles B. Inlander is a consumer advocate and health-care consultant based in Fogelsville, Pennsylvania. He was the founding president of the nonprofit People's Medical Society, a consumer-advocacy organization credited with key improvements in the quality of US health care, and is author or coauthor of more than 20 consumer-health books.

A controversial health insurance program is growing by leaps and bounds throughout the country. With "step therapy," your insurer requires your doctor to prescribe the cheapest effective prescription drug for your condition (lowest step) before allowing you to use more expensive drugs (higher step). It's not only being required by private insurance companies, it is also being used in Medicare prescription drug plans (Part D).

Latest development: As of January 2019, Medicare Advantage plans have the option of using step therapy for Part B drugs—those directly paid for by Medicare to practitioners (including oncologists and dermatologists) for treatment of such conditions as cancer or psoriasis.

Insurers argue that just because a drug is new or more expensive, that does not mean it is better or more effective than an older brand-name medication or its generic equivalent. In fact, for most people, the older drug probably does work just fine. However, while step therapy programs grow, research has uncovered many unintended consequences, such as patients getting sicker or not improving when forced to take a cheaper drug that is less effective than a more expensive one. Some insurance plans won't even cover newer, more expensive drugs.

The good news is, you can still get the benefits of the step therapy philosophy—

without losing out if there's a drug you really need. *Here's how...*

• **Check with your insurer.** If your employer's health plan covers your medications, ask the insurer if your doctors are required to use step therapy programs. The same applies if you have a Medicare prescription drug plan (Part D) or are a member of a Medicare Advantage plan. Terms of coverage may change from year to year, so carefully review all information about meds that the insurer provides.

Insider tip: Make sure you check your insurer's formulary (list of drugs covered) at least annually—and ask the insurer whether any drug you're taking is part of a step protocol. In addition to requiring step therapy, the insurer can add or drop drugs from the formulary at any time.

• **Don't hesitate to file an appeal.** Several states have passed legislation, or have pending legislation, allowing you to appeal an insurer's decision to deny coverage via a step therapy program. Your appeal will be considered within three days, but your doctor will need to make the case for a higher-step drug based on your response to a lower-step drug and/or other factors.

Insider tip: Even if your state has no specific laws regarding step therapy appeals, you can still appeal a negative decision through your state's insurance department or directly through Medicare (if you are in traditional Medicare or a Medicare Advantage plan).

• **Use caution if you're switching plans.** If you plan to—or must—switch your health plans and are already taking a high-step-level, expensive drug, make sure that your new plan both covers that drug and will allow you to stay on it. Even if you stay in a plan only to find that your insurer is dropping that expensive drug you are on, don't be afraid to file an appeal.

Step therapy has an upside, too: Even if you are not in a required step therapy program, ask your doctor whether you can be prescribed the lowest- cost drug that is effec-

tive for your condition. In most cases, it will do the job.

Are Your Medications Making Your Life Worse?

Barbara Farrell, PharmD, assistant professor in the department of family medicine and an adjunct assistant professor in the School of Pharmacy, both at University of Waterloo, Canada. She was named Pharmacist of the Year by the Canadian Pharmacist Association in 2011 and is cofounder of the Canadian Deprescribing Network. Follow her research team on Twitter (@deprescribing). Deprescribing.org

It happens for the best of reasons. Your cardiologist, say, prescribes one medication, then you see your endocrinologist and get another, and your rheumatologist gives you another—and the doctors don't talk to one another. Each is trying to help you—but collectively, they could be hurting you...possibly badly.

Polypharmacy—taking a combination of medications that does more harm than good—is a national epidemic, and it's getting worse. The truth is, our medical system is a lot better at prescribing medications than at stopping ones that are no longer needed—deprescribing. Yet doing so, carefully and under medical supervision, reduces the adverse side effects and often improves health. Would it help you to deprescribe?

A Sneaky Multiplication

Polypharmacy can happen before you know it. *Case in point:* Many medications, regardless of the conditions they're prescribed for, can have depression as a side effect. They include certain blood pressure drugs...heart drugs...drugs for heartburn (proton pump inhibitors)...even painkillers. The more of these drugs you take, the higher your statistical risk of developing depression.

Polypharmacy also is associated with a host of other adverse effects including an increased risk for falls and cognitive impairment that can lead to emergency room visits and hospitalization. The problem often gets worse as you get older—you're not only likely to need more medications, but your body's ability to process those medications declines. A drug or dosage that was appropriate when initially prescribed might no longer be safe or appropriate. However, polypharmacy can happen at any age.

A "Miraculous" Recovery

You now understand polypharmacy. For an idea of how deprescribing can work, consider this case study...

The woman sat slumped over in her chair—and then slid out onto the floor when she tried to stand. She had been diagnosed with dementia and was on the waiting list for a long-term-care facility, where she seemed likely to live out her remaining days. Instead, 10 weeks later, she was walking and living an active life. Her long-term-care stay had been canceled—her doctors realized that she did not even have dementia!

What changed? A medical team reviewed this woman's case and discovered that she was taking 32 prescription medications each day—and together, the medications that had been prescribed to help this woman instead were ruining her life. The review team gradually eliminated 15 of those drugs and reduced the dosages of several others.

For most, polypharmacy's effects are subtler. And to determine whether it's happening to you, you probably will need to press your doctor or doctors. Most physicians are far more likely to write prescriptions than to review and eliminate them. That's slowly changing, but for now it's up to you to take the lead. *Here's how...*

• **Make a medications list.** It's a good idea to put all your prescription drugs, over-the-counter medications, vitamins and other supplements in a bag and bring them to your doctor and ask for a review. But also bring a list of each of these, including dosages, to help your doctor review them accurately and

quickly. Group drugs together on the list by their purpose—heart drugs, pain drugs, etc.

Call your doctor's attention to medications that are likely to be problematic. *Certain kinds of prescription drugs, if used long term, are particularly likely to cause problems...*

• **Sleeping pills.**

• **Blood sugar drugs** (especially sulfonylurea drugs).

• **Blood pressure drugs** (especially if they lead to low-pressure episodes).

• **Narcotic pain drugs.**

• **Heartburn/GERD drugs** (proton pump inhibitors).

Ask your doctor—or doctors—to review all your medications. You might start a conversation this way—"I read an article about the dangers of polypharmacy, and I want to take a serious look at all of the medications I am taking..." For any particular medication, you might ask, "Is this prescription and dosage a problem to take for as long as I've been on it? Is it appropriate for my age? Could I be on a lower dose?" If you see several specialists, have this conversation with each one.

If you are prescribed medications after a hospital stay, follow up with your own doctor. According to a study of elderly patients discharged from 11 Veterans Affairs medical centers, 44% were prescribed one or more unnecessary drugs.

And even if the medications are appropriate for you at discharge, ask your doctor—or the hospital pharmacist—which ones you can stop taking a few weeks or a month later.

Avoid Future Unnecessary Prescriptions

To reduce your odds of being given unnecessary prescriptions in the first place...

• **If you develop a new health problem, raise the possibility that drugs are causing it.** Ask, "Could this be a side effect of any of the drugs I'm currently taking or the combination of drugs?" It might not be, but you'll ensure that your doctor considers that possibility.

Shorten Your Hospital Stay

Avoiding opioids after major surgery can shorten hospital stays. More than 75% of colorectal-surgery patients who were treated using multidepartment protocols, nerve blocks and carefully managed and administered non-narcotic pain relievers had shorter hospital stays than patients treated with opioids. Key elements included education about pain management before surgery, use of nonopioid general anesthetic during surgery and modified abdominal-nerve blocks. Patients treated with this method—known as Enhanced Recovery After Surgery—averaged 2.3 days in the hospital, compared with 2.7 days for patients treated with opioids.

Sophia A. Horattas, MD, Cleveland Clinic Akron General Hospital, Ohio, and leader of a study presented at the American College of Surgeons Clinical Congress 2018.

Ask the following questions about any new medication—how long should you take it… how will you know whether it's working… and what side effects should you watch for.

Explore lifestyle changes that can reduce the need for certain prescriptions.

Example: Consider relaxation techniques before resorting to sleeping pills. Jot down your questions before you see your doctor.

• **Talk to your pharmacist.** With any new prescription, raise the question of polypharmacy with your pharmacist. If he/she has a concern that your doctor did not bring up, ask him to call your doctor's office to resolve the situation.

Helpful: Use the same pharmacy for all your prescriptions. That increases the odds that the pharmacist will spot potentially problematic drug interactions even before you ask about them.

Be aware of the risks of stopping certain medications too quickly. Discontinuing certain prescription drugs can cause side effects—and some can be dangerous. This is especially true for certain classes of medications including antidepressants, blood pressure drugs called beta-blockers and sleeping pills. But there are others, too. So don't reduce or stop any drug without guidance from your doctor…and if a doctor does recommend ending a drug, ask for detailed instructions on how to do that properly.

A Woman's Guide to Overcoming Opioid Disorder

Leslie A. Hayes, MD, a family medicine practitioner who specializes in women's health and addiction at El Centro Family Health in Española, New Mexico. The study titled, "Women and Opioids: Something Different Is Happening Here," Yale University School of Medicine, published in *The Lancet*.

Opioids are an equal-opportunity health threat, yet women aren't getting their fair share of help to overcome this form of substance abuse. If you're a woman with an opioid addiction (or know someone who is), take these steps now. They could save your life.

Why Women Are at Greater Risk

Many people don't realize that the opioid epidemic is hitting women as hard as it is men, with troubling distinctions. Women are more sensitive to pain than men and, as a result, are more likely to start taking opioids and get hooked on them sooner than men. Women also are prescribed opioid pain pills more often than men are. In addition, women in general have a telescoped course for substance use disorder—with almost every substance, women get more complications sooner.

Women also are more likely than men to receive prescriptions for other medications such as benzodiazepines, tranquilizers with side effects that, when taken along with opioids, dramatically increase the chances of an overdose.

Yet because the "profile" of an overdose victim still is thought of as a young man, women often don't get the help they need in this kind of emergency. For instance, according to a report on opioid-related deaths in Rhode Island, EMTs were three times less likely to administer the overdose antidote *naloxone* (Narcan) to women.

This all translates to an alarming statistic: According to researchers from Yale University, the rate of overdose deaths from opioids among women jumped by 583 percent from 1999 to 2016 compared with a 404 percent increase among men over the same period—that means, women accounted for 50% more deaths than men.

How to Help Yourself Now

Take the following steps to save your life…

• **Don't wait any longer to get help for addiction.** Because of responsibilities at home and at work, many women wait too long to seek treatment for opioid abuse—well after they acknowledge that they have a problem. Every three minutes, a woman in the US arrives at an emergency room for prescription painkiller misuse or abuse. Don't put off getting treatment.

• **Choose a treatment program sensitive to the needs of women.** Look for a program that offers *Seeking Safety* with a trauma-based approach. It is not designed specifically for women, but since so many women with opioid use disorder have a history of trauma, it is a good option. Effective treatment often combines medical-assisted therapy with counseling. Ask your doctor or therapist for a recommendation if you're having trouble finding one on your own.

• **Keep lifesaving naloxone in your home.** Given as an injection or nasal spray, *naloxone* (Narcan) can reverse an opioid overdose. It's available in many states without a prescription at most major pharmacies. Everyone in the house should know where it is and how to use it.

Important: It does not replace getting immediate medical attention—call 911 right after using it.

Note: If you're still experiencing the condition that first led you to opioids, work with your doctor to control it, ask about alternative medications and consider other steps to conquer pain.

How to Get Off Dangerous Heartburn Drugs

Gregory P. Gaspard, MD, assistant professor of medicine at Tulane School of Medicine in New Orleans. He routinely works with his reflux patients to reduce or eliminate PPI usage.

If you've been taking a proton-pump inhibitor (PPI) to relieve heartburn/reflux symptoms for more than two weeks, it's time for an exit strategy.

Here's why: Chronic use of these over-the-counter acid-suppression drugs increases long-term health risks such as hip fractures and may increase risk for dementia and heart attacks. They are sold under the brand names Zegerid, Prilosec, Prevacid, Protonix, Nexium, AcipHex and Dexilant.

Here's the rub: Just stopping these pills abruptly often leads to hypersecretion, an increase in stomach acid that can make symptoms worse. Fortunately, there are research-backed ways to minimize this. No approach is perfect, but one of these methods can get you past the first few days or weeks until the hypersecretion wanes.

Cut your dose in half. Doing so has been shown to be highly unlikely to lead to a relapse in symptoms.

Example: If you're taking Nexium, step down from the 40-milligram (mg) pill to the 20-mg pill.

Downside: You're only reducing the long-term risks, but it's an easy first step.

Take a PPI only when you need one. Many people think that they need to take a PPI every day for it to work, but that's not true.

Downside: You'll still experience symptoms when you have a GERD episode until the PPI kicks in, but this is a safer way to use PPIs.

Switch to a different heartburn medication. These include "H2 blockers," sold under the brand names Pepcid, Tagamet, Axid and Zantac. Even plain old antacids can help.

Downside: You still may experience some symptoms.

Meanwhile, make lifestyle changes to minimize the need for medications. Avoid trigger foods…don't eat late at night…and, most effective of all, lose weight if need be (dropping 10 to 15 pounds often makes a huge difference). After you eat, don't lie down for a few hours. If you have night symptoms, elevate your head in bed by raising the head of the bed (put something under the bed's feet) or by using a reflux wedge pillow.

Important: Long-term PPI use may be appropriate for some patients with a significantly inflamed esophagus (esophagitis) as diagnosed by endoscopy…and patients with Barrett's esophagus, a potentially precancerous condition that can be brought on by chronic reflux (GERD). If you have severe GERD symptoms, see your doctor to make sure that you don't have one of these conditions.

Don't Miss a Drug Recall

Jack E. Fincham, PhD, RPh, professor of pharmaceutical and administrative sciences, Presbyterian College School of Pharmacy, Clinton, South Carolina.

If you take prescription medication—especially if it's for high blood pressure or heart problems—listen up!

The FDA recently announced a series of recalls for several lots of blood pressure medications that contain losartan, valsartan or irbesartan after tests found contamination with a suspected cancer-causing chemical.

Not all drug labels include lot numbers (used by pharmaceutical manufacturers to track medications). So anyone taking one of these medications should ask his/her pharmacist if the dispensed generic prescription drug is manufactured by one of the companies cited in the recalls.

Important: Don't stop this—or any—medication without checking with your doctor. The risk of stopping a drug cold turkey could be worse than the risk from any possible impurities it contains. *Also…*

• **Ask your pharmacist about the manufacturer of any drug you're taking.** If there's any question about the manufacturer's track record, ask the pharmacist to get the drug from a different manufacturer.

• **Search for drug recalls.** Go to the FDA website, FDA.gov, and enter a medication name in the search field to see if a drug you're taking has been recalled.

• **Sign up for e-mail alerts at FDA.gov/ safety/recalls.** The e-mails provide the latest recall information about drugs and other FDA-regulated products.

Medical Travel Companions Available

Medical travel companions can help people with health issues handle airports, flights and safe arrival at their destinations. Travel Care & Logistics (YourFlightNurse. com) provides trained medical companions and can help arrange for a caregiver throughout someone's entire out-of-town trip. Other firms offer door-to-door nonmedical assistance—Consider Flying Companions (FlyingCompanions.com)…Travel Helpers (GoTravel Helpers.com)…FirstLight Home Care (First LightHomeCare.com). All services are expensive, requiring purchase of an extra ticket for the companion, plus all of that person's expenses, plus a fee to the service provider. Be sure to ask exactly what each service's personnel can and cannot do.

Kiplinger's Retirement Report.

Chapter 8

HEART HEALTH FOR WOMEN

Avoid These Heart Attack Traps

The message is finally sinking in—men are not the only ones who have heart attacks.

However: Common medical mistakes are putting millions of middle-aged and older women at risk for a heart attack, the number-one killer of American women, with nearly 300,000 deaths every year.

To find out what women can do to protect themselves, we spoke with C. Noel Bairey Merz, MD, a renowned women's heart specialist.

An Overlooked Problem

A common scenario illustrates the problem women face. Let's say a woman sees a doctor and complains about persistent chest pain. The doctor orders an angiogram, a test that detects the plaque in the major arteries of the heart that can decrease or stop blood flow, triggering a heart attack. But the angiogram shows no blockages, so the doctor tells the woman she doesn't have heart disease. A week later, she has a heart attack.

Many women experience angina, which is marked by frequent and intense chest pain, even when they do not have blockages in the major arteries of the heart—the leading cause of heart attack in men. In women, the pain also can be caused by coronary microvascular dysfunction in the tiny arteries around the heart.

This condition poses a similar threat to a woman's heart as a blockage in the major arteries. But standard heart tests—such as an angiogram or an electrocardiogram (which detects abnormal heart rhythms and poor blood flow)—don't detect coronary microvascular dysfunction.

Troubling recent finding: Researchers from the Barbra Streisand Women's Heart Center, Smidt Heart Institute at Cedars-Sinai in Los Angeles asked 340 women who complained of chest pain but had no blockages in major coronary arteries to have a cardiac MRI, a highly detailed imaging scan of the heart. According to the research, the MRI found nearly one in 10 (8%) of the women

C. Noel Bairey Merz, MD, director of the Barbra Streisand Women's Heart Center, Linda Joy Pollin Women's Heart Health Program and Preventive and Rehabilitative Cardiac Center at the Smidt Heart Institute, all at Cedars-Sinai Medical Center, Los Angeles. She also is professor of medicine at Cedars-Sinai and chair of the National Institutes of Health–sponsored Women's Ischemia Syndrome Evaluation (WISE) initiative, which is investigating methods for more effective diagnosis and evaluation of coronary artery disease in women.

had already suffered a heart attack—in most cases, previously undetected.

Other sobering research: In a study conducted by researchers at the Yale School of Public Health, 62% of women having a heart attack were found to have three or more non–chest pain symptoms (see list at end of article)—and more than half of those women said their health-care provider did not think the symptoms were heart-related.

7-Step Plan

Because women with heart disease are routinely undertreated, it's crucial to develop a strategy to effectively diagnose the condition—and, if it's present, to effectively treat it. To do this, partner with your physician. Here's what you need to know…

STEP #1: **Take heart disease seriously.** It kills more women than any other disease—more women than all cancers combined. If you've got one or more risk factors for heart disease, ask your primary care physician for a cardiovascular workup (see below). Those risk factors include high blood pressure, high LDL cholesterol, smoking, excess body weight, a sedentary lifestyle, a poor diet (one that emphasizes sugary, fatty processed foods) and a family history of heart disease.

STEP #2: **Get a second opinion.** Perhaps your physician has conducted tests and told you that you don't have heart disease—but you have symptoms that make you suspect you do, such as shortness of breath or unexplained chest pain or pressure. Get a second opinion from a doctor who will listen to your concerns. It could be an internist or a cardiologist. Second opinions are covered by most health insurance and—given the seriousness of heart disease—it's a prudent action.

STEP #3: **Get the right stress test.** If your risk factors put you at high risk for heart disease, your doctor may order a stress test, also called a treadmill test, exercise electrocardiogram, graded exercise test or stress electrocardiogram. This test—in which you exercise at increasingly intense levels while hooked up to electrodes that measure the electrical

activity of your heart—determines blood flow to your heart and can detect abnormal heart rhythms.

Other options include a stress echocardiogram or nuclear stress test, both of which also generate images of the heart and can more accurately determine blood flow…and the dobutamine or adenosine stress test, a drug-based test used in people who are unable to exercise. If you have any questions about the right stress test for you, consult a cardiologist.

STEP #4: **Ask about a stress cardiac MRI or cardiac PET scan.** These tests have become more widely available only in the last 10 years. They are more sensitive, so they improve the detection of more subtle and female-pattern abnormalities in smaller hearts—which means they help women more than men. Either test would be particularly important in women with persistent chest pain and an abnormal stress test.

STEP #5: **If you're having unexplained heart symptoms, ask your doctor to investigate less common forms of heart disease.** One uncommon condition is spontaneous coronary artery dissection, a tear in the artery wall. This condition, which can lead to heart attack, is more often detected in younger women (half the time during or shortly after pregnancy), who have symptoms such as unexplained chest pain.

The other is stress-related cardiomyopathy (also known as "broken heart syndrome"), which can cause chest pain and shortness of breath. It is caused by severe mental stress or shock, such as the death of a spouse, or a near-miss automobile accident. The condition is usually treatable, and most patients recover, although recurrence can happen in 5% to 10% of cases.

STEP #6: **Demand standard therapy.** Studies show that women with diagnosed heart disease are significantly less likely than men to be treated with standard therapy. If you've been diagnosed with heart disease, talk to your physician about lifestyle changes (including smoking cessation, diet and exercise), along with the drugs you may need—

such as low-dose (81 mg) aspirin to prevent artery-clogging blood clots, a statin to lower high cholesterol and medication to reduce blood pressure.

STEP #7: **Go to the ER.** If you're having any of the symptoms of a heart attack that are common in women (see below), the emergency room is where you belong. And once you're there, don't let anyone tell you that you're not having a heart attack. Instead, insist on getting the troponin test, which detects protein in the blood generated by damaged heart cells…in other words, by a heart attack. This simple test—a sample of blood is all that's required—generates results in 15 to 20 minutes and provides incontrovertible evidence as to whether you are or aren't having a heart attack.

Important: Call 911 instead of driving yourself, and take a low-dose aspirin if you suspect that you are having a heart attack.

More from Dr. Bairey Merz…

Red Flags Women Should Watch For

Most women who are having a heart attack don't experience crushing chest pain, the "classic" heart attack symptom found in most men. *Instead, a woman might have…*

- **Sharp or burning pain or pressure in the chest.**
- **Pain or pressure in the neck, jaw, throat, abdomen or upper back.**
- **Shortness of breath.**
- **Indigestion and heartburn.**
- **Nausea and vomiting.**
- **Extreme fatigue.**
- **General upper-body discomfort.**

Doctors frequently fail to recognize these symptoms as red flags for heart attack. The result—heart disease and heart attacks are often misdiagnosed in women.

Don't Hesitate to Call an Ambulance for Yourself

Findings from the Polish Registry of Acute Coronary Syndromes (PL-ACS) presented at Acute Cardiovascular Care 2019, a European Society of Cardiology (ESC) congress.

The classic image of a heart attack victim is a man clutching his chest. Of course, women can be affected, too. In fact, more women than men die of heart disease each year in the US.

Now: New research shows that women who suffer heart attacks may be undermining their own survival, in part, because they are reluctant to call an ambulance for themselves. By underestimating the seriousness of their own symptoms—and prioritizing other people's needs—women could be depriving themselves of possibly lifesaving treatment.

Study details: In research presented at an Acute Cardiovascular Care conference of the European Society of Cardiology in Malaga, Spain, researchers tracked 7,582 men and women who suffered a heart attack caused by a major artery blockage. When treating this type of heart attack, known as an ST-elevation myocardial infarction (STEMI), the goal is to resolve the blockage as promptly as possible—restored blood flow means less heart tissue death…a lower risk for future heart failure…and a lower overall risk for death.

It's recommended that treatment (opening the blocked artery with a stent) begin within 90 minutes of diagnosis. The quickest way to diagnose a heart attack is via an electrocardiogram (ECG) that is administered in an ambulance as the patient is being transported to a hospital. In this study, 45% of patients were treated within that crucial 90-minute window, but fewer of them were women (41% compared with 47% of men).

The research also showed a disparity in the use of ECG during the ambulance transport. While 40% of men of all ages received an ECG, on average, only 34% of women age 54 and under got tested in the ambulance (45% of women age 75 and older were tested).

The treatment delay in women was due, in part, to women hesitating to call an ambulance for themselves, according to the researchers. Women put off making that call because they believed they minimized the seriousness of their symptoms and/or had too many responsibilities, including their work and child-care duties. The researchers noted that this is especially true of younger women (under age 55).

"In addition to running the household, women make sure that male relatives receive urgent medical help when needed," said research coordinator Marek Gierlotka, MD, PhD, associate professor of cardiology at the University of Opole, Poland. "It is time for women to take care of themselves, too." Even though the study was conducted in Poland, the researchers believe that the findings are likely to apply to women living in other countries.

Women may also fail to recognize their own symptoms as those of a heart attack. Chest pain and tingling in the left arm are the classic symptoms, but they may have pain elsewhere, such as the back, shoulder or stomach.

Takeaway: Don't wait! Call 911 if you or anyone around you experiences possible heart attack symptoms, such as pain in the chest, but also in the jaw, throat, neck, shoulders, back or stomach for 15 minutes or longer. Fast treatment benefits both sexes equally.

Think You're Having a Heart Attack? How Chest Pain Is Evaluated in the ER

Case study titled, "Improving Emergency Department Care for Low-Risk Chest Pain" by researchers at Kaiser Permanente Southern California and Oregon Health and Sciences University, published in *New England Journal of Medicine Catalyst*.

Chest pain is the number-two reason people go to the emergency department (stomach pain is number one).

While the vast majority of patients are not having a heart attack, the process for ruling out a heart attack can involve extensive testing and a hospital stay. But there's a better approach now gaining traction in the US—one that was developed more than a decade ago in the Netherlands...

The "Heart" of the Matter

For some patients, symptoms along with results from blood tests and an electrocardiogram (EKG) provide indisputable proof that a heart attack has occurred or is occurring. But, for many others, these first tests are inconclusive. It's then up to the ER doctor to make a judgment call about next steps to further investigate what's then termed "low-risk chest pain."

In the US, most patients with low-risk chest pain wind up being admitted to the hospital for observation and further testing, such as a cardiac stress test, to be certain that a heart attack wasn't missed. Yet the "miss rate," or amount of heart attacks that were missed, is just 2.1% of these patients. That means that nearly all of them are having unnecessary and expensive procedures.

As hospitals try to use evidence-based guidelines to improve cost and quality of care, some emergency departments are starting to use the Dutch-developed 10-point scoring system called HEART, an evidence-based, decision-making tool designed to reduce miss rates and unnecessary admissions. HEART is an acronym for the five markers that are evaluated—history, EKG, age, risk factors and troponin.

This is how the scoring works...

History: Patients are given 2 points if they have high-risk symptoms such as heavy chest pain, sweating, nausea and vomiting, relief after taking nitroglycerin or pain that gets worse with exertion...1 point if the chest pain is sharp rather than heavy and is not accompanied by other symptoms...and 0 if symptoms are mostly low-risk for heart attack.

EKG: Patients are given 2 points if they have signs of decreased blood flow and other changes…1 point if there are EKG changes that are not specifically indicative of heart disease…and 0 if normal.

Age: Patients are given 2 points if 65 or older…1 point if between 45 to 64…and 0 if under 45.

Risk factors: Patients are given 2 points if they have a history of coronary heart disease, peripheral artery disease, stroke or three or more heart attack risk factors such as obesity, diabetes, high blood pressure, high cholesterol or a family history of heart disease…1 point for one or two of these risk factors…and 0 for no risk factors.

Troponin: Troponin, a protein involved in muscle contraction, is measured with a blood test. It can signal heart muscle damage. Patients are given 2 points for a high troponin level…1 point if it is borderline…and 0 if it is within the normal range.

A score that totals 0 to 3 means there's low risk for heart attack, and patients are likely to be sent home and told to follow up with their primary care provider.

A score of 4 to 6 signals moderate risk, and patients will be admitted for observation and possible cardiac stress testing.

A score of 7 to 10 is high risk, and these patients are admitted to the hospital and referred to a cardiologist for treatment.

The US Gets Heart Smart

While there have been a few other scoring systems available to doctors, international studies have consistently shown that HEART outperforms them all.

Kaiser Permanente Southern California, a large health-care organization, decided to adopt HEART at 14 of its area hospitals and review the results. An analysis of all 12,000 patients given HEART scoring found that, rather than the expected 2.1% miss rate, it was just 0.18%. (A "miss" is defined as any patient sent home without a diagnosis of heart attack and who went on to have a heart event in the following 30 days.) Drilling down even further, among the subgroup of patients with low HEART scores who were sent home with-

out a hospital admission, the miss rate was only 0.09%. The results were so positive that Kaiser Permanente plans to adopt the system in other areas of the country that it serves. It may be coming to an ER near you.

Important: If you experience chest pain, always assume it's medical emergency and call 911. Don't try to diagnose yourself with HEART or any other system, and never drive yourself to the ER.

Women More Likely to Die

Women are more likely to die in the year after a heart attack occurs than men. The death risk for these women is 60% higher than the risk for men. After the first year, death rates for men and women are the same.

Georg Schmidt, MD, professor of cardiology, Technical University of Munich, Germany, and leader of a study published in *PLOS ONE*.

The Overlooked Heart Danger for Women

Erin D. Michos, MD, MHS, associate director of preventive cardiology at Johns Hopkins Ciccarone Center for the Prevention of Heart Disease and associate professor of medicine at Johns Hopkins Medicine, both in Baltimore.

When it comes to women's equality, this type is not a good development. Women are having heart attacks at younger and younger ages—putting their heart attack risk closer to that of men. In fact, nearly one-third of the women in the US who have heart attacks are now between 35 and 54 years old.

On top of that—perhaps because women traditionally have not had heart attacks as frequently or as young as men have—the level of care given to women having heart attacks is not as good as the care given to men. According to research published in *Journal of the American Heart Association*, women get neither the correct diagnostic tests nor the needed lifesaving drugs as often as men do. Women also experience delays in treatment in the emergency department compared with men, waiting, on average, an extra 13 minutes...when every minute counts.

To protect yourself (or a loved one who is a woman), understand that women are just as vulnerable to heart disease as men...but women's heart attack symptoms often are not as obvious as men's. Women's symptoms more often include a cold sweat, nausea, vomiting, fatigue or pain in the arm, back, neck or jaw and not necessarily the gripping chest pain that men tend to get. Don't let fear of embarrassment if it turns out to be a false alarm or any other reason keep you from calling 911 if you experience such symptoms. Another dangerous statistic: Compared with men, an extra 27 minutes elapse, on average, before women having heart attacks even get to the emergency department. So do everything you can to get there, and insist on appropriate testing and medications. Afterward, if you're prescribed drugs, make sure you take them—women are less likely than men to do so.

Little-Known Heart Disease Risk Factors

Being *short:* Genes determining height also are associated with cardiac risk factors. *Living near noisy roads:* Heavily trafficked roads raise air pollution nearby, and this can make heart conditions worse. *Pessimism:* It is associated with depression, which, if untreated, is linked to heart disease. *Living at sea level:* Those living at higher altitudes, where there is less oxygen, appear to have better-functioning lungs and cardiovascular systems. *Failing to eat breakfast:* Consuming a morning meal regularly is associated with lower rates of heart disease.

Not getting a flu shot: Heart attack risk is six times greater in the week after infection with influenza virus than in the year before or after—the shot may prevent the infection.

Roundup of experts on heart attack risk factors, reported at BHF.org.uk and Health.com.

6 Heart Disease Prevention Myths: About Aspirin, Omega-3s, Statins and More

Erin D. Michos, MD, MHS, associate director of preventive cardiology at Ciccarone Center for the Prevention of Heart Disease at The Johns Hopkins University School of Medicine in Baltimore.

Heart disease remains the number-one killer of both men and women in the US today, so prevention is paramount. But conflicting news stories make it tough to figure out what to do. Should you take a baby aspirin...a fish oil supplement...a statin? Since everyone is different, is the risk for some people actually overblown? *Here's what's true about preventing heart disease... what's false...and how to know what you should do...*

MYTH: A baby aspirin a day keeps heart disease away. A number of recent studies conducted at major medical research institutions have confirmed that most healthy people without known heart disease shouldn't be taking daily aspirin to prevent heart attacks. The ARRIVE trial looked at more than 12,500 men (age 55 or older) and women (age 60 or older) who were at moderate risk for heart attack, while the ASPREE study included more than 19,000 healthy, low-risk adults over age 65. Both studies were designed to determine whether a daily low-dose aspirin would prevent a first heart attack or stroke. Not only did the low-dose aspirin not reduce that risk in either study—it also increased the risk for major gastrointestinal bleeding. Even more alarming, in ASPREE, the group randomly assigned to take aspirin experienced more deaths from cancer.

Important: Aspirin still is recommended for patients who have had a heart attack already to prevent a second one. But if you're healthy and popping a daily aspirin, my advice is to ask your doctor about stopping your aspirin.

MYTH: Over-the-counter omega-3 supplements prevent heart disease. A recent review of major studies found that over-the-counter supplements did not reduce the risk for heart disease or stroke in the general population.

But one type of high-dose omega-3 prescription drug may help certain patients.

New research: The REDUCE-IT trial, conducted at Harvard Medical School, studied Vascepa, a purified form of eicosapentaenoic acid (EPA) given in a high dose (4,000 mg) to patients already treated with statins who were at high risk for cardiovascular disease or diabetes and who had high triglyceride levels. In early results, Vascepa reduced cardiovascular events such as heart attacks and strokes by 25% over five years. (The full results will be presented at the American Heart Association annual meeting in November 2018.) While this may turn out to be an effective prescription for certain patients, these results shouldn't prompt healthy people to take over-the-counter fish oil supplements.

MYTH: The higher your level of HDL "good" cholesterol, the more protected you are from heart disease. HDL is the so-called "good" cholesterol because it helps remove "bad" LDL cholesterol from your bloodstream. And studies have found that people with high HDL seem to have lower risk for heart disease. But new research casts doubt on whether it's truly protective.

Example: No drug therapies that boost HDL have been shown to reduce heart disease risk.

And too high a level of HDL actually may be harmful. Two recent studies have shown an association between very high levels of HDL (above 80 mg/dL) and increased heart attacks and death from all causes. We don't

Heart Disease and...

...Parkinson's Disease

About 60% of people with Parkinson's experience serious damage to nerve connections in the heart—before they develop tremors or other symptoms of the neurological disorder. Imaging tests called radioligand scans could detect heart damage and allow treatment at an earlier stage, and possibly offer earlier diagnosis of Parkinson's.

University of Wisconsin-Madison.

...Type 2 Diabetes

New heart risk found in people with type 2 diabetes.

Recent study: Researchers analyzed data from two studies, one done in Scotland and the other in Spain. Despite the different lifestyles and diets of the two groups, participants from the two countries shared a common trait—those with type 2 diabetes and low iron had a 217% greater risk of developing heart disease than those with normal iron levels. Taking steps to prevent iron deficiency, especially if you have diabetes, could benefit your heart.

Milton Fabian Suárez-Ortegón, PhD, Usher Institute of Population Health Sciences and Informatics, University of Edinburgh, Scotland, UK.

know why this is, but it may be that very high HDL indicates that your HDL is not functioning properly. Until more is known, focus on the heart disease risks that you can control, such as increasing physical activity, optimizing body weight and keeping triglycerides, LDL cholesterol, blood pressure and blood sugar under control.

MYTH: If your cholesterol is too high, you need a statin. Actually, some people with high cholesterol don't benefit from a statin—and some people with low cholesterol actually do. While high cholesterol, especially "bad" LDL cholesterol, is a major risk factor for heart disease, it's not the whole story. Many other factors matter—age, gender, race, blood pressure, family history and whether you smoke, have diabetes or are sedentary. So doctors evaluate your overall risk factors for heart disease to help determine whether to treat you with a statin. They do so by calculating your 10-year risk of having a heart attack or stroke. A score of 7.5% or higher means that a statin is "recommended"—whatever your cholesterol number.

Even if your score is 7.5% or higher, however, you still may not need a statin. Why? The calculator, developed by the American Heart Association and the American College of Cardiology, may overestimate risk, some studies find.

What to do: If your score is high, ask your doctor about a coronary artery calcium (CAC) scan, which detects calcium deposits in arterial plaque. If your CAC score is zero, there's no need for a statin. If it's high (typically 101 or above), that means you have a high risk for heart disease, and a statin generally is recommended. What if it's in the middle, between one and 100? That's a decision to make with your doctor, considering your other risk factors—along with your personal preference about whether you want to start taking a statin.

MYTH: Reducing inflammation is a healthy goal, but we don't know whether it will reduce heart disease risk. Actually, we do. Cardiologists have suspected for some time that chronic inflammation—a state in which your immune system is in overdrive—can fuel the development of clogged arteries (atherosclerosis)...and trigger plaque to rupture and cause a heart attack. But we didn't know until recently whether tamping down inflammation could really help prevent heart attacks and strokes.

Now we know that it can. Last year, the CANTOS study, conducted at Brigham and Women's Hospital in Boston, showed that *canakinumab*, a type of drug called a monoclonal antibody that reduces inflammation, reduces the risk for a new heart attack or stroke by a significant 15% in people who already have had a heart attack.

While the drug still is experimental (and likely will be very expensive if/when it's FDA-approved), the good news is that we already know how to substantially reduce chronic inflammation with healthy habits. These include not smoking...keeping your waist size no more than 40 inches for men and 35 inches for women, regardless of your body weight...eating a Mediterranean-type diet...exercising regularly...getting six to eight hours of sleep every night (the sweet spot for heart health)...and reducing stress (meditation, yoga).

MYTH: Unless I have diabetes, my blood sugar levels won't affect heart health. Blood sugar that's consistently even just a little above normal means that you have prediabetes. As a result, you're not only at greatly increased risk for diabetes but also heart disease. It's a wake-up call to improve your lifestyle, including weight loss (often losing 10 pounds is enough to bring blood sugar back to normal)...increasing dietary fiber...eliminating sugar-sweetened drinks and processed meats...and exercising. Simply by taking a 30-minute daily walk, you can reduce the risk that prediabetes will turn into diabetes by 30%.

Is High HDL Cholesterol Always Good?

Michael D. Ozner, MD, medical director Center for Prevention and Wellness, Baptist Health South Florida, Miami, and author of *Heart Attack Proof* and *The Complete Mediterranean Diet*.

The thinking on high-density lipoprotein (HDL) cholesterol has recently undergone a dramatic shift. HDL has traditionally been known as the "good" cholesterol. That's because it generally carries harmful fats in the artery wall to the liver for processing.

Women have been told to aim for an HDL level of at least 50 mg/dL because lower levels are linked to a higher risk for cardiovascular disease (CVD). (In men, a level of 40 mg/dL or below is associated with increased odds of developing CVD).

Once a patient has met the minimum threshold for HDL, doctors have long-assumed that the higher the level of this cholesterol, the better.

However, scientists have now learned that the function of HDL is more important than the level of HDL. In fact, high HDL levels may not always help protect against CVD.

Here's why: As more has been discovered about the structure and function of HDL, it's become clear that HDL can be either helpful by playing an anti-inflammatory/antioxidant role…or harmful by possibly promoting inflammation and oxidation. In addition, the ability of HDL to remove cholesterol from the artery wall can be variable. Research conducted by scientists at the University of Copenhagen, published in the *European Heart Journal*, shows this dichotomy.

In the study, which analyzed health records for 116,000 adults, the researchers found that women with extremely high levels of HDL had a 68% higher risk of dying during the six-year study period than those with normal levels…for men, extremely high HDL was linked to a 106% higher risk for death.

Also, while epidemiology research confirmed the well-established risk for extremely low levels of HDL, the risk or benefit of HDL is dependent on HDL function rather than absolute levels.

So how can you tell what your HDL level means? When looking at one's risk for CVD, the key is to remember that your HDL level is only one way that doctors assess this. More important are your levels of low-density lipoprotein (LDL) cholesterol, the so-called the "bad" cholesterol, and blood fats known as triglycerides—both of which must also be factored into your CVD risk profile.

While most guidelines recommend an LDL level of less than 100 mg/dL, clinical studies show that optimal levels are below 70 mg/dL. The optimal level for triglycerides is less than 100 mg/dL. Your level of the inflammation marker C-reactive protein (CRP) is also helpful in assessing your risk for CVD—2 mg/L or above is associated with increased odds of having a heart attack or stroke.

What I also recommend: A test for a key protein known as apolipoprotein-B (Apo-B). It appears on the surface of all cholesterol particles that can enter the artery walls and potentially lead to dangerous plaque buildup. Patients should aim for an optimal level of less than 60 mg/dL. A high apoB level more accurately predicts CVD risk than elevated LDL levels. You can ask for this test along with your standard lipid panel. Some health insurers will cover the cost.

Bottom line: Especially if you have risk factors for CVD, such as high blood pressure, diabetes and/or a family history of early heart disease, talk to your doctor about the best tests to monitor your levels of cholesterol and other lipid levels.

It's wise for everyone to follow well-established heart-healthy habits to keep CVD risk in check. Eat a healthful diet, such as a Mediterranean-style plan with lots of fruits, vegetables, fatty fish and whole grains…exercise for at least 30 minutes on most days…maintain normal body weight…avoid smoking…manage stress…and get good-quality sleep.

Depending on your overall risk for CVD, you may also require medication, including a statin and/or newer types of lipid-lowering drugs such as cholesterol absorption inhibitors—for example, *ezetimibe* (Zetia)—and PCSK9 inhibitors, such as *alirocumab* (Praluent) or *evolocumab* (Repatha).

Seed Oils Lower Cholesterol

In a recent meta-analysis that ranked fats, including oils, for their effectiveness at controlling blood lipids, sunflower, rapeseed, safflower and flaxseed oils did the best job at controlling LDL "bad" cholesterol. Olive oil, a staple of the heart-healthy Mediterranean diet, came in at the middle of the pack.

Lukas Schwingshackl, PhD, postdoctoral researcher, department of epidemiology, German Institute of Human Nutrition, Potsdam-Rehbruecke, Nuthetal, Germany.

The Heart Tests You Really Need—It's Not Cholesterol

Andrew Rubman, ND, founder and medical director, Southbury Clinic for Traditional Medicines, Southbury, Connecticut. He writes the Bottom Line blog "Nature Doc's Patient Diary." SouthburyClinic.com

When you think about your heart health, you probably think of your cholesterol numbers…and maybe whether your "good" cholesterol (the HDL kind) outweighs your "bad" cholesterol (the LDL kind). However, the trouble with just knowing the numbers from standard cholesterol tests is that they don't tell enough about your risk for heart attack or stroke. To get a better picture, you need more.

What's wrong with the cholesterol tests we've all come to know and trust? To better understand, it helps to know what cholesterol is and does. Cholesterol is a waxy, fatty substance produced in the liver (small amounts come from diet) and found in every cell. Among other functions, it is the prime material the body uses to make sex and adrenal hormones. Cholesterol circulates to and from cells via the bloodstream by combining with protein to form lipoproteins—hence, high-density lipoprotein (HDL) and low-density lipoprotein (LDL).

It might be helpful to picture this protein as a truck and the cholesterol as its load. With HDL, the load is light, so the "truck" can pick up (scavenge) more cholesterol from arteries on its way back to the liver—why it's called "good." With LDL, the load is heavy—so cholesterol tends to be dropped off along the way as plaque on artery walls, clogging arteries.

The problem: The numbers you get from traditional cholesterol tests tell only how much cholesterol is circulating in your blood. They don't tell whether cholesterol is being deposited on your artery walls, which is the real danger. This is why some people with perfectly fine blood cholesterol numbers turn out to have serious heart disease (sometimes discovered too late)…and why some people with what look like alarming blood cholesterol numbers are not developing heart disease. The "enabler" of cholesterol-clogged arteries is inflammation. Inflammation roughs up the surface of artery walls, causing cholesterol to stick. Without inflammation, the surface of arteries remains smooth…and cholesterol has a better chance of flowing by without depositing plaque.

Because of these limitations of traditional cholesterol blood tests, many health-care professionals are turning to other tests that give a more comprehensive picture of heart health—including whether inflammation is a problem. These cardio tests are not part of a standard checkup, so you may need to ask your doctor for them specifically. While many labs do cardiovascular testing, the panel of tests that I find most useful are done by Boston Heart Diagnostics in Framingham, Massachusetts, who also provide an interpretation of the results and suggestions for treatment strategies based on overall results.

Note: To order the tests from Boston Heart Diagnostics, your doctor will need to register with the lab first. The tests are also available from other labs, but the names of the tests may be different—your doctor will know which tests to order from the descriptions in this article. The tests may be covered by your insurance carrier, whether you have them done by Boston Heart Diagnostics or another lab, but check first whether you need preapproval.

The Boston Heart Diagnostics tests include…

•**Test for fatty-acid balance.** The balance of fatty acids, such as omega-3 and omega-6, affects cholesterol and triglyceride (blood fat) levels and is important for heart health. The typical US diet tips toward too much omega-

6 and not enough omega-3—an imbalance that contributes to inflammation and sets the stage for plaque depositing in arteries. This test shows whether dietary adjustments are needed to improve fatty-acid balance.

• **Statin-induced myopathy genotype test.** Statin drugs, prescribed to reduce LDL cholesterol, sometimes cause statin-induced myopathy—muscle aches, cramps and in rare cases a life-threatening condition of severe muscle breakdown called rhabdomyolysis. This test looks for a gene that increases the risk of statin-induced myopathy by up to 17-fold.

• **Prediabetes Assessment.** This assessment uses a patient's blood glucose level along with height, weight and certain medical history information to predict the patient's 10-year risk for developing type 2 diabetes. Since diabetes is a direct contributor to heart disease and inflammation, identifying a patient's diabetes risk (and reducing it if necessary) is an important part of protecting heart health.

• **HDL Map Test.** HDL is not all "good"—there's a kind of HDL called apoA-1 that is associated with lower cardiovascular disease risk and a kind of HDL called prebeta-1 that is associated with higher cardiovascular risk. Knowing the balance of these HDL subgroups is one of the best predictors of whether plaque is depositing in arteries. This test helps estimate disease risk far better than knowing just the total HDL number…and helps doctor and patient determine a treatment strategy and track how well it's working.

• **Test for cholesterol balance.** This measures markers of LDL cholesterol that can determine whether cholesterol-lowering drugs are likely to be effective for the patient.

The results from these tests give you and your doctor a detailed picture of the current state of your cardiovascular health. The results also can help your doctor decide whether further testing, such as a coronary artery calcium scan or a test for C-reactive protein (CRP), might be appropriate…and if treatment is needed, what options, including medication and lifestyle changes, are most likely to work for your health profile and physiology.

Statins for Older Folk

Statins do not prevent heart disease in healthy people over age 75. They do reduce cardiovascular disease and death from any cause in older people with heart disease or type 2 diabetes. But they are not effective for primary prevention—reducing the risk for a first heart attack in healthy older adults.

Study by researchers at Jordi Gol Institute for Research in Primary Care, Barcelona, and Girona Biomedical Research Institute, Girona, Spain, published in *The BMJ*.

Turn Up Your Thermostat

For every one-degree decrease in indoor temperature reading, there was a 0.48 point rise in systolic (top number) blood pressure readings and a 0.45 point rise in diastolic (bottom number). This study, based on nearly 5,000 people in their homes, may help explain the spike in hypertension rates in the winter.

To help prevent winter increases in blood pressure: Keep the inside of your home at a minimum temperature of 69.8°F, particularly if you have hypertension or a family history of heart disease.

Stephen Jivraj, PhD, associate professor in quantitative science, epidemiology and public health, University College London, UK.

Clean Air Reduces Blood Pressure

Car exhaust, fires and cigarette smoke are harmful pollutants in our outdoor and indoor air. In a study of 40 older adults living in urban areas, exposure to indoor air pollution was reduced by 40%—and systolic (top number) blood pressure dropped 3.4 points—after only three days of using a true HEPA or HEPA-type air purifier. The air purifiers used in the study are available in home stores for as little as $70.

Masako Morishita, PhD, associate professor of family medicine, Michigan State University, East Lansing.

Dietary Supplements Can Affect Blood Pressure

Andrew Rubman, ND, founder and medical director, Southbury Clinic for Traditional Medicines, Southbury, Connecticut. SouthburyClinic.com

Seasoning your food with herbs and spices generally doesn't have much effect on blood pressure. But the concentrated forms of herbs used in supplements can raise blood pressure...or lower it. It depends on what supplements you're using.

Among the herbal supplements that can raise blood pressure are...

•**Licorice,** found in formulas to relieve indigestion, heartburn, menstrual disorders, canker sores, cold symptoms and sore throat, among others. This refers to whole licorice. There's another form, called deglycyrrhizinated licorice, that is less likely to raise blood pressure for most people (some people may be sensitive even to the DGL form of licorice).

•**Bitter orange,** used in weight-loss formulas and, ironically, also to improve appetite...and used for upset stomach, constipation, diarrhea, intestinal gas, nasal congestion and chronic fatigue syndrome. While generally safe in foods and beverages, bitter orange can cause potentially severe adverse cardiovascular effects in some people.

•**Ginkgo biloba,** found in supplements to improve memory, cognition, anxiety, cardiovascular function and eye health.

•**Senna,** used as a natural laxative and in supplements for irritable bowel syndrome (IBS), hemorrhoids and weight loss and used as a bowel prep before colonoscopy.

•**Guarana,** used in supplements for weight loss and to enhance athletic performance, reduce mental and physical fatigue and boost sexual desire.

•**St. John's wort,** well-known as a natural treatment for mild-to-moderate depression, also used to treat anxiety, stomach upset, insomnia and fluid retention.

Supplements that can reduce blood pressure include those that contain cinnamon, garlic, ginger and/or cat's claw (Uncaria tomentosa). Vitamin D-3, as well as the citrate forms of calcium and magnesium, also can reduce blood pressure. People with high blood pressure who want to try managing it naturally may have success with calcium, magnesium and/or vitamin D-3. (It's best to ask your doctor about the best dosages.)

Herbal supplements aren't the only common, everyday culprits that can affect blood pressure. Coffee, tea, energy drinks and other beverages with caffeine can raise blood pressure. So can nonsteroidal anti-inflammatory drugs (NSAIDs) such as indomethacin and ibuprofen...monoamine oxidase inhibitor drugs used to treat depression and Parkinson's disease...tricyclic antidepressants...and decongestants that contain pseudoephedrine or phenylephrine.

Many product labels include warnings about effects on blood pressure—so read labels carefully and take what they say seriously. Of course, not all products, including many herbal supplements, come with any warnings at all. Herbal supplements have a "health halo" in some people's minds. Play it safe by letting your doctor know everything you take, including supplements that you may think are not worth mentioning because they're "just herbs." That's especially important if you're being treated for a medical condition.

Under Age 40? Your High Blood Pressure Is More Harmful Than You Might Imagine

The study "Association of Blood Pressure Classification in Young Adults Using the 2017 American College of Cardiology/American Heart Association Guideline with Cardiovascular Events Later in Life," led by researchers at Duke Health in Durham, North Carolina, and published in *Journal of the American Medical Association*.

Is there a point in life at which high blood pressure is "OK" to have—say, when you're relatively young and your body is quite resilient?

Researchers from Duke Health in Durham, North Carolina, wanted to learn about the effect of high blood pressure when it starts relatively early in life, and they set about this in a novel way. Instead of starting with people who are young today and then following them for many years, they examined existing health records going back to 1985 on nearly 5,000 American adults who had blood pressure readings taken twice before age 40. And then, instead of using the definition of "normal" blood pressure that was in effect decades ago when those readings were taken, they applied today's more stringent definition of normal blood pressure to categorize each of those 5,000 people as having normal, elevated or high blood pressure.

Then they looked at which of these people suffered serious cardiac events during the ensuing years—and the news was not good, not even for those young adults who had had mildly elevated blood pressure. The message for today's people under age 40? The new blood pressure guidelines (details below), published in 2017 by the American College of Cardiology and American Heart Association, should be taken seriously—and taken seriously now, not just later when you're older.

The Damage Done

Prior to the new guidelines, high blood pressure was diagnosed when a person's blood pressure was 140/90 or above. But the Duke researchers categorized study subjects' (mostly untreated) blood pressure readings based on the 2017 guidelines—normal (systolic, or top number, of less than 120 and diastolic, bottom number, of less than 80)...elevated (systolic 120 to 129 and diastolic less than 80)...stage 1 hypertension (systolic 130 to 139 or diastolic 80 to 89)...or stage 2 hypertension (systolic 140 or greater, diastolic 90 or greater or taking high blood pressure medication).

Results: Study participants whose blood pressure readings were defined as elevated, stage 1 hypertension or stage 2 hypertension before age 40 had a significantly higher risk for a serious cardiovascular event, including coronary heart disease, stroke, heart failure and peripheral artery disease, over the next 19 years than those whose readings were normal.

The risks increased with the degree of hypertension. For example, those with elevated blood pressure had a 67% higher risk of having some type of cardiovascular event than the normal blood pressure group...those with stage 1 hypertension had a 75% higher risk. Not surprisingly, stage 2 hypertension was associated with the most significant risk—people in this group were three-and-a-half times more likely to have a future cardiovascular event.

Bottom line: The new guidelines are useful in identifying young people who have a higher risk of developing heart problems as they age so they can begin early treatment. People under age 40 should follow the same advice as older adults to reduce their risk for hypertension, such as maintaining a healthy body weight...getting regular exercise...reducing stress—and giving up cigarettes if they smoke. For further blood pressure management strategies, consult your physician.

High Blood Pressure? Hold Off on That Medication

James P. Sheppard, PhD, research lecturer and Sir Henry Dale fellow in the Nuffield Department of Primary Care Health Sciences at the University of Oxford in the UK and lead author of the study "Benefits and Harms of Antihypertensive Treatment in Low-Risk Patients with Mild Hypertension," published in *JAMA Internal Medicine.*

There's no doubt that high blood pressure is a major risk factor for cardiovascular disease. But there's plenty of doubt about when to start blood pressure medication in someone with low-risk, mild hypertension.

Mild hypertension is typically considered a systolic blood pressure between 140 and 159 or a diastolic blood pressure between 90 and 99. The most recent guidelines from the American Heart Association and the American College of Cardiology state that anyone with risk factors for cardiovascular disease and a blood pressure of 130/80 or higher should be treated. They also say to treat everyone with a blood pressure of 140/90 or higher even without any risk factors.

The problem? These guidelines are primarily based on the Systolic Blood Pressure Intervention Trial (SPRINT). SPRINT was a large study, but most of the patients were already being treated and they were not low risk. "Low risk" usually means no history of cardiovascular disease, family history of early heart disease and no evidence of heart enlargement, atrial fibrillation, diabetes or chronic kidney disease.

To specifically investigate the risks and benefits of treating low-risk, mild hypertension, researchers from Oxford University in the UK used data extracted from the UK Clinical Practice Research Datalink between 1998 and 2015, a database of electronic medical records that represents the entire population of the UK. They focused on a group of more than 38,000 patients who fit the description. Half of the patients were treated with hypertensive medications within 12 months of diagnosis and half were not. The researchers followed them for about six years to see how the risks and benefits of treatment compared between the two groups.

The results: There was no evidence of benefit for the patients taking medication. Treatment was not associated with a lower risk for death, heart attack, stroke or heart failure.

Treatment was, however, associated with significantly higher risk for low blood pressure, syncope (dizziness), electrolyte imbalances and sudden kidney damage. Although the overall risk of such adverse events was low, they were about 30% to 70% more likely to occur in the treated patients.

The dilemma: US guidelines recommend drug treatment to lower blood pressure more quickly than other countries. In the UK, low-risk patients with mild hypertension are given lifestyle advice rather than medication. Elsewhere in Europe, lifestyle advice is recommended for a number of months before medication is considered. This study has some limitations, namely that patients were not randomly allocated to a treatment or no treatment group, which could bias the results. However, it would take even larger and longer studies than this one to arrive at a treatment consensus, and the cost of conducting such a trial would be so high that it may never be undertaken.

So how can you use this new information? If you or a loved one is trying to figure out the best treatment for mild, low-risk hypertension, first recognize that there is no one-size-fits-all approach. Weigh the pros and cons of treatment in view of your personal risk factors, including your age. Recently, a separate study done in the US found that people with elevated blood pressure in their 40s had greater heart risks later in life if they didn't take early steps to lower it. (The average age of patients in the UK study was 55.)

The one "treatment" that should be part of every person's plan to manage blood pressure involves adopting known lifestyle changes—a more healthful diet, not smoking, exercising more and reducing stress, none of which are associated with the risks of medication.

To Keep Your Blood Pressure Under Control, Think of Your Sweetheart

Study titled, "The Impact of Physical Proximity and Attachment Working Models on Cardiovascular Reactivity: Comparing Mental Activation and Romantic Partner Presence" was conducted by researchers at University of Arizona, Tucson, and published in *Psychophysiology*.

When your stress levels get ratcheted up, it's comforting to have your spouse or partner by your side...but of course that's not how life works. Most of us are on our own when we're racing to meet a deadline at work, for example, or undergoing an uncomfortable medical procedure.

But don't despair. In a study recently published in *Psychophysiology*, simply imagining your loved one's presence during stressful situations can be just as good as the real thing...at least when it comes to keeping your blood pressure under control. *Here's how the research unfolded...*

Study details: Researchers recruited 102 volunteers who described themselves as being in a committed, high-quality romantic relationship. To test the participants' stress responses, they were asked to submerge one of their feet in three inches of water chilled to just above freezing (38°F to 40°F) for four minutes. The participants' blood pressure, heart rate (beats per minute) and heart rate variability (the changes in time between heartbeats) were measured before, during and after the task.

During the big chill, one-third of the volunteers were randomly chosen to have their romantic partner in the room with them...

one-third were asked to focus on a mental image of their partner...and the remaining participants (the control group) were instructed to think about what had happened or would happen during their day.

When measuring heart rate and heart rate variability, there was no variability among the three groups. However, the participants with a partner who was physically present and those who simply imagined their loved one had a lower blood pressure response to the stress test than those who were told to think about their day.

The real kicker: Thinking about the romantic partner was just as effective at minimizing the participants' blood pressure reactivity as actually having the person physically present. The study results may help explain why quality romantic relationships are linked to better health in a significant body of scientific evidence.

"Life is full of stress, and one critical way we can manage this stress is through our relationships—either with our partner directly or by calling on a mental image of that person," explains Kyle Bourassa, lead study author and a University of Arizona doctoral student in psychology.

Give it a try: The next time you feel the stress building, close your eyes and create a detailed mental picture of your romantic partner. Concentrate on an image of his/her face...and think of a meaningful experience you two have shared. With that image in mind, you're likely to have a better shot at keeping your blood pressure under control.

Your Heart and Your Gut

Improving gut health may lower heart disease risk. Arterial hardening raises cardiovascular risk and is closely related to inflammation, both of which are connected to the balance of gut microbes. In a recent study, nearly 10% of arterial hardening could be explained by gut microbes. Eat a diet rich in omega-3 fatty acids and fiber found in fruits, vegetables and nuts. Supplementation with omega-3s (fish oil) and probiotics also may help.

Ana M. Valdes, PhD, is associate professor of musculoskeletal genetics at University of Nottingham School of Medicine, UK, and coauthor of a study published in *European Heart Journal*.

Too Much Caffeine Can Stress the Heart

In 2017, a 16-year-old boy died of a heart arrhythmia after drinking too much caffeine. The Food and Drug Administration recommends keeping daily caffeine consumption to 400 milligrams (mg)—the amount in two to three cups of coffee, depending on brand and roast. Consuming 500 mg or more can lead to feeling jittery or nauseated and can lead to irregular heartbeat, high blood pressure, anxiety and irritability—all of which can have adverse effects on cardiovascular health.

Robert Glatter, MD, assistant professor of emergency medicine, Northwell Health and Lenox Hill Hospital, both in New York City, quoted at Forbes.com.

New Antioxidant Supplement Supports Blood Vessel Health

MitoQ is a form of coenzyme Q10, a heart-health supplement, with an added molecule so that it accumulates in cell mitochondria. Otherwise healthy older adults with reduced blood vessel function did better on artery health measures when they took MitoQ for six weeks versus when they took placebos—evidence that daily supplementation may improve vascular disease.

Matthew Rossman, PhD, is a postdoctoral researcher in the department of integrative physiology at University of Colorado, Boulder, and lead author of a study published in *Hypertension*.

Is Daily Aspirin Helping Your Heart?

Your dose of daily aspirin to prevent heart attack and stroke might not be helping you. New study: The benefits of low-dose 81-mg aspirin, including lower risk for heart disease and colon cancer, are limited to people weighing up to 154 pounds. If you weigh more, a higher dose may be needed—but higher doses increase bleeding risk. Work with your doctor to find the right balance.

Peter M. Rothwell, MD, PhD, is head of the Centre for the Prevention of Stroke and Dementia, University of Oxford, UK, and lead author of a study published in *The Lancet*.

Surprising Deadly Danger from Cipro Antibiotics

US Food and Drug Administration Safety Announcement, "FDA Warns About Increased Risk of Ruptures or Tears in the Aorta Blood Vessel with Fluoroquinolone Antibiotics in Certain Patients," December 20, 2018.

Cipro and other widely prescribed antibiotics may put certain people at increased risk for a potentially deadly aortic aneurysm, the FDA now warns. Even if you're not currently taking one of these antibiotics, you might need to call it out with a loved one, since the risk is higher in males. *Reading this could save a life…*

Cipro is one of a class of antibiotics called fluoroquinolones. You've probably taken a fluoroquinolone—which also includes Avelox, Floxin and Levaquin—at least once, since they've been around for more than 30 years. These are broad-spectrum drugs, meaning that they can treat a wide range of bacterial infections—including infections of the lungs, skin and urinary tract.

Now case reports and four studies show that for people at risk for aortic aneurysm (AA), taking a fluoroquinolone doubles their risk. AA is a bulge in a weak spot in the wall of the large artery that carries blood from the heart down through the chest and belly to the rest of the body. An AA can lead to dissection—the layers of the artery separate, allowing blood to leak between the layers—and possibly to rupture, which is a medical emergency that is usually fatal without immediate surgery.

The US Food and Drug Administration (FDA) issued a warning in December 2018 that applies to all fluoroquinolone antibiotics that are taken as pills or injections. The FDA says these antibiotics should not be used unless there are no other antibiotic options for people at risk for AA. *Risk factors include...*

•**Being elderly** (some studies found increased risk in people over age 65 while other studies found risk increased over age 70).

•**Having a history of aneurysm in any artery of the body.**

•**Having a history of "hardening of the arteries" (atherosclerosis).**

•**Having high blood pressure.**

•**Having a genetic condition that weakens arteries** (such as the genetic connective-tissue disorders Marfan syndrome and Ehlers-Danlos syndrome).

•**Being male and a current or former smoker.**

Overall risk for AA is still relatively small, even for people at increased risk. Per every 100,000 people, there are about 300 cases of AA per year among those at highest risk, compared with about nine cases among the general population. But because AA is potentially deadly and can happen quickly, a doubled risk needs to be taken seriously.

The FDA advises patients to let their doctors know if they have any risk factors for AA before taking a fluoroquinolone, and to discuss whether a safer antibiotic can be prescribed instead. If a fluoroquinolone is still the best—or only—option, patients and doctors need to be aware that the increased risk for AA continues for 30 days after taking the drug.

Important: Get to an emergency room or call 911 immediately if you have severe, sudden and steady pain—which may feel like throbbing and/or feel deep—in your chest, belly or back. You also may have trouble breathing or swallowing.

And if you are a man age 65 to 75 and have ever smoked, the US Preventive Services Task Force recommends that you have a onetime ultrasound screen for AA. Screening can discover an AA early, when it can be corrected surgically to prevent rupture.

The current warning is the latest among several issued recently for fluoroquinolones. Earlier in 2018, the FDA warned of a risk for low blood sugar and mental health changes that can include insomnia, anxiety and paranoia. There also was a previous warning of higher risk for nerve damage and tendon ruptures.

Winter Heart Attack Deadlier

The risk of having a heart attack is the same throughout the year. However, the risk of dying within 30 days of a severe attack was 50% higher in the six coldest months, according to data on more than 4,000 heart attacks.

Possible reasons: Winter-associated infections, such as pneumonia...and ambulance delays.

Arvindra Krishnamurthy, MD, cardiologist, Leeds General Infirmary, Leeds, UK.

Smartphone ECG for AFib

Mark Houston, MD, MS, MSc, director, Hypertension Institute, Nashville. HypertensionInstitute.com

If you are concerned about an irregular heartbeat, or atrial fibrillation (AFib), see your doctor for an evaluation. Risk factors include high blood pressure, coronary heart disease, congestive heart failure, sleep apnea, COPD, asthma, thyroid issues, diabetes and/or a family history of AFib. Symptoms can include palpitations, a fast heart rate (150 beats per minute or higher), dizziness, breathlessness, fainting and/or fatigue. AFib can cause serious problems such as stroke.

If AFib is suspected, your doctor will most likely have you wear a cardiac-event monitor, such as a seven-day Holter monitor, which performs electrocardiograms (ECGs) in order to detect heart-rhythm abnormalities. Treatments for AFib include blood thinners, heart-rate control medications and cardioversion or ablation, procedures that disrupt faulty signals in the heart. If AFib is diagnosed, a system, such as the KardiaMobile ECG monitor (Alivetec.com) for smartphones and tablets, would be helpful.

AFib Dangerous in Minority Populations

A common heartbeat irregularity threatens minority populations. Atrial fibrillation is more common in whites, but it is more likely to cause dangerous complications in blacks and Latinos—who may benefit from increased monitoring and genetic testing that can detect hidden risk and allow for preventive strategies.

JAMA Network Open.

Still Under Stress After a Heart Attack? If You're a Woman, Your Life Is in Jeopardy

Hawkins Gay, MD, MPH, fellow in cardiovascular medicine at the Northwestern University Feinberg School of Medicine and a coauthor of "Mental Stress–Induced-Myocardial Ischemia in Young Patients With Recent Myocardial Infarction; Sex Differences and Mechanisms" along with researchers at the Emory University School of Medicine published in *Circulation*.

E xperiencing a heart attack is scary enough. But if you're a young or middle-aged woman and you don't address the stress in your life, you're leaving yourself vulnerable to a second heart attack—very vulnerable.

New study: Researchers at Emory University School of Medicine studied about 300 men and women, ages 22 to 61, who had suffered heart attacks. The researchers found that the women in this group were twice as likely as the men to experience myocardial ischemia—in which the heart doesn't get enough blood—brought on by mental stress, which places them at much higher risk of having more heart attacks.

The Stress Connection

Stress impacts the smallest blood vessels in the body, and this effect happens more in women than in men. That may be why women are more vulnerable to stress-induced heart attacks even though they often have less obstructive heart disease than men. Complicating the emotional element further, young and middle-aged women who survive heart attacks are likely to feel depressed or traumatized by the event...on top of any lifestyle stress, worsening their prognosis.

Add Stress Control to Your Life

After suffering a heart attack (or even when trying to avoid one), you'll typically talk to your doctor about diet, exercise and other positive lifestyle changes to make, such as quitting smoking and drinking less alcohol. But discussing how to reduce stress in your life—and how important this is—doesn't get as much attention as it should. Cardiologists should recommend that every female heart attack patient be screened for high levels of stress.

The American Heart Association's *Go Red for Women* program offers many ideas for managing stress (GoRedforWomen.org...click on "Healthy Living").

How you respond to stress matters, too. Rather than diving further into upsetting situations—perhaps with the goal of settling them as soon as possible—it's often less stressful to walk away, for the time being at least, and then revisit the situation once you've had a chance to reflect and calm down.

Quick Hits: 6 Ways to De-Stress in a Flash

Create a personal game plan to follow when stress escalates with options you can do anywhere, any time. *Your list might include...*

• **Meditate with a three-minute guided program on your smartphone.**

• **Do five minutes of yoga.**

• **Take a 10-minute walk.**

• **Listen to your favorite music and tune out everything else.**

• **Read a relaxing or engrossing book.**

• **Watch a favorite happy movie clip on YouTube.**

MINOCA: The Heart Attack You've Never Heard Of

"Population-Level Incidence and Outcomes of Myocardial Infarction with Non-obstructive Coronary Arteries (MINOCA): Insights from the Alberta Contemporary Acute Coronary Syndrome Patients Invasive Treatment Strategies (COAPT) Study," by Kevin R. Bainey MD, assistant professor of medicine in the division of cardiology, and colleagues at the University of Alberta in Edmonton, Canada, and published in *International Journal of Cardiology.*

You know the risk stemming from completely blocked arteries—heart attack. But did you know that a minor blockage is enough to cause a heart attack in some people...and that doctors tend to minimize the severity of this type of heart attack? Now, a recent study finds that there is definitely cause for concern, especially among women.

We're talking about MINOCA, the acronym for a myocardial infarction (heart attack) with non-obstructive coronary arteries, somewhat of a mystery compared to more common

heart attacks...and under-researched...but dangerous.

Typically, MINOCA has been thought of, and treated, as a less serious type of heart attack. It's not unusual for MINOCA patients to be reassured and sent home from the hospital after experiencing one without the level of care prescribed to other heart attack victims and without a real focus on preventing another heart attack.

But when researchers at the University of Alberta in Canada reviewed the medical records of almost 36,000 patients admitted to hospitals for any type of heart attack, they found startling results...

• **Only 6% of these heart attack patients did not have blocked blood flow to the heart**—meaning their heart attacks were MINOCA. Yet, during the next five years, 11% of these MINOCA patients went on to have second heart attacks or died, showing just how strongly MINOCA can influence future health.

• **Only 25% of heart attack patients with blocked arteries were women,** but 50% of MINOCA patients were women.

• **Only about 40% of MINOCA patients were put on medications to prevent future heart attacks.** And women with MINOCA were likely to be treated with hormone replacement therapy—which does not help to reduce heart attack risk—or antidepressants instead.

• **The average age of MINOCA patients was 59,** about 4 years younger than for a blockage heart attack.

Clearly, there's a heart danger stalking middle-aged people that is not being taken seriously enough, especially with female patients. The key takeaway from this study is that MINOCA is a serious type of heart attack and should be approached that way by both patients and doctors. Although the exact cause of MINOCA remains a mystery, possibilities include a temporarily blocked artery due to a blood clot or a spasm of an artery due to atherosclerosis. In reality, people who get a MINOCA do have diseased coronary arteries. They may have plaques like other heart attack patients and some narrowing of a coronary artery but not enough to cause a complete blockage.

Why women are more affected by MINOCA remains another part of the mystery. Researchers suspect that female hormones may cause a weakening or dysfunction of the inside lining of heart arteries, making them more susceptible to atherosclerosis spasms, but more research needs to be done.

How to Protect Yourself

Risk factors for MINOCA are similar to risk factors for other heart attacks—high blood pressure, high cholesterol, diabetes, smoking and a family history of heart attack. So, according to the American College of Cardiology, you can reduce your risk of MINOCA with the same heart-healthy lifestyle habits everyone should be following, such as eating healthy, staying active, managing stress and not smoking.

Also, keep in mind that a MINOCA heart attack can feel like any other heart attack with severe chest pain, but it doesn't have to—women, for example, often have milder symptoms such as shortness of breath, nausea, vomiting, dizziness and back or jaw pain. Man or woman, if you have these symptoms, call 911 right away.

The strongest takeaway from this eye-opening study concerns what to do if you do have a MINOCA heart attack: Treat it seriously and do not let your doctors do otherwise. Tell them about this article if that's what it takes. Then, the good news is that you should respond to the same prevention strategies used by people who have had more traditional types of heart attacks, including medications such as statins, beta-blockers and others. But if your doctor persists in telling you that your MINOCA was not that serious, get another opinion.

Is Robotic-Assisted Heart Surgery Right for You?

Husam H. Balkhy, MD, professor of surgery and director of Robotic and Minimally Invasive Cardiac Surgery at University of Chicago Medicine & Biological Sciences. A pioneer in the field of robotic cardiac surgery, Dr. Balkhy performs more than 200 of these procedures a year.

Every year in the US, heart surgeons perform more than 300,000 coronary artery bypass operations. This procedure is no small feat—it restores blood flow to a person's heart when the coronary arteries are severely narrowed or blocked (atherosclerosis).

But "open-heart" surgery also is quite invasive. The breastbone (sternum) is literally sawed in half to expose the heart. The heart is stopped, and blood is circulated using a heart-lung machine. The surgeon then removes one or more healthy blood vessels from other parts of the body—usually the saphenous vein in the leg, which runs from the groin to the ankle—and creates a "graft" to bypass the blocked arteries of the heart. Mortality rates within 30 days of surgery are 1% to 2%.

What many people don't realize: There's another possible choice. If you have severe atherosclerosis—and medication, stents or other treatments aren't an option—robotic-assisted coronary bypass surgery may be worth considering.

Facts you should know...

The Minimally Invasive Option

Even though minimally invasive, robotic-assisted coronary bypass surgery was approved by the FDA more than a decade ago, it has only recently become more widely available throughout the US with at least a dozen hospitals now offering the procedure.

Known as "closed-chest" heart surgery, the robotic procedure does not require the breastbone to be split in half. Instead, the surgeon sits at a console and uses his/her hands to remotely control thin, flexible robotic "arms" equipped with a miniature camera. (This type of endoscopic device is used for many operations, from knee replacements to gallbladder removal.)

The robotic arms reproduce the surgeon's movements with total accuracy—but because the arms are more flexible and precise than a human hand, they enhance the surgeon's manual dexterity. A second surgeon is positioned at the patient's bedside to help exchange the robotic arms and assist in the procedure.

The high-definition, 3-D camera on the robotic arms—controlled by foot pedals, which allow the camera to zoom in and out—provides magnification five times greater than the magnifying visor (loupes) worn by a doctor performing open-heart surgery—and 12 to 15 times greater than the naked eye.

Smaller incisions are a big benefit: Using the robotic arms, the surgeon makes four to five fingertip-size incisions in the chest, between the ribs, rather than the eight- to 10-inch incision required by traditional open-heart surgery. The sternum is untouched.

The surgeon then "harvests" one or both healthy internal mammary arteries (two arteries that run along either side of the breastbone and feed the chest wall), rather than veins from the leg, and uses them for the bypass. Benefit: Research shows that internal mammary artery grafts last longer than grafts from the leg and also increase the odds of postsurgical survival. Note: Mammary artery grafts also can be used with open-heart surgery.

Recent Scientific Evidence

With robotic-assisted coronary bypass surgery, most cases do not require the heart to be stopped during the procedure, eliminating the use of the heart-lung machine. There's less blood loss, which reduces the need for transfusions. Because the aorta is not manipulated and the heart is not stopped, the risk for ischemic stroke is less with robotic-assisted coronary bypass surgery (less than 0.5% in our experience) compared with traditional open-heart surgery (1% to 2%).

Because the breastbone isn't split open, there's less risk for postsurgical complications and infection. Postsurgical pain is less and goes away faster. In fact, it's often managed using *acetaminophen* (Tylenol) or aspirin instead of narcotics once the patient is discharged home.

The postsurgical hospital stay is typically one to three days versus five to seven with the open-heart procedure. This allows patients to return to work and other normal activities much faster—usually within a couple of weeks, compared with about 10 weeks after open-heart surgery.

Important recent findings: Research shows that two groups of people who typically have trouble with open-heart surgery do better with robotic-assisted coronary bypass surgery...

•**Women.** Even though women usually have more complications from open-heart surgery, poorer long-term pain relief and lower rates of survival compared with men, women had identical outcomes to men when they had robotic-assisted coronary bypass, based on a study I conducted with colleagues at University of Chicago Medicine & Biological Sciences and published in *Innovations*.

•**Morbidly obese people**—those with a body mass index (BMI) greater than 35.

Examples: A 5'10" person who weighs 250 pounds has a BMI of 35.9...a 5'5" person who weighs 215 pounds has a BMI of 35.8. In another study I conducted with colleagues, and published in *The International Journal of Medical Robotics and Computer Assisted Surgery*, we looked at results from 234 patients who had robotic-assisted coronary bypass, 43 of whom were morbidly obese. We found no difference in postoperative complications or mortality rates between those who were morbidly obese and those who weren't.

When It's Not the Best Option

Even with the advantages described above, robotic-assisted coronary bypass surgery isn't the best choice for everyone. *Examples*...

More Than Just Bypass

Bypass surgery isn't the only type of heart surgery that can be robotically assisted. Robotic heart surgery also is used for valve repair...to correct atrial fibrillation (irregular heartbeat)...to implant pacemakers...to remove heart tumors...and to repair congenital heart defects. In fact, with the exception of heart transplants and ventricular assist devices, nearly any heart operation can be done robotically.

• **A person who needs quadruple bypass.** There are only two internal mammary arteries to use for grafts.

• **If you've had major lung surgery.** Scar tissue from the surgery might interfere with the procedure.

The main risks involved in robotic-assisted coronary bypass are related to inexperienced surgeons. Patients can protect themselves by not having any kind of surgery (robotic or otherwise) by a surgeon who is inexperienced (see below).

Making the Decision

If your cardiologist says that you need heart surgery, ask if you're a candidate for robotic-assisted coronary bypass surgery. If the answer is no, consider getting a second opinion from a surgeon who specializes in minimally invasive and robotic-assisted coronary bypass

surgery. Prominent institutions that perform such surgery include University of Chicago...Emory Healthcare in Atlanta...Mayo Clinic in Rochester, Minnesota...Johns Hopkins Medicine in Baltimore...Lankenau Hospital in Philadelphia...Lenox Hill Hospital in New York City...and Medical City Dallas.

If you decide on robotic-assisted coronary bypass surgery, be sure to find a surgeon who has a lot of experience. Ask the surgeon how many procedures he/she has performed and what the outcomes were. Surgeons and teams who have done 50 to 100 cases are beyond the learning curve for robotic-assisted coronary bypass.

Pump Iron for Heart Health

Weight training improved cardiovascular risk factors, including high blood pressure, diabetes and elevated cholesterol, more than walking or biking, according to a study of more than 4,000 women and men.

Best: Combine weight training—often done at a higher (more heart-protective) intensity—with aerobic activity, which is also beneficial for heart health.

Maia P. Smith, PhD, MS, statistical epidemiologist and assistant professor, department of public health and preventive medicine, St. George's University School of Medicine, Grenada.

Chapter 9

INFECTIOUS DISEASE

Do You Still Douche? Try These Much Healthier Alternatives to Vaginal Health

Why are there still so many douching products still on the market? Douching is supposedly bad for women.

Despite the advice doctors have been giving for years now, many women continue to douche and purchase vaginal douching products. In fact, the US Department of Health & Human Services reports that nearly one in five women between the ages of 15 and 44 douches.

Douching involves flushing the vagina with fluid—typically vinegar and water, plus other additives like baking soda, iodine, fragrance or even antiseptic with store-bought douches.

Reasons why women douche: To achieve a "clean" feeling…to eliminate odor…soothe itching…wash away menstrual blood after a period…wash away semen after sex…and avoid a sexually transmitted disease. But doctors don't advise douching for any of these reasons.

Why douching is not healthy: The vagina is naturally acidic and, just like the intestinal tract, is host to billions of beneficial bacteria that help fight off infection and keep the vagina healthy. If you douche, the healthy bacteria in the vagina are disturbed and harmful bacteria can take over. What's more, store-bought douches are usually alkaline and, as mentioned above, can contain fragrance and other additives that can negatively affect the healthy bacteria in the vagina.

Bottom line: Douching can lead to more yeast infections and bacterial vaginosis (bacterial overgrowth)…pelvic inflammatory disease, an infection of the reproductive organs…cervicitis (inflammation of the cervix)…increased risk for sexually transmitted diseases…and pregnancy complications.

Other reasons not to douche: Symptoms for which women would commonly douche, such as unusual vaginal odor or discharge, itching or irritation and discomfort during sex, need to be evaluated by a gynecologist instead of being self-treated and possibly masked by douching. Also, douching before

Anna Cabeca, DO, a board-certified obstetrician/gynecologist based in St. Simons Island, Georgia, and author of *The Hormone Fix: Burn Fat Naturally, Boost Energy, Sleep Better and Stop Hot Flashes the Keto-Green Way.* DrAnnaCabeca.com an appointment with your doctor will make it more difficult for him/her to provide a correct diagnosis and may make an infection worse or spread it to other areas.

Proper Care for "Down There"

The vagina is self-cleaning, so women do not need to douche for cleanliness—it's designed to eliminate semen and other fluids through natural discharges. However, you can keep your outer vaginal area healthy by gently cleansing with mild soap and water.

All vaginas have a natural odor, but if you're looking to minimize it, you can try soaking in a hot bath with a few drops of lavender essential oil. Also, wear 100% cotton underwear during the day—cotton absorbs moisture that can lead to excess odor, itching and infection. If you regularly wear panty liners, opt for organic cotton varieties. And at night, let air circulate around your genitals by going commando (without underwear).

Eating a diet that minimizes sugar and carbohydrates and includes healthy fats, such as omega-3 fatty acids (found in salmon), olive oil and avocados, is also beneficial for vaginal health. Additionally, I recommend taking a daily probiotic, especially during a course of antibiotics or soon after. And if you have a history of yeast infections, you may want to ask your doctor about trying a probiotic that's inserted vaginally.

Hidden Dangers of Feminine Hygiene Products

Kieran C. O'Doherty, PhD, associate professor, department of psychology, and researcher on the human microbiome, University of Guelph, Ontario, Canada. He is lead author of the study "Vaginal Health and Hygiene Practices and Product Use in Canada: A National Cross-Sectional Survey," published in *BMC Women's Health*.

Women, listen up! You may love those feminine creams, lubricants and wipes, but are these products doing more harm than good? Perhaps so, according to new research.

Background: It's been known for some time that douching can disrupt the vaginal flora—the balance of "friendly" and "unfriendly" bacteria in the vagina. When this occurs, it increases a woman's risk for bacterial vaginosis, a mild vaginal infection that commonly results in a fishy-smelling discharge.

To learn more about other vaginal health practices, researchers from University of Guelph in Ontario asked 1,500 Canadian women about their use of vaginal hygiene (aka "feminine hygiene") products, such as anti-itch creams, sanitizing gels, moisturizers/lubricants and feminine wipes, during their lifetimes and in the last three months. These over-the-counter (OTC) products are used for everything from vaginal dryness to smelly female parts.

Study results: A whopping 95% of the women surveyed reported that they had used vaginal hygiene products. The study, published in *BMC Women's Health*, further revealed big differences in the rates of infection between users and nonusers of vaginal hygiene products.

Biggest offender: Women who applied vaginal gel sanitizers (sometimes known as "vaginal deodorizers") reported having eight times as many yeast infections and almost 20 times as many bacterial infections as those who didn't "sanitize."

The use of feminine washes or gels was associated with three-and-a-half times higher odds of having bacterial vaginosis compared with nonusers. Among women who used these products, there was two-and-a-half times higher odds of having a urinary tract infection (UTI).

There were similar findings among those who used feminine wipes and lubricants/moisturizers. Women who used these products reported having a UTI twice as often and a yeast infection two-and-a-half times as often, respectively.

Even though the researchers can't say for sure that these products caused any of the infections, the study results do provide a reason to further investigate whether these gels, creams, wipes, etc., disrupt the natural vaginal environment and inhibit the growth of healthy bacteria.

Without enough healthy bacteria, a woman's body is less capable of fighting off infections. In addition to UTIs and yeast infections, this could theoretically mean that women are also increasing their risk for other conditions linked to unhealthy vaginal flora—such as pelvic inflammatory disease, cervical cancer and sexually transmitted diseases. If additional research supports the findings, these products could indeed be doing more harm than good.

Bottom line: The body naturally produces secretions that clean the vagina from the inside. To play it safe, it's best for women to limit their cleansing and freshening routine to a once-a-day wash (maybe more than once if you're menstruating) with warm water and perhaps a mild, unscented soap.

Your vagina doesn't need to smell like lavender or jasmine or a tropical rainstorm to be healthy. In fact, those added scents may just add to your problems. It's seems that this part of a woman's body can take care of itself just fine—thank you very much!

Another Mosquito-Borne Virus

Another mosquito-borne virus has been identified in northern Florida. The Keystone virus, known to be widespread among animals, has been confirmed in a human. Like the Zika virus, it may cause severe infections including brain inflammation, but doctors don't know to look for this virus.

Prevention: Wear long-sleeved clothing… use DEET spray…and stay inside at dawn and dusk. Symptoms include rash and flu-like symptoms.

John A. Lednicky, PhD, is research professor, department of environmental and global health, College of Public Health and Health Professions, University of Florida, Gainesville, and lead author of a study published in *Clinical Infectious Diseases*.

HPV: The Killer That We Don't Talk Enough About

Diane M. Harper, MD, MPH, MS, a professor in the departments of family medicine and obstetrics and gynecology at University of Michigan and physician director for Community Outreach, Engagement and Health Disparities at University of Michigan Rogel Cancer Center. She is one of the country's leading experts on HPV.

It's a fact that still flies under the radar for many people…the majority of anal and cervical cancers—and most cancers affecting the penis and oral cavity (mouth, throat and sinus cavities)—are linked to the human papillomavirus, or HPV, the most common sexually transmitted infection in the US.

Each year in the US, about 6,000 cases of anal cancer, approximately 11,000 cases of cervical cancer, 3,300 cases of vaginal or vulvar cancer, 900 cases of penile cancer and 13,000 cases of oropharyngeal cancer are attributed to HPV.

Why you should be informed about HPV: Even if you've been in a monogamous sexual relationship for years, you may unknowingly be carrying the potentially deadly virus. An estimated 80% of all sexually active men and women in the US (that's about 79 million people) will be infected with HPV at some point in their lives, and about 14 million people become newly infected each year.

Cancer-Causing HPVs

There are more than 100 strains of viruses in the humanpapilloma family. HPV is a well-known cause of warts on the genitals and elsewhere on the body (such as on the hands or feet). Two strains of HPV—type 6 and type 11—lead to genital warts, while more than 30 strains can cause warts on other parts of the body.

Important: Even though genital warts may be emotionally disturbing, they do not turn into cancer.

There are 14 high-risk HPV types that are associated with cancers in humans. HPV 16 causes most cases of cancers of the cervix, anus, penis, vagina, vulva, head and neck and esophagus. Together, HPV 16 and 18 cause about 70% of all the cervical cancers.

A Hidden Threat

Infections due to cancer-causing strains of HPV usually go undetected because they do not cause warts or any other signs or symptoms.

Both women and men who are infected can unknowingly transmit the virus—usually during sexual encounters (vaginal, anal or oral sex). The virus enters the body through cuts or tiny tears in the outer layer of the skin in the vagina, cervix, penis, anus and mouth. Because HPV is spread through skin-to-skin contact, it's possible that skin-to-skin kissing (not saliva transmission) leads to head and neck cancers and that oral sex leads to esophageal cancer.

The good news is that the body's immune system effectively eliminates the cancer-causing virus in about 90% of HPV infections—usually within two years. When the virus stays in the body beyond two years, it is considered persistent and the risk for cancer of the genitals, cervix, anus or oral cavity rises.

Are You at Risk?

Most HPV infections are transmitted through sexual activity, but about 10% to 15% of the population become infected via nonsexual sources that have not yet been identified. In general, the risk for HPV infection is higher for people with impaired immunity—for example, anyone undergoing chemotherapy or those with diabetes or an autoimmune disease, such as lupus or rheumatoid arthritis, and for people who have many sexual partners or who use devices that cause tears (even very tiny ones) in the skin of the genitals, anus or mouth.

A common ingredient in many vaginal spermicides, nonoxynol-9, triples a woman's risk for HPV infection. It damages the lining of the vagina and makes it easier for the virus to enter through the skin.

Testing and Diagnosis

For decades, the Pap test has been used to detect precancerous changes to cells in the cervix. If a woman's Pap results were described as atypical, she was advised to undergo a test that checks for one or more of 14 cancer-causing HPV types.

The US Preventive Services Task Force recently released guidelines that reversed this course. Now women 21-to-29 years old are screened every three years with a Pap test alone, but those 30-to-65 years old can get the HPV test to screen for cervical cancer. If the test is positive, then a Pap test is done. If the test is negative, a woman can safely wait five years to be screened again. The two older options for Pap testing every three years or co-testing with both the HPV test and the Pap test are also valid ways to screen.

The HPV Vaccine

Gardasil has replaced the original Gardasil vaccine. It prevents infection from seven of the 14 high-risk strains of HPV associated with cancer (the original protected against just two, HPV 16 and HPV 18). It was recently approved by the FDA for men and women up to age 45.

How it's used: The Centers for Disease Control and Prevention (CDC) recommends two doses given six to 12 months apart for young people getting the vaccine before their 15th birthday and three doses for everyone over age 15 with the second dose given one to two months after the first dose and the third dose six months after the first dose.

Safety profile: A controversial 2006 report published in *JAMA* found some serious adverse effects, including death, after Gardasil use. However, repeated studies done in the US and internationally since then and reviewed by the World Health Organization have found it safe. It is not yet known if it poses any risks to women given the vaccine while pregnant. Discuss the risks and benefits of the vaccine with your physician.

Other Preventive Steps

Using a condom reduces—but does not eliminate—risk for HPV infection in women and men. This is because the virus can occur in areas that aren't covered by a condom, and it can be spread by hand-to-mouth contact. Being in a mutually monogamous relationship with someone who has had few or no previous partners also curbs risk.

Women who use spermicides that contain nonoxynol-9 (including male condoms that use this ingredient) to prevent pregnancy should consider switching from this form of birth control to some other method, such as oral contraceptives or cervical caps. Both men and women should ask for an oral cancer check during each dental visit. And men should regularly check for signs of penile cancer, such as visible bumps or ulcers.

The HPV Test: Why It's Better Than the Pap for Cervical Cancer Screening

Diane Harper, MD, MPH, MS, professor in the departments of family medicine and obstetrics and gynecology at University of Michigan, physician director for Community Outreach, Engagement and Health Disparities at University of Michigan Rogel Cancer Center and one of the country's leading experts on HPV.

Guidelines for how to screen and when to screen for cervical cancer had been a moving target until late 2018, when the US Preventive Services Task Force clarified very simply what techniques work and how often screening needs to happen. But those guidelines are different depending on age. *Here's what you need to know…*

For Women Ages 30 to 65

The guidelines state that you can choose between…

- **Having the HPV (human papilloma virus) test every five years**
- **Having the Pap test every three years**
- **Co-testing with the Pap and HPV tests every five years**

Why all the choices? Although research has shown that for women 30 years and older the HPV test picks up more suspect lesions sooner than the Pap test does and with fewer false positives, it will take time for the medical community to adopt such a landmark change (some doctors are still doing annual Pap tests even though the move to every three years is already over a decade old—know that since insurance reimbursement follows the current guidelines, patients may then be billed for screening too frequently). So, for the time being, the Pap is still one of the stand-alone options. It is also used after a stand-alone HPV test if that test comes back positive. The most expensive way to use the Pap test is to do it at the same time as the HPV test (co-testing)—it may provide a convenience but at a cost.

Discuss all three options with your doctor to find the most appropriate one for you. Your unique personal or family health history might lead your primary care physician to recommend one over another.

How HPV Testing Works

Many experts believe that, ultimately, the HPV test will be the one standard. It looks for 14 high-risk strains of HPV including HPV-16 and HPV-18, the two responsible for 70% of all cervical cancers.

If you choose to have the HPV test and…

- **The test is negative,** you won't need any cervical cancer screening for five years.
- **The test is positive,** it does not mean you have cancer, but does mean you'll need to follow it up with a Pap test to give your doctor more information—whether the virus

has caused any changes in your cervix or is just sitting there.

Your doctor may just be able to use the liquid from your HPV test to do the Pap test and not need to call you back for an exam.

What typically happens next...

•**If that Pap test is normal or shows that any changes are minor,** in a year you'll repeat the HPV test to see if the virus cleared on its own and if not, have a repeat Pap to check for any further changes to the cervix.

•**If the changes on your Pap are more severe, then you'll likely have a colposcopy with biopsy.** A colposcopy uses a lighted instrument to look for precancerous changes or lesions in the tissue of your cervix—a lesion is an indicator that there is usually more disease than is showing. Biopsies, or tissue samples, will be taken from both the outside and the inside of your cervix and examined.

•**If all the results are negative,** you'll need to have two normal tests (a negative HPV and a normal Pap) six months after the biopsy and again six months later before you can return to every five-year screening.

•**If the biopsies show severe changes,** then you'll have another procedure called LEEP, which uses electrical current to remove the abnormal cells from the cervix.

Note about the HPV test methods: Both the Pap and HPV tests can be done during a gynecological exam. However, you can also collect your own HPV sample at home with a swab and send it to a lab for testing.

Two recent studies looked at the effectiveness of self-collected HPV tests and found that the results were comparable to those done in a doctor's office. These kits are already available online—examples include Selfcollect.com and Mylabbox.com and can be a good option for women without easy access to screening clinics.

For Women Ages 21 to 29

The guideline for this age group is for only the Pap test to be done every three years.

Why is there a difference based solely on age? Most sexually active young women have been exposed to at least one strain of HPV. The body will usually be able to rid itself of the virus on its own in two or three years. During that time, women will automatically test positive for HPV even though it's unlikely that there's any cancer. For those under 30, the Pap test is the more sensitive way to screen for cervical cancer.

For Women Over Age 65

Although the guidelines don't recommend screening for women in this age group who had adequate prior screening and are not at high risk, if you're very sexually active—or your partners could be, talk to your doctor about continuing HPV screening.

For Women with Certain Health Conditions

All the above guidelines are for women at average risk of cervical cancer. They don't address women who have a high risk for cervical cancer because of HIV-1, having had an organ transplant or their mothers took the drug DES to prevent miscarriage. If you're in any of these situations, talk to your doctor about how often you should be screened and what tests are most appropriate.

Note: The BRCA gene is not associated with cervical cancer, so cervical cancer screening recommendations are independent of BRCA status.

Testing for Other HPV-Associated Cancers

HPV is also associated with head and neck and anal cancers...and for women, vaginal and vulvar, and for men, penile cancers. There are no guidelines for routine screening for these cancers, but there are tests that can look for them. For instance, there's an anal version of the Pap test that can look for precancerous changes...if you have itching or bleeding from your anus, talk to your doctor about this right away. The main warning sign for head and neck cancer is laryngitis that doesn't seem to go away.

To understand more about the HPV infection, read "HPV: The Killer That We Don't Talk Enough About" on page 189. And to help keep your immune system strong and able to clear the virus, practice these essentials: Eat a healthy diet…exercise regularly… drink alcohol in moderation…get appropriate screenings…and if you smoke, quit. Smoking makes your immune system less effective and speeds up the transition from healthy cells to cancerous ones.

More Grown-Ups Should Get the HPV Vaccination That Used to Be for Kids—Are You One?

Anna Wald, MD, MPH, head of the allergy and infectious diseases division, professor of medicine, laboratory medicine and epidemiology, University of Washington, Seattle.

You may have heard that the age limit for getting the HPV vaccine was increased to 45, but what does that really mean if you're over the previous ceiling of age 26? After all, when the vaccine was first introduced, the idea was to offer protection against key strains of the virus before people became sexually active. The answer is simple—it can still be a lifesaver. And the reason is that the vaccine can prevent reinfection as well as new infections.

The CDC estimates that 80 million Americans carry one or more strains of HPV (human papilloma virus), a dangerous family of viruses that can cause not only genital warts but also cervical, vaginal and vulvar cancers in women…penile cancer in men…and throat cancer in both sexes. Research shows that, unlike with most other viruses, contracting one strain of HPV may not confer immunity—not only can a person still be in-

fected by other HPV strains (there are more than 100 in all), but also reinfected by the same initial strain.

While it's ideal to be vaccinated during the preteen years, people up to age 45 still will benefit from the vaccine's primary goal—protection against the most dangerous strains of the HPV responsible for the cancers mentioned above.

How the Age Change Came About

The FDA extended its approval of the Gardasil 9 vaccine up to age 45 for both sexes after a groundbreaking study of more than 3,000 women, ages 27 to 47, for whom Gardasil was found to be 88% effective in preventing HPV infection, genital warts, vulvar and vaginal precancers, cervical precancers and cervical cancers related to the virus. Because men have been shown to have the same immune response as women, experts anticipate that the vaccine will also offer men in this age group protections against genital warts and cancer. This is especially important considering the recent steep rise in HPV-related cancers in men.

Why this should matter to you: HPV is the most prevalent sexually transmitted disease in the US—the CDC states that nearly all men and women will get at least one type of HPV at some point within their sexually active lifetimes. If you have new sexual partners or if there's any chance that you and your current partner aren't completely monogamous, you're at risk of being infected with one or more HPV strains and should consider getting vaccinated. Note that teens age 15 and older and adults need a total of three shots unlike younger teens, who need only two.

People over age 26 may not be able to have the vaccine covered by insurance. Despite FDA approval, most clinicians and insurance companies are following the recommendations from the Centers for Disease Control and Prevention, which states that the vaccine is more effective at younger ages.

About the vaccine: There are no serious or long-lasting side effects of the vaccine. As with any shot, you might have soreness, swelling and/or redness at the injection site. Some people have reported getting a headache soon afterward.

Also, there is more to learn about the vaccine, including how long its protection lasts.

Important: Even if vaccinated, women still need regular tests to identify cervical cell changes. The vaccine does not replace these screening measures.

Flu Can Be Missed...and Become Deadly

Leslie Kernisan, MD, MPH, a geriatrician and founder of the aging health podcast and website, BetterHealthWhileAging.net. Study titled "Underdiagnosis of Influenza Virus Infection in Hospitalized Older Adults," by researchers at Vanderbilt University School of Medicine in Nashville, Tennessee, published in *Journal of the American Geriatrics Society*.

D id you know that you can have the flu without having flu symptoms? It's particularly true for people over age 65—and it can be really dangerous.

To understand why, consider the H3N2 flu strain that circulated during the 2018–2019 flu season. It was so fierce that it overwhelmed many people, even many of those who were vaccinated against it. Hospitals were packed, hundreds of people died, and many more became seriously ill while the season continued into the spring. As always, people over 65 were more vulnerable than younger people to flu-related serious illness (such as pneumonia), hospitalization and death.

Here's the shocker: A new study found that older people going to hospitals with respiratory illnesses—during flu season—were less likely than younger people to be tested for the flu! *Here's what the study found—and how to protect yourself...*

Undercover Operation

Researchers analyzed how often flu tests were ordered for 1,422 patients who were admitted to four Tennessee hospitals during several of the past flu seasons. Many, but not all, had symptoms that can signal the flu, including cough or fever. The researchers looked at the rates of testing for the flu according to doctors' orders. They also independently—and surreptitiously—tested each patient for the flu themselves.

Results: Doctors flu-tested only 28% of patients, and were only about half as likely to order flu testing for patients 65 or older than they were for patients who were younger.

Important finding: More than one-quarter of the older people with confirmed influenza infection in this study did not have classic influenza-like signs such as cough and fever.

Here's why: Older people often don't develop the cardinal signs of infection from the flu—their immune systems do not respond as vigorously as younger people's. For example, they're less likely to develop a fever, which is one of nature's defenses against many viruses and bacteria. Plus, older people may have lower normal temperatures, so the typical definition of fever (above 100.4°F) may not be the right guide.

As a result, in older people with the flu, it might initially seem like a worsening of symptoms of chronic conditions they already have, such as asthma, congestive heart failure or chronic obstructive pulmonary disease (COPD). Or they might just feel fatigued and under the weather. But doctors should know better—especially during flu season—because these patients are actually in grave danger.

Why Prompt Diagnosis Matters

Knowing that you have the flu is critically important. Even though early symptoms of the flu may appear less worrisome in older people than in younger people, the flu can—and often does—ultimately come roaring forth in these older people and turn very serious very quickly. Research suggests that in people who are "high risk"—and everyone age 65 or older is considered high risk—early use of antiviral medications can significantly reduce the risk for serious complications of the flu, including bronchitis, pneumonia and death.

Important: The 15-minute rapid-flu test often used in doctors' offices and hospitals frequently results in "false negatives," meaning you may have the flu but the test doesn't detect it. So if your rapid test is negative, ask your doctor to also give you a follow-up test, which can take a few hours.

If you've already had the flu shot and you feel ill during flu season, ask to be tested for the flu anyway. Especially in difficult years, when the vaccine is not a great match for the actual flu that is circulating, it is quite possible to get the flu even though you've been vaccinated.

Get Tested—But Protect Yourself First

Because the flu resulted in such serious illness and risk for death during the 2018–2019 flu season, the Centers for Disease Control and Prevention issued an emergency update that said that people at high risk who are suspected of having the flu should be started on antiviral medications immediately—even before an influenza test confirmed the presence of the virus. It's best to start antiviral medications within the first two days of having symptoms, and the earlier they're started, the better they work. But the drugs may still be beneficial when treatment is started later. (*Note*: It's still important to get accurate test results to find out if you do indeed have the flu, since that knowledge can guide your continued treatment.)

Bottom line: If you are over 65 and you don't feel well, get tested for the flu even if you do not have a fever or cough. Don't wait to see what happens or until you get much sicker—anti-influenza medication works best the sooner you start it and can help you avoid

hospitalization. It's possible that doctors and hospitals may be more attuned to flu testing in a bad-flu year, but if it is not offered, ask to have the test.

More ways to protect yourself…

• **Make sure to get the flu shot.** It's not 100% effective, but it's better than not getting it at all.

• **Ask your doctor about getting vaccinated against pneumococcal disease to protect you against pneumonia and other illnesses that can make the flu particularly deadly.** The one-time-only vaccination series (usually two shots administered one year apart) is recommended for all people age 65 and older.

How to Survive a Dangerous Flu Season

The 2017–2018 flu season was the worst in the US since the 1970s—49 million people got sick…960,000 were hospitalized…and nearly 80,000 died. It was a perfect storm—a particularly nasty influenza virus…a vaccine that was less effective than usual…and a growing population of older people, who are most susceptible to the flu and related complications. About 70% of flu hospitalizations and 90% of deaths were among people age 65 and older.

It's hard to know how bad a flu season will be (even with predictions), so it makes sense to protect yourself. We interviewed an infectious-diseases expert and an integrative physician to bring you a powerful toolkit to help you avoid the flu—and if you do get sick, to help you get better fast.

Flu Shots, Booze and Shut-Eye

Infectious-diseases specialist William Schaffner, MD, advises everyone to…

• **Get an annual flu shot even if you're skeptical.** If you've already gotten one, bravo. But fewer and fewer Americans are doing so. Now research from the Centers for Disease Control and Prevention (CDC) shows that skipping the shot was a significant contributor to the record-high hospitalizations and deaths during the 2017–2018 flu season. According to the CDC, only 37% of US adults got vaccinated—down significantly from more than 43% the year before. If you're skeptical about the flu shot based on what happened during a bad-flu season—the vaccine was less effective than usual—keep in mind that things would have been even worse without it. If you are vaccinated and still get the flu, you're likely to have a milder infection. It also will be shorter in duration, and you'll be less likely to get pneumonia, to be hospitalized—or to die.

• **If you're age 65 or older, make sure that you get one of the vaccines licensed for use in older adults.** There are two—the high-dose flu vaccine and the adjuvanted flu vaccine. Either one is fine and will give you a bigger immune response than the standard shot. I don't recommend the nasal vaccine for older people. September is the best time to get vaccinated, but if you forget, January and February are not too late because flu season often lasts through March.

• **Get extra protection if you think you've been exposed to the flu.** If flu is rampant in your community or a family member brought it home, your doctor can prescribe an antiviral medication (see "If You Do Get the Flu" on next page). These not only help reduce flu symptoms, especially if taken within 48 hours of the start of symptoms but, according to the FDA, also may help prevent flu if you are exposed. It's still important to get a flu shot, of course, but an antiviral medication can provide additional protection if needed.

Tip: If you're planning a trip between now and spring, ask your doctor about prescribing an antiviral for you to have on hand in case you find yourself surrounded by people with the flu. Cruise ships, in particular, are hotbeds for the flu.

• **Cut back on or avoid alcohol during flu season.** Alcohol negatively affects the body's immune response and can increase the likelihood of getting an infection as well as the severity of an infection. Do stay hydrated, though—that helps your immune system function at its best.

• **Stay active.** Regular exercise boosts immunity, so keep up your fitness routine throughout the winter even when you feel like hibernating.

• **Keep a solid sleep schedule.** Healthy men and women who average less than seven hours of sleep per night are three times more likely to catch a cold, compared with those who get eight hours or more of sleep, and good sleep likely helps ward off the flu, too.

• **Be smarter about hygiene.** Besides frequently washing your hands and using an alcohol-based hand sanitizer, regularly sanitize shared surfaces such as those in bathrooms and kitchens…and doorknobs throughout the house. Don't get too close to sick people if you can help it—viruses can be spread not only by sneezes but also by simply breathing. And stay home if you're sick so that you don't become a dreaded spreader of germs.

William Schaffner, MD, professor of preventive medicine in the department of health policy and professor of medicine in the division of infectious diseases at Vanderbilt University School of Medicine, Nashville.

Natural Ways to Prevent Flu

Integrative medicine practitioner Fred Pescatore, MD, often prescribes dietary supplements for the fall and winter to help his patients prevent colds and flu. *It's fine to take one, two or all three of the following…*

• **N-acetyl cysteine (NAC).** This antioxidant can help prevent the flu, and clinical studies have found that it helps ward off flu symptoms even in people who already are infected with the virus.

Typical dose: 500 milligrams (mg) per day.

• **Olive leaf extract.** This supplement contains a bitter compound called oleuropein that has strong antiviral properties.

Typical dose: 500 mg per day.

•**Monolaurin.** This antiviral is derived from lauric acid, one of the main fats in coconuts. It destroys viruses by breaking down their outer membranes.

Typical dose: 300 mg per day.

Other natural preventives…

•**See the light.** Sunlight helps your body produce vitamin D, a potent immune booster. Some scientists think that the lack of sunlight and reduced vitamin-D production in the darker months help explain why flu is so common then. For extra protection, give yourself some full-spectrum light inside your home, too. Light therapy has been shown to enhance the immune system in the winter, and a full-spectrum light box is well worth the investment for this purpose.

Fred Pescatore, MD, a practitioner of natural and integrative medicine in New York City, author of several books including *The A-List Diet* and former associate medical director of the Atkins Center for Complementary Medicine.

If You Do Get the Flu

From Dr. Schaffner…
Antiviral drugs can make your illness milder…shorten the duration of the time you are sick…and may prevent serious flu-related complications that can lead to hospitalization. It's best to take an antiviral within 48 hours of symptom onset, so call your doctor the minute you start to feel sick. Classic flu symptoms include sudden onset of fever, aches, chills and tiredness.

Even if you've had the flu for more than a few days, an antiviral drug still may lessen symptoms. That's especially important for people at high risk for flu-related complications, which includes people who are age 65 or older and people with medical conditions such as heart disease, diabetes or asthma.

Oseltamivir (Tamiflu) is the standby, and it's still effective, but now there's a new option—*baloxavir marboxil* (Xofluza), which was approved by the FDA in October 2018. Unlike Tamiflu, which is taken over the course of five days, it's a single dose. It also dramatically cuts "viral shedding," so you're less infectious (Tamiflu hasn't been shown to do this). Overall, Xofluza and Tamiflu are about equally effective, and their costs are very similar.

From Dr. Pescatore…
The following remedies can help reduce the severity and duration of the flu. *It's fine to use one or any combination of these remedies…*

•**Oregano oil gargle.** Put two drops of oregano oil in one-quarter cup of water, gargle and spit. It is fine to gargle up to four times a day. Keep in mind—it has an intense flavor, and you'll smell like pizza!

•**Active hexose correlated compound (AHCC).** This mushroom extract has been shown to shorten the duration of flu and ease symptoms. It also improved the immune response in people who took it right after getting a flu shot.

Typical dose: 500 mg three times a day.

•**Elderberry tea** is an antiviral that's effective for treating flu symptoms and shortening the duration of the illness. Drink one cup a day. You also can take it as an extract or a syrup.

•**Robuvit, an antioxidant supplement derived from French oak wood,** helps people recover more fully after flu symptoms have passed. In a study, people who took the supplement daily for three weeks after their flu symptoms subsided had better post-flu strength, sleep quality and attention span, compared with people who didn't take it.

Typical dose: 200 mg three times a day.

Stylish Flu Protector?

Miryam Z. Wahrman, PhD, professor of biology, William Paterson University, Wayne, New Jersey. Dr. Wahrman is author of *The Hand Book: Surviving in a Germ-Filled World*.

You may have seen ads for a product called the Scough, which looks like a scarf or bandanna but contains an activated carbon insert that the manufacturer claims filters out germs and viruses and neutralizes them. While activated carbon can bind to some volatile organic compounds, such as formaldehyde, and some gases in cigarette smoke, it does not filter bacteria or viruses. Another ingredient mentioned is "silver nanoparticle impregnated filtration." Silver is known to inhibit bacterial growth, but the manufacturer doesn't specify the extent of the silver coating or provide any proof, such as independent testing, that supports its effectiveness in reducing disease risk for the wearer.

My advice: If you're worried about exposure to germs in crowded places, consider wearing a surgical mask, which is well-documented to be effective. If you don't like the look, place your own bandanna or scarf over it.

Plus: Don't forget to wash your hands often!

Natural Remedies to Bounce Back from the Flu

Jamison Starbuck, ND, is a naturopathic physician in family practice and producer of *Dr. Starbuck's Health Tips for Kids*, a weekly program on Montana Public Radio, MTPR.org, both in Missoula. DrJamisonStarbuck.com

If you get the flu, you may assume that you're down for the count and just have to wait it out. A medical doctor may prescribe an antiviral medication, such as *oseltamivir* (Tamiflu), if you talk to him/her within 48 hours of your symptoms starting. That's the window when the drug should be started for it to be most effective, which means lessening fever and symptoms and shortening your illness by about a day. But even in the midst of misery, you can start a bounce-back program—therapies designed to hasten your recovery from the flu beyond what you can get from over-the-counter pain and congestion

medications…and speed your body's overall healing by boosting your immune system.

What I recommend (regardless of whether you're taking a prescription antiviral) during and soon after a bout of the flu…*

• **Drink flu-fighting tea.** A tea made from equal parts elder (flowers and berries), linden and chamomile has antiviral properties and is relaxing to the mind and body. Steep two teaspoons of the mix in eight ounces of water, then strain. Drink five cups per day (as hot as you can tolerate to encourage blood flow to your lungs) and preferably 30 minutes before or after meals. If tea is not available, take one-quarter teaspoon of a tincture of one or more of these herbs in a cup of hot water four times a day during your illness and for a few days afterward.

• **Try homeopathy.** To shorten your recovery time, take two pellets of homeopathic Influenzinum 30 C, twice a day for three days while you are battling flu symptoms. Put the pellets under your tongue and let them dissolve. Take 30 minutes before or after eating. Influenzinum sparks an immune response to the flu virus.

• **Add an adrenal-boosting regimen.** When you are really sick, your body uses lots of cortisol, a stress hormone that helps defend against illness and restore well-being afterward. Depending on your health, your age and the severity of the illness, supplies of cortisol can run low during a bout of the flu. That's why my bounce-back protocol includes adrenal support—herbs and nutrients that help your body produce cortisol. For this, I often prescribe vitamin B-5, also known as pantothenic acid (250 mg, twice daily with food)…vitamin C (1,000 mg, twice daily with food)…and a tincture of Panax ginseng (one-quarter teaspoon in two ounces of water, twice daily, 15 minutes before or after eating). I recommend taking this regimen throughout the course of the flu and for one week after your symptoms subside.

* Talk to your doctor before trying these remedies if you have a medical condition or take medication.

•**Get moving!** When you've just come down with the flu and have a fever and significant pain, get your rest. But as soon as these symptoms pass—even though you may still be sniffling, tired and suffering from stiff muscles—try to take a short walk outside to get a few deep breaths of fresh air. If possible, do this every two to three waking hours. If you have chronic lung disease, use caution—cold air can cause shortness of breath. Gentle walking promotes circulation, and deep breathing increases the amount of oxygen that fuels your body.

Be aware: The flu often causes muscle weakness, which can linger following the illness. Pay attention to your balance and muscle strength, and take precautions, if needed.

Important: If you have the flu and develop a high fever, painful cough or shortness of breath, see your doctor right away. The flu increases risk for pneumonia, which can be deadly.

Mint Herbs Cure Winter Ills

Jamison Starbuck, ND, is a naturopathic physician in family practice and writer and producer of *Dr. Starbuck's Health Tips for Kids,* a weekly program on Montana Public Radio, MTPR.org, both in Missoula. DrJamisonStarbuck.com

Few of us make it through winter without coming down with a cold, cough or sore throat. But popular over-the-counter (OTC) medications are notorious for causing side effects such as drowsiness, blood pressure spikes and dry mouth.

For common winter ailments, I often recommend what I call "mint medicine." Even though the mint, or *Lamiaceae,* family is most widely recognized for culinary spices, such as basil, rosemary, thyme and marjoram, it also includes several medicinal herbs. You probably know about peppermint and spearmint, but many lesser-known yet effective medicinal herbs also should be on your radar—especially during winter cold-and-cough season. My three favorites...*

•**Horehound might be familiar to some as an old-fashioned candy/cough drop.** For centuries, it has been used to treat ailments of the respiratory tract, including bronchitis, colds, sore throat and cough. Horehound is especially useful because it has expectorant and decongestant properties, so it helps the respiratory tract rid itself of mucus or phlegm. Because horehound dries up mucus, you should use it when you are blowing your nose a lot or coughing up or spitting out phlegm many times throughout the day. Don't use horehound if your cough is dry or if your throat is raw. Even though horehound candy has traditionally been used as you would a cough drop, many brands contain a lot of sugar. The tincture, however, doesn't have sugar and it's more potent—thus more effective—for respiratory ailments.

Typical dose: 30 drops, in two ounces of water, taken on an empty stomach, four times a day until symptoms improve. If it's too bitter for your taste buds, stir the tincture into a teaspoon of honey.

•**Hyssop, like horehound, is best used with colds and respiratory conditions that lead to congestion and lots of mucus.** Hyssop works synergistically with horehound, so if you're looking for a stronger effect, try combining the two herbs. For example, you can combine hyssop tincture with equal parts horehound tincture and take 30 drops of the mix in two ounces of water four times a day until the illness is gone.

Great gargle for sore throat: Hyssop tea, sweetened with honey, acts as an antiseptic and soothes inflammation. Gargle with hyssop tea as often as desired. Hyssop tea also can reduce a fever, especially when combined with peppermint. For this, steep one teaspoon of dried hyssop and one teaspoon of dried peppermint leaves in eight ounces of boiled water for five minutes, then strain. Sweeten, if desired, with honey, and drink

*As with any herbal medicine, talk to your doctor before trying if you have a medical condition or take medication.

one cup of tea every two waking hours until you have had four cups. Do not exceed four cups in one day—astringent herbs can slightly irritate the stomach if you overdo it.

• **Catnip is widely used in Europe for colds.** Like horehound and hyssop, it has a drying effect but also is calming and gentle on the stomach. Catnip is a good bedtime tea if you have trouble sleeping because of a productive cough or nasal congestion.

What to do: Pour eight ounces of boiling water over two teaspoons of dried herb. Cover and steep for 10 minutes, then strain. Drink up to four cups daily, including a cup at bedtime, if needed, until you feel better.

How to Soothe a Summer Cold

Murray Grossan, MD, ear, nose and throat specialist, Tower Ear, Nose & Throat, Cedars-Sinai Medical Center, Los Angeles. DrGrossansLibrary.com

Having a cold in the summer can be more miserable than having one in the winter. But there are things you can do to feel better faster even during summer's hot, sticky temps.

The first thing to know is that it isn't only hot weather that makes colds feel worse in the summer—summer colds are often medically worse because they are caused by a different kind of virus. While the various viruses that cause colds are present year-round, rhinoviruses are most prevalent in winter, and enteroviruses are more common in summer. Both kinds cause muscle aches, fever, sore throat, sneezing and a runny, stuffy nose, but enteroviruses also can cause mild respiratory problems, nausea, vomiting, diarrhea, pinkeye and, in rare cases, endanger the heart (myocarditis) and the brain (encephalitis). And while both kinds of viruses are transmitted by coughs and sneezes, enteroviruses also are spread by fecal matter. (Think contaminated bathroom surfaces at highway rest stops, beach and park portable restrooms,

amusement park restrooms and all those other favorite summer hangouts.)

Another reason summer colds can seem worse than winter ones is psychological. If everyone else is out having summer fun while you're stuck inside with a box of tissues, it can feel particularly unfair…and lonely. Research shows that feeling lonely can make physical stressors—such as cold symptoms—seem more intense. This is a good time to Skype, Facebook, text and telephone to catch up with family and friends!

Time-honored winter cold remedies work just as well for summer colds, including drinking plenty of liquids, such as tea and chicken soup, and eating foods that are easy to digest. If hot drinks don't appeal when outside temperatures are in the 80s and 90s, room-temperature drinks are OK. But give icy-cold beverages a miss because they can make a summer cold worse. A hot or warm drink first thing in the morning can mitigate morning cold symptoms and may even lessen symptoms for the rest of the day. Ideally, sip the beverage before getting out of bed. (Avoid coffee and alcohol, which can be dehydrating when you have a cold.)

Your ability to handle temperature changes is reduced when you have a cold. Going in and out of air-conditioning can make symptoms worse, as can having cold air blasting directly at you, such as in a movie theater. Getting chilled also can make you more vulnerable to other viruses besides the one you already have. If you can't avoid frigid AC drafts, cover up with a jacket, sweater, long pants, etc.

Good sleep is especially important when you're trying to get over a summer cold (or a winter one). Try a little Benadryl (take half a 25-mg tablet)—it will make you drowsy and reduce your symptoms.

Whether to exercise depends on what you feel up to doing. Hard workouts are not generally a good idea when you have a cold, but the most important thing is to dry yourself off after you exercise to avoid getting chilled. A gentle walk outside in sunlight—you can avoid the hottest time of day, of course—helps kill viral infections.

What else helps…

• **Bromelain.** Taking 500 gelatin-dissolving units (GDU) twice a day of bromelain, an enzyme found in pineapples, can help relieve the pain of a sore throat and achy muscles. Bromelain is generally considered safe, but check with your doctor.

• **Humming.** Humming a low tone or an "oooommmm" sound deep in your throat helps the nasal cilia move the virus out of your nose and throat. Try 15 minutes every hour.

• **Honey.** Take one teaspoon of honey twice a day to thin mucus and speed healing. Processed honey is better in order to avoid possible allergies from raw honey.

• **Wading in the waves at the water's edge on a beach or walking in early-morning dewy grass helps fight infections**—if you're up to it, give these outings a try. You'll probably meet some people to chat with and feel less isolated in the bargain!

How to Survive Sepsis

Steven Q. Simpson, MD, professor of medicine at University of Kansas, Kansas City, and chief medical officer of the Sepsis Alliance, Sepsis.org. He was among the authors of the *2016 International Guidelines for Management of Sepsis and Septic Shock.*

When it comes to medical emergencies, we all know that heart attack, stroke and asthma attacks are among the most serious. But there's a medical emergency that most people don't know about even though it kills 270,000 people in the US each year. That's one death every two minutes…and more deaths than those caused by breast cancer, prostate cancer and AIDS combined.

This runaway killer is known as sepsis. It is a life-threatening condition that occurs when the body goes into overdrive to fight an infection, such as pneumonia, the flu or even a urinary tract infection.

Sepsis causes a deadly cascade of events when the chemicals that the immune system releases into the blood to fight infection trigger inflammation throughout the body that leads to tissue damage, organ failure and death. If not recognized and treated promptly, sepsis can worsen—and kill—within a matter of days…or even hours.

Latest development: New efforts are under way to help people identify sepsis more quickly and get the right treatment promptly so they can survive this devastating illness.

What you need to know to protect yourself and your family…

The Danger Signs

While anyone who is battling a bacterial, viral or fungal infection can develop sepsis, the old and very young are at particular risk. So are people with chronic diseases such as diabetes, cancer, chronic obstructive pulmonary disease (COPD) and kidney disease.

Sepsis is commonly misdiagnosed because its symptoms—including fast breathing (greater than 20 breaths per minute—the normal rate is 12 to 20)…a racing pulse (above 90 beats per minute)…the chills…pale, clammy skin…and extreme fatigue—can be mistaken for any number of health problems such as heart attack, stroke, pulmonary embolism, exacerbations of chronic lung disease or heart failure.

Misdiagnosis also can occur because there is no definitive test for sepsis—it is diagnosed based on a checklist of signs and symptoms.

To help people identify the red flags of sepsis, the Sepsis Alliance has created the TIME acronym…

Temperature: It can be either above normal (such as 100.4°F or higher) or below normal (such as 96.8°F or lower). Severe chills or burning fever are common.

Infection: It may be obvious, such as the flu or an abscess, or there could be less obvious signs and symptoms, including intense pain in some part of one's body, profound weakness or loss of appetite for both food and water.

Mental decline: People with sepsis are often confused or disoriented. They may be very sleepy and hard to rouse.

Extremely ill: Sufferers often experience intense, sharp pain in the chest, belly or elsewhere. They may be short of breath. Many survivors recall, "I felt like I was going to die."

If you think you may have sepsis, seek immediate medical attention. If your doctor isn't available, call 911 or get to an emergency room.

Important: Whether you're seeing your own physician or an ER doctor, make sure he/she knows your concerns. *Ask straight out*: "Could this be sepsis?" Don't be shy about pushing for tests for impaired organ function such as creatinine for kidney function, lactate (lactic acid) level, platelet count, bilirubin and liver enzyme studies.

Keep in mind that the diagnosis of sepsis is missed completely about half of the time—and a delay in treatment can be fatal. Untreated sepsis can rapidly turn into shock, in which blood pressure plummets and tissues are starved for oxygen and nutrients. For every hour that treatment is delayed, the likelihood of septic shock increases.

Newest Treatment Options

The latest sepsis practice guidelines, jointly issued by American and European critical care medicine societies, more strongly emphasize the urgency of sepsis diagnosis and treatment.

Under these guidelines, a main goal is to eradicate infection with antibiotics that cover a wide variety of bacteria. Equally important is raising blood pressure to restore delivery of oxygen and nutrients to the organs and normalize their ability to function. This means intravenous fluids and, if needed, vasopressor drugs, such as norepinephrine, that stimulate the heart and tighten blood vessels to improve function.

Drugs to reduce immune system activity, once a mainstay of treatment, are no longer standard, reflecting a better understanding of the complex biology involved. Instead, researchers are exploring the use of anti-inflammatory drugs early in the condition's course and immune-stimulating drugs later.

Another change involves medical centers' adoption of highly organized procedures to bring optimal treatment to their patients in the shortest time.

For example, in New York State, which mandates this approach, patients who were diagnosed and treated for sepsis after three hours (and up to 12 hours) of an exam were 14% more likely to die in the hospital than those treated within three hours, according to a 2017 study published in *The New England Journal of Medicine*.

To be alert for possible sepsis: If you have a loved one in the ICU, ask the doctors every day if there are signs of infection, especially if the person is on a mechanical ventilator.

Lingering Ailments

Scientists are discovering increasing evidence that the effects of sepsis can linger. Up to half of survivors suffer "post-sepsis syndrome" (PSS). Physical aspects of PSS reflect damage to vital organs and other tissues. There can be impaired breathing and liver and kidney function, which are often irreversible. Gangrene due to tissue death caused by infecting organisms can necessitate amputation. Fatigue and muscle and joint pain are sometimes disabling.

Recent discovery: The long-term mental impact has only recently been recognized. This may include insomnia, hallucinations, panic attacks, poor concentration, impaired memory and even post-traumatic stress disorder (PTSD).

While the reasons for such mental effects are not yet known, it's believed that sepsis may disrupt the protective blood-brain barrier, leaving the brain vulnerable to damaging inflammation.

Medications used in the ICU—especially sedative agents, including benzodiazepines such as *midazolam* (Versed)—also may have negative effects on mental functioning, sometimes lasting for years.

Much remains to be learned about PSS, but it seems likely that quick action early in the course of sepsis could cut the risk.

Avoiding Sepsis

The key to preventing sepsis is to prevent infection. *To do this…*

•**Get recommended vaccinations,** including yearly flu shots and vaccination against pneumonia.

Also: Sepsis can occur with shingles if the skin becomes infected with bacteria. This is an additional reason to consider getting the shingles vaccine.

•**Practice good hygiene.** Wash your hands frequently and thoroughly (for at least 20 seconds).

•**Clean any cut, scrape or burn quickly and apply antiseptic or antimicrobial cream.** If a wound shows signs of a worsening infection—redness, swelling, red streaks radiating up the arm or leg—seek immediate medical attention.

Note: Sepsis is not generally contagious, but some infections that cause sepsis are, such as plague or meningococcal meningitis.

The Growing Danger of Antibiotic Resistance

Cindy M. Liu, MD, PhD, MPH, associate professor in the department of environmental and occupational health and chief medical officer of the Antibiotic Resistance Action Center at the Milken Institute School of Public Health at George Washington University in Washington, DC.

We've all heard that antibiotic resistance—the ability of some bacteria to resist even the strongest drugs—is on the rise. In fact, it's been said that the "antibiotic era" may be coming to an end. But what does this mean for you?

For answers, we spoke with Cindy M. Liu, MD, PhD, MPH, a leading expert on the use and misuse of these powerful drugs.

Is antibiotic resistance truly a serious health threat?

Absolutely! Every year, about two million infections from drug-resistant organisms occur in the US, and "superbugs," such as methicillin-resistant S. aureus (MRSA), are causing more serious illnesses.

The list of such drug-resistant bacteria just keeps growing. The most recent threats include carbapenem-resistant Enterobacteriaceae, which lead to infections that occur primarily in hospitals, nursing homes and other health-care settings…and antibiotic-resistant gonorrhea, a sexually transmitted disease. Antibiotic-resistant infections cause at least 23,000 deaths per year in the US.

Why does antibiotic resistance continue to be such a big problem?

Bacteria have an innate ability to develop resistance. And the frequent use of antibiotics—both by individual patients and by society as a whole, including agriculture—gives bacteria even more opportunities to develop resistance.

When a person takes an antibiotic for an infection, the antibiotic penetrates the individual's entire body, not just at the site of infection. This puts pressure on one's normal bacteria (called the microbiome).

If you happen to be carrying a superbug in your gut or nose, on your skin or anywhere in the body, then that superbug can thrive as the antibiotic kills off your resident bacteria. So even if the antibiotic kills the original infection, you could become the source of a superbug that you could pass on to other people.

This happens frequently in hospitals, where there are lots of sick people taking lots of antibiotics, but it probably also happens in our homes and workplaces. This is one of the reasons why it's so important to wash your hands frequently and thoroughly. Proper hand hygiene can prevent you from picking up superbugs and can also prevent you from spreading them if you happen to be carrying one.

But we won't get a real handle on the problem until doctors change their prescribing habits and people stop demanding antibiotics when they don't need them. The Centers for Disease Control and Prevention (CDC) estimates that one-third to one-half of all antibiotic prescriptions are unnecessary or used inappropriately.

How might an antibiotic be used inappropriately?

The most common inappropriate use of antibiotics is for upper-respiratory-tract infections. Most of the time, these infections are caused by viruses, and antibiotics don't kill viruses. So why are people getting antibiotics for viral infections? Part of the problem is that people (including many doctors) still think that there's no harm in taking an antibiotic, so they use them "just in case." However, now we're learning that antibiotic use puts us at increased risk for all kinds of negative side effects—from drug allergic reactions to being infected by potentially deadly C. difficile, a toxin-producing bacterium that kills tens of thousands of people in the US each year.

We mostly hear about antibiotic resistance as a public health threat. Are individuals personally at risk if they take antibiotics frequently? Some people—those with diabetes, women with recurring urinary tract infections (UTIs), older adults, etc.—are prone to frequent infections. The more they take antibiotics, the higher their risk of developing an antibiotic-resistant infection. But it's not just these people who are at risk. We are all at risk for superbug infections and negative side effects when we take antibiotics.

Should I ask my doctor not to prescribe antibiotics?

When a doctor is giving you (or your child) an antibiotic, I think everyone should at least ask whether the medication is really needed—and if it should be taken right away or if you can wait for a few days to see if the

symptoms clear up on their own. The treatment guidelines for infections tend to favor drug therapy, even when the evidence suggests that no treatment or watchful waiting might be a better choice in some cases.

Some clinicians feel pressure to prescribe antibiotics, even when the medication is not necessarily indicated, to hedge their bets and help them to have shorter visits. And some actually may prescribe unnecessary antibiotics just because they think that's what the patient wants, not what the patient needs. It's important for doctors to hear from you that you don't want an antibiotic unless it's truly necessary.

Is it true that patients who stop antibiotics early increase the risk for resistance, both for themselves and for society as a whole?

The conventional wisdom is that stopping an antibiotic before a prescription is completed will give bacteria the opportunity to mutate and become resistant. But some experts aren't so sure.

A British team of scientists reported that there's little real evidence to support this idea. They concluded that lengthy antibiotic treatments—including those in which prescriptions are followed to the letter—are more likely to cause resistance than prevent it. That's because each day that you are on antibiotics, you are disrupting your microbiome and potentially fueling the growth of superbugs.

The disruption of your microbiome can also put you at risk for other infections. Antibiotic-related changes to vaginal bacteria, for instance, can lead to the overgrowth of fungal cells and yeast infections, while antibiotic-related changes to the gut microbiome greatly increase the risk for infection by C. difficile. The risk for these kinds of infections increases with frequent and lengthy antibiotic use.

The paper from the British team, published in the prestigious *BMJ*, is controversial, since it goes against most of the messaging that's been promoted over the past several decades. Even the CDC website says to finish your prescription. Clearly, we need a lot more research into this, and we need to develop evidence-based messaging for the general public.

I believe that shorter antibiotic treatments might be better for some patients, depending on the type of infection, the drug being used, the patient's medical history, etc. For example, it's probably relatively low risk for someone who's being treated for a UTI to stop the antibiotics after the symptoms have resolved. It's certainly reasonable to ask your doctor if it's OK to stop the drug when your symptoms improve, even if you haven't finished the full prescription. (*Important*: Do not just stop taking an antibiotic on your own because you feel better.)

What else can we do to combat resistance?

People get tired of hearing it, but hand hygiene is one of the most important things you can do for your health—and the health of those around you.

It's particularly important when you've been in a hospital or doctor's office. Your health-care providers are constantly being exposed to drug-resistant organisms...and they don't always wash their hands.

One study found that 75% of the cell phones carried by health professionals were contaminated with disease-causing germs, including MRSA.

My advice: Wash your hands with soap and water (or at a minimum, use an alcohol-based hand sanitizer) when you arrive at your doctor's office and when you leave... after being in public places...and after handling meats. And don't forget to wash your knives, cutting boards and countertops after handling meats/poultry.

You don't need to go out and buy special antimicrobial soaps. These products are no better than regular soaps at getting rid of superbugs and actually may help fuel the problem when they are flushed into the environment.

How to Tell If You're Hooked on Antibiotics

David Hyun, MD, senior officer, Antibiotic Resistance Project, The Pew Charitable Trusts and coauthor of study titled, "Comparison of Antibiotic Prescribing in Retail Clinics, Urgent Care Centers, Emergency Departments, and Traditional Ambulatory Care Settings in the United States," published in *JAMA Internal Medicine*.

You feel sick enough to drag yourself to a doctor...and leave clutching a prescription for an antibiotic. Hold on! There's a one-in-three chance that this drug won't help you—and a decent chance that it will hurt you.

Studies done in 2016 and 2018 by The Pew Charitable Trusts in partnership with the CDC found that's the case. Although the studies did not investigate the root causes for this antibiotic Rx explosion, the researchers believe that there are many factors at work. Some are "social," meaning that patients expect and demand antibiotics when they feel sick, influencing doctors' decisions to prescribe them.

Example: You mention to your doctor that the last time you had these same symptoms, you took a particular antibiotic (you even mention it by name) and it did the trick. Whether or not it was the intention behind your comment, the doctor may infer that you expect to be prescribed the same antibiotic this time.

This is not to say that medical doctors don't know when an antibiotic is truly indicated—they know that antibiotics kill only bacterial infections. But sometimes it's hard to diagnose whether an infection is caused by bacteria or a virus. Some doctors may decide to prescribe an antibiotic just to be on the safe side.

But "the safe side" has a downside. Treating with unnecessary antibiotics accelerates the emergence of antibiotic resistance—the development of bacteria that are no longer sensitive to the antibiotics currently available.

This is an extremely dangerous situation: It's estimated that, every year 2 million Americans get an antibiotic-resistant infection and 23,000 people die from one.

It's also possible to have adverse reactions to antibiotics, ranging from minor symptoms such as rashes and gastrointestinal discomfort to severe complications including Clostridium difficile, a bacterial infection that can result when the drug kills off healthful bacteria in your body, and the potentially deadly epidermal necrolysis, a disorder that starts with a severe skin reaction.

Illnesses That Do and Don't Need to Be Treated with Antibiotics

Some bacterial illnesses are very unlikely to go away without antibiotics. Two common ones are bacterial pneumonia and urinary tract infections.

Conditions that are often inappropriately treated with antibiotics include…
- **Viral upper respiratory tract infections, including the flu**
- **Viral pneumonia and bronchitis**
- **Asthma**
- **Allergies**
- **Sinus infections**
- **Sore throat**
- **Middle ear infections**

However, complicating things is the fact that sometimes sinus infections, sore throats and middle ear infections are caused by bacteria and do require antibiotics. But there is no good way to collect samples from the sinuses or the ears in a typical doctor's office to culture to find out whether bacteria are present. These are situations when prescribing antibiotics to be safe might make sense.

On the flip side, some scientists are reevaluating the common procedure of treating acute uncomplicated diverticulitis (inflammation of small bulging pouches that can form in the lining of the digestive system, especially the colon) with antibiotics. Two studies published in the British Journal of Surgery concluded that antibiotics didn't speed up recovery time or prevent complications or recurrence of the infection. With the growing concern over antibiotic resistance, some European guidelines have started to recommend managing acute uncomplicated diverticulitis without antibiotics.

Doctors in the US have not yet reached this conclusion. A review published in 2018 in *The American Journal of Gastroenterology* found that not treating diverticulitis with antibiotics appears to increase the need for elective surgery, and surgery carries its own set of risks. More study is needed before doctors should stop prescribing antibiotics for this infection.

How to Avoid Taking Unnecessary Antibiotics

It helps to recognize that your expectations and approach to your medical visit play a significant role in whether a health-care provider prescribes an antibiotic.

When an illness lands you in your doctor's office or at an urgent care center, go without the preconceived idea of needing an antibiotic. Ask questions about your diagnosis so that you can help make an informed decision about your treatment. If the doctor thinks that an antibiotic is necessary, ask why so that you're confident it's the right course of action.

If you have a condition for which it's not possible to confirm a bacterial cause, such as a sinus infection, you might work out a treatment-and-follow-up plan with your doctor that puts off taking an antibiotic while you wait to see if other remedies help.

To keep your need for antibiotics to a minimum, double up on efforts to stay well. Antibiotic use increases in the winter and throughout flu season because the flu can look like a bacterial infection or can lead to one. Take all the preventive steps you can, including getting vaccinations that are appropriate for you and frequent hand washing.

On Antibiotics? Don't Reach for Probiotics Just Yet

Eran Elinav, MD, PhD, Bill & Melinda Gates Foundation International Research Scholar and professor and chair of immunology at Weizmann Institute of Science in Rehovot, Israel, and coauthor of the study "Post-Antibiotic Gut Mucosal Microbiome Reconstitution Is Impaired by Probiotics and Improved by Autologous FMT," published in *Cell*.

For some people, taking a course of antibiotics may cause digestive upset and diarrhea. That's why so many people now take probiotic supplements after antibiotics. The probiotics will replenish the "friendly" bacteria that are killed by the antibiotics, restoring the "microbiome"—the balance of gut bacteria that we all need for good health (and good digestion).

But surprisingly, proof of the effectiveness of this strategy has been highly debated. Now two large studies have taken a closer look—and the argument for using over-the-counter probiotics after antibiotics does not look strong.

In the latest study, researchers treated 21 volunteers with a seven-day course of commonly prescribed wide-spectrum antibiotics. Some volunteers were randomly assigned to take an 11-strain probiotic mixture after the course of antibiotics.

Result: The microbiomes of the volunteers who didn't take probiotics recovered within three weeks of the cessation of antibiotics, while those in the probiotic group did not recover even five months after stopping antibiotics.

While the generic, store-shelf-type probiotics didn't help in this study, the future may hold an effective solution. In the same study, participants who received their own mixture of gut bacteria after finishing antibiotics—a procedure called autologous fecal microbiome transplantation—reconstituted their microbiomes within days of the procedure. This technique is not widely offered, but a time may come when doctors either routinely offer it to patients after antibiotics or can in some other way prescribe a probiotic formula that is precisely personalized to each patient...rather than using the current and ineffective one-size-fits-all approach.

The "New" and Dangerous Sexually Transmitted Disease HTLV-I

Robert Gallo, MD, professor of medicine and of microbiology-immunology and cofounder and director of the Institute of Human Virology at the University of Maryland School of Medicine, and cofounder and international scientific director of the Global Virus Network, and Yutaka Tagaya, MD, PhD, assistant professor at the Institute of Human Virology at the University of Maryland School of Medicine, both in Baltimore.

A very old viral infection in humans is becoming a substantial threat. It is devastating people in central Australia, among other locations. Could it be the second coming of HIV...and headed for the US and everywhere else, too? For answers, we turned to Robert C. Gallo, MD, the scientist who with his colleagues reported the discovery of this virus, HTLV-1, in 1980, but whose attention turned to HIV/AIDS when that virus swept across the globe.

A Deadly "New" Disease That Isn't New

Most people have never heard of HTLV-1, and it was even off the radar of many health professionals until quite recently. But researchers renewed the alarm about HTLV-1—that stands for "human T-cell leukemia virus Type 1"—at the 2017 international meeting of Dr. Gallo's Global Virus Network in Melbourne, Australia. HTLV-1 had already been identified as the first human virus known to directly cause a human cancer, specifically an adult T-cell leukemia and lymphoma, and the first human retrovirus ever shown to cause disease at all. Later a French group showed that it also causes a severe paralytic neurological disease. But now, it's also been found to cause a deadly lung infection, called bronchiectasis, and it is killing one particular group of people in far less time than the decades it takes for those cancers to develop, Dr. Gallo said.

HTLV-1 is a retrovirus. It's not as immediately infectious as most other viruses, such as the flu virus, but rather it takes some time to find a way into the DNA of people exposed to it. An astonishing 45% of the indigenous people in Alice Springs, Australia, are infected with HTLV-1. And that's not the only place. Other pockets of rampant HTLV-1 infection around the world are in New Guinea, Japan, Haiti, Jamaica, Peru, Chile, Brazil, Colombia, West Africa and Florida, primarily involving immigrants from the Caribbean region. There is an important difference between the outbreaks in Australia and elsewhere, according to Yutaka Tagaya, MD, PhD, a colleague of Dr. Gallo's. The virus currently affecting Alice Springs is a different subtype than the one seen in the other hot spots and may be more infectious— the lung infection is killing more people and doing so much faster than any other illness caused by HTLV-1. But the how and why of the rampant lung infection are still mysteries.

Important note: According to a study on HTLV-1–infected patients in Florida published in Blood Advances, the leukemia/lymphoma caused by the disease is very aggressive and ultimately fatal. There are currently trials of antiviral drugs under way and anti-CCR4 antibody therapy is approved in Japan to combat the disease.

Do You Need to Be Worried?

Other than a few news headlines that followed the Global Virus Network meeting, we haven't heard much about HTLV-1 in the US because it is still relatively rare here—less than 0.1% of Americans overall are infected. But it is disproportionately hitting certain groups—while very few Americans of European descent have been infected, 1% to 2% of African Americans have been infected, a comparatively huge number.

Being infected does not mean a particular person will necessarily develop cancer or another illness—some people are just carriers. But because HTLV-1 is similar in important ways to its cousin HIV, it's important to be aware of it. Like HIV, HTLV-1 is a sexually transmitted disease and can be spread through exposure to infected blood and from mother to child through breastfeeding.

The US, Australia, Japan, Peru, Brazil and most European countries test their blood banks for the virus, but not all countries do. Medical centers in the US used to, but no longer do, test transplant organs for HTLV-1, the government's rationale being that there are too few cases of HTLV-1 to justify the cost, especially in view of a high rate of false positives from the test. Dr. Gallo points out that the risk may need to be reevaluated in light of recent studies in Japan in which the HTLV-1 infection associated with organ transplants was shown to substantially increase the chances of developing aggressive neurological disease.

As one of the scientists who first connected the dots between HIV and AIDS, Dr. Gallo is advocating for HTLV-1 to be added to the list of sexually transmitted diseases maintained by the World Health Organization, which recognizes it but has not given it the importance of other diseases. Greater recognition by the WHO would almost certainly speed up efforts around the world for development of treatments and a vaccine and for additional countries to test their blood supplies and transplant organs. Dr. Gallo believes that if all focus hadn't completely shifted to HIV when it was discovered, science could have prevented what's happening now to the indigenous people of central Australia.

Until this all happens, he suggests the following to protect yourself from being infected by HTLV-1, particularly if you're a world traveler…

• **Practice safe sex, get tested and ask any partners to be tested for the virus,** as many people do for the HIV virus.

• **Be aware of the blood-testing practices of the country you're in,** and if there's any way to avoid it, don't get a blood transfusion in a country that does not test its blood supply for HTLV-1.

●**If you need an organ transplant, ask that the organ be tested for HTLV-1.**

Note: If you're pregnant, get tested for HTLV-1 and, if you test positive, don't breastfeed.

Could HTLV-1 take us by surprise and become a ubiquitous killer the way HIV did in the 1980s? Both Dr. Gallo and Dr. Tagaya think that type of global epidemic is unlikely because HTLV-1 is not nearly as easily transmitted as HIV. It's an older virus, and mankind has already somewhat adapted to it biologically. But more and more people are being exposed to it. For instance, HTLV-1 hotspots in Japan used to be only in the southwest and northern parts of the country, but now there is one in Tokyo as well. Both Drs. Gallo and Tagaya said that we're probably seeing the early stages of what will become a global problem, but not with the speed or prevalence of HIV.

Gut Acting Up?

Don't assume that it's something you ate. *New discovery:* Some viruses (including the Zika and West Nile viruses) damage nerve cells in the intestine as well as the brain.

Result: Abdominal pain and constipation. *Cell.*

What to Do If Your Dog Bites Your Hand

William Schaffner, MD, professor of preventive medicine in the department of health policy and professor of medicine in the division of infectious diseases at Vanderbilt University School of Medicine in Nashville.

As a general rule, dog bites on the hand need to be attended to medically unless they are very minor and superfi-cial—and seeing just any health-care provider won't be enough.

There's a tendency to want to minimize a bite, especially when it's your own dog, explained infectious disease specialist William Schaffner, MD, but that's a mistake.

The reasons: Even when there isn't a lot of pain, a dog bite can result in serious injury to soft tissues and tendons. It can cause nerve damage as well as infection and leave you with limited motion in your hand if not properly—and quickly—treated, and it doesn't matter whether it's your dog, a neighbor's or a stranger's.

Dog bites are not just puncture injuries but also "crush injuries," and either way, they can be more serious than they look. The amount of force from a dog's jaw can be substantial, so a bite can mash tissue well beyond any broken skin. If the dog grabbed you and then moved its head side to side while holding on—an instinctive attack behavior—it can worsen the injury.

What about germs? Dogs' mouths tend to be somewhat cleaner than people's mouths, but they are still teeming with bacteria. Your dog's bite is therefore also an injection of bacteria. If those germs are injected deeply enough, they can easily cause not only a local infection but also a dangerous systemic infection. People with weakened immune systems or diabetes are even more susceptible, but no one is immune.

Here are the steps that should be taken if your dog bites your hand…

●**Wash your wound with soap and water immediately,** wrap it with some gauze or, in a pinch, a clean towel and head to the ER.

Why the ER? Your primary care provider and even a typical "urgent care" facility aren't equipped to handle the protocols for a dog bite.

Tip: Don't go alone—getting bitten by your own dog is a traumatic experience, and you'll likely be shaken up, so if possible, let someone else drive even if you think you can drive yourself. Don't waste time rummaging around for your dog's rabies certificate—if you're sure that it's been vaccinated, you don't need it.

• **At the ER, your care may include X-rays to make sure there are no broken bones,** an exam to determine the depth of the injury, cleaning and debriding the wound (removing any damaged tissue to promote healing) and any needed surgery. (If you were bitten on the face, the emergency department can also bring in a plastic surgeon.) The doctor will also make sure that the injury didn't involve a compartment—the various tendons in the hand that enable the muscles to make your fingers move are separated into compartments. If you get an infection in a compartment, it can injure the corresponding tendon.

• **Since it's impossible to isolate the type of bacteria that got from your dog's mouth into the wound, a weeklong course of broad-spectrum antibiotics is the standard treatment.** If you don't remember when you had your last tetanus shot, you'll likely be given a booster, possibly the Tdap vaccine, which protects against tetanus, diphtheria and pertussis (whopping cough) and is commonly the one used.

• **You may need a follow-up visit with a specialist if you had surgery or rehab after your hand heals.** If the emergency department you go to isn't part of your healthcare provider's electronic network, you'll likely be told to let your doctor know about the incident and the care you received…and to give his or her office a call if you see signs that your wound is getting worse—swelling, pain, redness (especially if it's extending beyond the area of the bite), discharge and/or a low-grade fever.

• **Also consider whether you need to call your vet to discuss the situation.** Ask yourself if this was a provoked bite—were you playing roughly with your dog, did he get startled or was a stranger involved? In these cases, it was likely an isolated incident. But do be more concerned if your dog became aggressive spontaneously and talk to your vet about steps to take.

Don't Let Your Cat Make You Sick

C at-scratch disease is a bacterial infection that happens when a cat bites or scratches hard enough to break a person's skin or licks an open wound. The bacteria that cause the disease are found in 40% of cats. Felines rarely have symptoms, but affected people can have swollen lymph nodes for months and may need antibiotic treatment or even hospitalization.

Self-defense: Wash your hands after any contact with a cat. Keep cats' claws trimmed. Wash any bites or scratches well with soap and running water. In case of any bite, seek medical attention.

HealthLetter.MayoClinic.com.

Why Are Probiotics in Some Hand Sanitizers?

Philip M. Tierno, PhD, clinical professor of microbiology and pathology, New York University School of Medicine, New York City.

S ome alcohol-based hand sanitizers now contain probiotics. Does this make the product more effective?

It's hard to tell. Alcohol-based hand sanitizers claim to kill 99.99% of the bacteria on our hands. Probiotics, of course, are the beneficial bacteria that are introduced into the body (typically via the gut). These "friendly" bacteria help offset the harm from disease-causing bacteria and other pathogens. A hand sanitizer that contains probiotics is formulated to kill harmful bacteria while protecting beneficial bacteria, according to one manufacturer.

How it works: Almost all germs on your hands—both good and bad—are destroyed by alcohol (or by some other antibacterial product) in hand sanitizer. With the use of a new encapsulation technique, the manufacturer has devised a way for the hand sanitizer to protect the good bacteria by "walling them off" so that they are not destroyed by these active ingredients. After the freshly applied hand sanitizer has evaporated, the encapsulated probiotics "break open" and recolonize your hands with beneficial bacteria, according to swab tests done by the manufacturer.

However, I would be skeptical of any manufacturer's claim that this new encapsulation technology actually allows good bacteria to repopulate the skin. There are hundreds of strains of bacteria that colonize on our hands, and we don't know which ones are being preserved via this process. Even so, the normal skin flora of the hands is more complex than previously thought. The manufacturer must prove that the correct strains have been chosen to repopulate the hands and that these would not cause any harm to people, including immunosuppressed individuals (such as those receiving chemotherapy).

My takeaway: Studies on this new technology need to be published in a peer-reviewed journal before any sound conclusions can be made. Strong research confirms that hand washing with soap and water is the best way to remove germs. According to the Centers for Disease Control and Prevention, soap and water are more effective than hand sanitizer at removing common pathogens, including those that cause common gastrointestinal ailments, such as Cryptosporidium infection, norovirus and Clostridium difficile (all three of which are not killed by alcohol)...rhinovirus, which causes about half of the cases of the common cold...flu viruses...and even certain superbugs such as methicillin-resistant Staphylococcus aureus (MRSA).

Don't make these mistakes: To ensure that you don't expose your hands to germs after washing, don't touch the faucet with your bare hands. Instead, use a tissue or paper towel to close it and to open the door when exiting the bathroom. Also, if there are automatic dryers available, don't hit the edges of the device when drying your hands.

If you have no access to soap and water, using an alcohol-based hand sanitizer that contains at least 60% alcohol is an effective way to kill most bacteria, viruses and other pathogens on your hands. Apply hand sanitizer (a quarter-size dollop) to the palm of one hand, then rub it all over both sides of both hands until the alcohol evaporates and your hands feel dry.

Epstein-Barr Virus Cured—Naturally

Andrew Rubman, ND, founder and medical director, Southbury Clinic for Traditional Medicines, Southbury, Connecticut. SouthburyClinic.com

---

The patient: Shelly, a single mother of two high schoolers who was passionate about being there for her kids, both athletes.

Why she came to see me: For the past two years, after her divorce, she had been suffering bouts of terrible fatigue that would "come on like a flu" and then seem to partially go away but leave her dragging for many months afterward. She was particularly troubled because she couldn't keep up with her children's field hockey and basketball activities. Her Ob/gyn, whom I had lectured with and co-managed a number of patients and pregnancies, suspected a chronic herpetic virus and found evidence of Epstein-Barr Virus (EBV) in a screening test.

How I evaluated her: I reviewed Shelly's bloodwork and ordered a more complete EBV panel, which showed evidence of a chronic recurrent reactivation of the virus. I explained to her that we had been taught to believe that the virus was incurable and that the best we could hope for was to improve her immune function so that she could limit the frequency and intensity of the reoccurrences.

How we addressed this problem: We discussed all of the pertinent factors contributing to improving immune function, from adequate sleep and stress management to changes in diet and nutritional supplements.

I prescribed a number of antioxidant and immune-stimulating vitamins, mineral, and botanicals. One in particular that I had had great success with in the past is a little-known botanical called *Lomatium dissectum*, which had been used historically as an anti-viral. An isolate of the tincture had been prepared and studied by the renowned naturopathic physician Ed Alstat, ND, and found to possess this property and avoid some of the side effects that had been reported by some with its use.

The patient's progress: I saw Shelly two weeks later and she appeared to be recovering nicely from her most recent bout of viral reactivation. I cautioned her to go "slow and steady" and continue the regimen, and let me know if she experienced a reoccurrence. After six months of being free of symptoms, we retested her blood and found no evidence of her even having the virus. As my MD friend quipped, "This isn't supposed to happen!" She remains healthy to this day.

Mysterious Earache...

Your ear is suddenly swollen, itchy and hurting. Is this just an earache or something else?

It's most likely an infection in the outer ear canal called otitis externa or swimmer's ear. Swimmer's ear develops when too much moisture gets in the ear canal, such as after swimming or shampooing your hair, allowing bacteria to grow. To confirm this, see your doctor. He/she may prescribe an antibiotic eardrop. I've also recommended to my patients with swimmer's ear an antihistamine such as *diphenhydramine* (Benadryl) to help ease the itching and swelling.

In the future, you may be able to prevent swimmer's ear by wearing earplugs or applying baby oil to your ear canal before you shampoo your hair or go swimming. Do not try this if your eardrum could possibly be perforated.

Murray Grossan, MD, ear, nose and throat specialist, Cedars-Sinai Medical Center, Los Angeles. GrossanInstitute.com

Chapter 10

KIDNEY, BLADDER AND LIVER HEALTH

The Best Checkup for Your Kidneys

When you see your doctor for a regular checkup, your kidney health may be getting short shrift. You may think your doctor is staying on top of all the tests you need…but not necessarily.

Screening for chronic kidney disease (CKD)—when it's performed—has traditionally involved a select group of blood and urine tests. But in today's busy doctors' offices, it's common for the urine test to not be ordered. This means that any testing you do receive may be inadequate. Now that's about to change.

Latest development: To simplify testing, the National Kidney Foundation has collaborated with the American Society for Clinical Pathology and other leading laboratory societies and laboratories to identify a combination of specific tests now called the Kidney Profile. When performed together, these tests—a urine sample for albumin-to-creatinine ratio (ACR) and a blood test for estimated glomerular filtration rate (eGFR)—streamline the testing process. These are the two tests recommended by the National Kidney Founda-

tion and the American Diabetes Association to test individuals at risk for kidney disease.

Pairing the results from these tests makes the Kidney Profile more accurate and comprehensive than receiving just one test. The combination not only detects CKD but also identifies the stage of kidney disease and provides a stronger prediction of one's risk for kidney failure, heart disease and other chronic conditions.

If CKD is detected, the test results enable doctors to better determine how a patient's individual case should be managed—typically with medications for those at earlier stages… and with dialysis or even a kidney transplant for people who have later-stage disease.

For example, high blood pressure with high levels of albumin in the urine, or ACR, should be treated with a blood pressure medication that also protects the kidneys—this could be an angiotensin-converting enzyme inhibitor, such as *benazepril* (Lotensin) or an

Joseph Vassalotti, MD, chief medical officer of the National Kidney Foundation, Kidney.org, and associate clinical professor of medicine in the division of nephrology at Icahn School of Medicine at Mount Sinai in New York City. His research has been published in peer-reviewed journals such as *American Journal of Nephrology, Kidney International* and *American Journal of Kidney Diseases*.

angiotensin receptor blocker, such as *losartan* (Cozaar).

Who Should Get the Kidney Profile?

The people for whom CKD testing is recommended haven't changed—they're the same individuals who should have been getting annual kidney screenings all along. *This includes people in specific high-risk groups for CKD, such as...*

• **Anyone who is age 60 or older.**

• **Adults with diabetes and/or high blood pressure**—chronic conditions that increase risk for CKD.

• **Adults of certain racial or ethnic backgrounds,** including those of African-American, Hispanic, Native American, Asian or Pacific Islander descent.

Why Testing Matters

If you're wondering whether testing for kidney disease really is that important, the answer is a resounding "Yes!" The condition, which impairs the kidneys' ability to remove wastes and regulate crucial chemical levels in the blood, such as sodium, potassium and calcium, is far more common than most people realize.

Startling statistic: An estimated 30 million Americans have CKD, but only 3.6 million are aware of it, while the others have no inkling that anything is amiss.

Worse yet, more Americans than ever before are now considered to be at risk of developing CKD due to diabetes or high blood pressure. This escalating number stems, in part, from the aging population and the obesity epidemic, both of which drive high blood pressure and type 2 diabetes.

The real danger: Once your kidneys are damaged, the harm that is done usually cannot be reversed. More than 450,000 Americans are now on kidney dialysis. The only other treatment for late-stage kidney failure is a transplant—an option that is limited by the relative lack of available kidneys.

The Kidney Profile Can Help Prevent This Scary Scenario

When it comes to annual screening for CKD, cost has never been an issue for most people. The Kidney Profile's blood and urine tests cost under $50 and are routinely covered by health insurance. They are easy to get—if your primary care doctor orders both types of tests for the most complete kidney assessment.

Because the Kidney Profile streamlines and simplifies CKD testing for doctors, patients will get the benefit of more complete testing. With leading labs adopting the combination of CKD tests under the heading of "Kidney Profile" on request forms and electronic health records, doctors won't need to search for and order each test separately...and they also can find the results in one place.

Let's face it: When one less click of a computer mouse or check mark on a handwritten form is needed to expedite proper care, your doctor's job gets easier...and the odds of effective care go up.

Important: If you have one of the risk factors (such as diabetes or high blood pressure), be sure to ask your doctor about getting the Kidney Profile. If it's not yet available in your community, ask for the blood (eGFR) and urine (ACR) tests to be ordered individually.

Hitting the Numbers

CKD can be present if one or both tests are abnormal over a period of 90 or more days. *Here are the numbers you should look for in the Kidney Profile (or in the following tests if ordered separately)...*

• **ACR urine test.** *What's being measured:* Albumin is a type of protein that may signal early kidney disease when it appears in the urine. Creatinine, a product of normal muscle metabolism, is filtered by the kidneys as a waste product.

Target numbers: The ACR is a highly sensitive indicator of kidney damage. If you have ever scrambled an egg, you might notice foam on the surface that represents albumin in the egg. Similarly, individuals with high levels of albumin in the urine may notice foamy urine, but the ACR test is more accurate than looking for foam. The ACR test result should be less than 30 mg/g. Higher levels indicate kidney damage, which in turn increases risk for kidney failure and heart disease.

•**eGFR blood test.** *What's being measured:* Creatinine levels are used in a formula that also incorporates your age, weight, race and gender to calculate your eGFR. The number indicates how well your kidneys are filtering blood to remove natural waste products and excess fluid.

Target numbers: You can think of eGFR readings as a percentage of kidney function. A reading of 60 or higher is considered normal, while a reading less than 60 is considered reduced kidney function. The lower the kidney function, the higher the risk for kidney failure and cardiovascular disease. Many people are diagnosed with stage 3 (or moderate) kidney disease when the eGFR result is 30 to 59. A result below 30 is considered severe CKD.

In general, people who have an eGFR of less than 30 should see a nephrologist (kidney specialist). Patients who have an eGFR of less than 15 usually need to be prepared for dialysis or a kidney transplant.

Note: Low kidney function should be considered when prescriptions are being ordered—some drugs should be avoided, and others need to have the dose adjusted if the drug is eliminated from the body via the kidneys. Approximately half of FDA-approved medications are cleared by the kidneys.

Important: People at risk for kidney disease should be tested at least once every year, but more frequent testing may be advised for more severe kidney disease. Speak to your doctor about the most appropriate testing schedule for you.

For more information, consult the National Kidney Foundation at Kidney.org/CKDinter cept/laboratoryengagement.

Kidney Stone Danger

People taking sulfa antibiotics (such as Septra and Bactrim) were more than twice as likely to develop kidney stones within three to 12 months as those not taking oral antibiotics, according to an analysis of 286,000 children and adults covering 21 years. Four other classes/types of antibiotics—*cephalosporins* (Keflex)…*fluoroquinolones* (Cipro)…*nitrofurantoin* (Macrobid)/methenamine (Hiprex) …and broad-spectrum penicillins—also increased kidney stone risk but to a lesser degree.

Gregory Tasian, MD, pediatric urologist, Children's Hospital of Philadelphia.

The Toxin Hiding in Superfoods

Sally K. Norton, MPH, researcher, nutrition consultant and author of the study "Lost Seasonality and Overconsumption of Plants: Risking Oxalate Toxicity" published in *Journal of Evolution and Health*. Sally Knorton.com

Oxalate is a compound in most plant-based foods and one that can cause kidney stones. But kidney stones may be just the tip of the iceberg, according to Sally K. Norton, MPH, a nutrition consultant and educator and an oxalate researcher.

It almost sounds like a trick by Mother Nature. Oxalate is found in foods we think of as extremely healthy, foods ranging from spinach and Swiss chard to almonds to chia seeds, yet it's often called an anti-nutrient because it limits your body's ability to absorb good-for-you minerals, especially calcium.

Norton emphasizes the diversity of oxalate's forms and harmful effects. They come in foods both as as sharp-edged crystals that can irritate your gut and as smaller molecules that can be absorbed and travel around the body. In addition to causing direct toxic effects when absorbed, oxalates can bind minerals and build up in nearly every type of body tissue, such as bones, tendons, joint fluid, skin, and especially the kidneys. But this is not widely known, even among researchers.

These deposits in your body can grow more damaging over time. In your kidneys they can turn into those painful kidney stones. Getting more, not less, calcium in your diet can actually help you avoid these stones, allowing the calcium to bind the oxalate and reduce how much you absorb in the first place.

An Unrecognized Problem

Many health care professionals believe that all plant foods are good for you, says Norton, and that other than causing kidney stones in some people predisposed to them, oxalates aren't a problem. But eat enough of them, and they can lead to a range of health issues.

A kidney stone can cause obvious symptoms such as intense pain. Signs of oxalate accumulation in other areas aren't as obvious, says Norton. There's no single set of symptoms that point to having too many oxalates in your system. But, she adds, there are clusters of problems that, for many people, improve when they carefully cut back on oxalate consumption.

Consider limiting your intake of foods containing oxalate if you experience two or more of the following…

- **Repeated kidney infections.**
- **Urine that's often cloudy.**
- **Irritable bladder** with frequent urination.
- **GI problems** such as leaky gut, constipation or diarrhea.
- **Joint pain** that comes and goes without obvious cause or that affects different parts of your body on different days.
- **Persistent or recurring back stiffness or pain.**
- **Difficulty getting restful sleep** and feeling fatigued because of it.
- **Cognitive issues** such as brain fog, memory loss or poor concentration.

- **Sensitive or achy teeth** without infection or cavities.
- **Persistent or lingering symptoms after an injury or operation.**

If you've had bariatric surgery, a malabsorption syndrome, or chronic gut inflammation, you'd be wise to watch your oxalate consumption. All these conditions cause excessive absorbtion of oxalate, Norton says.

Putting a Limit on Oxalate

Norton explains that a safe level of oxalate in food depends on how healthy a person's kidneys and digestive tract are. If you don't have any health issues, a safe limit might be as high as 200 to 300 mg a day. Otherwise, you'd be smart to cap oxalates at 150 mg per day or less. A low-oxalate diet is usually defined as 50 mg per day or less.

To give you an idea how quickly you can get into high levels of oxalate, consider this sample from Norton's "worst offenders" list…

- **Rhubarb,** 1,000 mg in one-half cup stewed or canned.
- **Swiss chard,** 900 mg in one-half cup.
- **Cooked spinach,** 500 mg in one-half cup.
- **Chia seeds,** 380 mg in one-quarter cup.
- **Baked white potato,** 120 mg in one medium.
- **Almonds,** 115 mg per ounce (20 nuts).

Other high-oxalate foods include cashews, peanuts, beets, okra, soy, pinto beans, black beans, figs, kiwi, prunes, bran cereals, chocolate, black or green tea and the spices turmeric and cumin. Norton adds that vitamin C can turn into oxalate in the body, so supplementing with more than 250 mg of C per day could make an oxalate problem worse.

No one need give up on plant foods. If you eat a lot of high oxalate foods and have symptoms that could be due to oxalates, try some smart substitutions. Safer yet very nutritious veggies include cabbage, cucumbers, lettuce, radishes, pumpkin seeds, squash and turnips. Heating does not remove oxalate from foods. However, boiling can leach out some of the oxalate.

Norton suggests learning more about oxalate toxicity at two non-profits that focus on conditions that could be worsened by high oxalate intake, the VP (Vulvar Pain) Foundation and the Autism Oxalate Project's Trying Low Oxalate Group that helps families use the low-oxalate diet (click on Find the Support Group).

Natural Cures for a Leaky Bladder

Jamison Starbuck, ND, is a naturopathic physician in family practice and writer and producer of *Dr. Starbuck's Health Tips for Kids*, a weekly program on Montana Public Radio, MTPR.org, both in Missoula. She is a past president of the American Association of Naturopathic Physicians and a contributing editor to *The Alternative Advisor: The Complete Guide to Natural Therapies and Alternative Treatments.* DrJamison Starbuck.com.

Most women (and many men) have had that "oh, no!" feeling of leaking urine when lifting a heavy object or laughing a little harder than usual. The occasional incontinent moment isn't a big deal. But when it happens daily, it's a problem. Prescription drugs such as *oxybutynin* (Oxytrol) and *tolterodine* (Detrol) can relieve symptoms of this condition but often cause side effects, including dry mouth and constipation. Natural medicine is safer and can offer long-term relief. *The main types of incontinence…*

• **Stress incontinence and urge incontinence.** If you lose urine when the bladder is stressed—as with a big sneeze—that's stress incontinence. If you have a sudden urge to urinate and lose urine if you can't get to the toilet almost immediately, that's called urge incontinence. With both of these types of incontinence, weak pelvic-floor muscles are often to blame. *My advice…*

• Urinate on a schedule. I suggest urinating every two hours while you are awake, whether you feel the urge or not. If your bladder is emp-

tied more regularly, you're less likely to leak. If nighttime incontinence is a problem, stop liquids four hours before bed. Instead, have a piece of fruit—it's watery and refreshing but won't fill your bladder the way a beverage will.

• Tone up. If your pelvic muscles are weak, Kegel exercises are the go-to solution…for both women and men.

What to do: While you're sitting or even standing, contract the muscles you would use if you suddenly wanted to stop the flow of urine. Do 10 contractions in a row, three times daily. You should notice a benefit within 10 days. If you hold a lot of tension in your lower abdomen or hip muscles—which often occurs in those who are sedentary—focus on gentle stretching, abdominal massage and deep breathing to help reduce incontinence.

• Check for food allergies. Food allergies cause irritation and inflammation. When the bladder wall is irritated, it's more sensitive and reactive, and this can lead to incontinence. Dairy, wheat and eggs are common triggers. If you suspect that you have a food allergy, ask your doctor about IgG blood testing to check.

• **Temporary incontinence.** Excess caffeine, alcohol, smoking, a diet high in salt and even acidic and spicy foods can irritate the bladder and cause incontinence, along with such symptoms as urinary frequency and urgency. Avoid the potential irritants above one at a time until you find the culprit(s).

Try botanicals: Corn silk and gravel root soothe bladder tissue and calm the urge to urinate. A typical dose is one-quarter teaspoon (in tincture form) of an equal blend of these herbs, added to two ounces of water and taken three times daily (15 minutes before or after meals) until your incontinence improves. These herbs can be used for a long time, but it's best to talk to your doctor if you plan to take any herb for more than a month or so.*

*Consult your doctor before using corn silk if you take medication for diabetes, blood pressure or inflammation, or if you take *warfarin* (Coumadin) or diuretics…and before taking gravel root if you have liver disease or take a seizure drug or the antibiotic *rifampin* (Rifadin).

Drink enough water: It may seem odd to drink more water if you're running to the bathroom all the time, but if you don't drink enough, your urine becomes concentrated, which aggravates the bladder and leads to incontinence. Drinking too much water can do the same. Use this formula—one-half ounce of water per pound of body weight daily. Your bladder will thank you!

Is the New Kegel Throne the Answer to Your "Gotta-Go" Problem?

Kevin Jovanovic, MD, an obstetrician/gynecologist in New York City. DrJovanovic.com

If that "gotta-go" urge is ruling your life and you're afraid to leave home without first mapping out all the restrooms on your route, you might want to sit down…on the kegel throne, that is—a device that sounds improbable at first, yet has helped many of the women who've tried it.

Whether due to age, pregnancy, childbirth or menopause, millions of women have poor bladder control. This includes the overwhelming urge to urinate even when your bladder isn't full (urge incontinence) or leaking urine (stress incontinence) when you jump, cough or laugh, making your favorite Zumba class risky business. Chances are you've tried doing the Kegel exercises that your doctor recommended to stimulate pelvic floor muscles and regain control of bladder function. But sometimes it's just not possible to do enough of them to make a difference. That's where the Emsella chair comes in.

The Emsella transmits magnetic resonance technology (similar to an MRI) to stimulate and contract pelvic floor muscles in a noninvasive way and without pain. It delivers the equivalent of 11,200 Kegels in a 28-minute session—most women fail to do even the recommended 30 Kegels in a day. The chair itself doesn't move (it does make a funny sound, though not as loud as an MRI machine), but how you sit on it—leaning forward or leaning back—allows the appropriate area to be targeted.

Unlike incontinence itself, the treatment is anything but embarrassing. All you do is sit on the cushioned chair fully clothed (you must remove all of your jewelry and part with your keys and cell phone).

Suggested treatment is twice-weekly sessions for three weeks. You may start to notice improvement after a single session. Once you strengthen these muscles, your pelvic floor will feel stronger, and this may encourage you to keep up with Kegels on your own.

Does it work? According to three studies done in the US, the UK and Bulgaria involving a total of 80 women, nearly all noticed an improvement in quality of life. On average, two-thirds were able to reduce their use of incontinence pads, some completely. Many also reported being better able to continue with Kegels on their own at the six-month follow-up.

In fact, doing 100 to 200 Kegels a week on your own is the best way to prolong the results. Right now, with limited use in this country, practitioners are suggesting a once-a-year Emsella maintenance visit.

Note: The chair may also improve sexual satisfaction in men and women because it boosts blood flow to the genital area, important for sexual response. It's also being looked at for improving bladder control in men. Studies are ongoing.

Important: You can't be pregnant and use the Emsella. Insurance does not cover the cost of treatment as of now, which runs an average of $2,000 for the six suggested sessions.

Keep in mind that although the Emsella is an FDA-approved device for female urinary incontinence, research on its effectiveness is in its early stages. Some people in the medical community are still skeptical, preferring more traditional methods such as a pessary (a device that's inserted to support the bladder and prevent leaking), pelvic physical therapy and/or medication or injections to more innovative ideas such as biofeedback. Also, because the chair is relatively new, you may need to hunt to find a gynecologist, urologist or urogynecologist who's offering it. You might start with the search function on the Emsella website (BodybyBTL.com, click on Solutions).

A Lasting Solution for Recurring UTIs

Laurie Steelsmith, ND, LAc, licensed naturopathic physician and acupuncturist in private practice in Honolulu. She writes Bottom Line's "Natural Healing Secrets for Women" blog and is coauthor of three books—the best-selling *Natural Choices for Women's Health*, the critically acclaimed *Great Sex, Naturally* and her latest, *Growing Younger Every Day*. DrSteelsmith.com

The patient: Andrea, a 33-year-old software engineer. *Why she came to see me:* Two weeks before walking into my office, Andrea had been feeling fantastic. Recently back from her honeymoon, she and her husband had just started training for their first triathlon—an endeavor that had her on the trails or in the water five to six days a week. In the last week, however, she'd begun experiencing a range of disconcerting symptoms, from vaginal itching and irritation to an increased urge to urinate that was often accompanied by pain.

At first these symptoms seemed "mild," but her face disclosed what she quickly reported: They'd intensified to the point that the mere thought of going pee left her anxious. Certainly, no stranger to urinary tract infections, Andrea was determined to prevent future infections so that she could compete in the upcoming race with her husband…and relish her life as a newlywed.

How I evaluated her: I started off with an in-office urine test. Besides looking for bacteria itself, I also look for the presence of white cells (which indicate an infection), red cells (which indicate blood in the urine—another sign of an infection), and nitrites (which

indicate bacteria in the urine). In addition, I sent her urine sample off to be cultured, including a sensitivity test to determine the best antibiotic if results indeed show abnormal bacteria growth.

I also checked Andrea's kidneys by doing a kidney punch (also called a Murphey's percussion test), which is a gentle punch to the area near where her kidneys are. Tenderness and/or pain indicates a person may have a kidney infection. (UTIs can become kidney infections if not treated promptly.) No pain after the thump means no kidney infection.

Because she complained of vaginal itchiness and irritation, I sent in a vaginal culture too.

Finally, I conducted an in-depth discussion of Andrea's lifestyle and general well-being.

What my evaluation revealed: While Andrea's kidneys weren't tender (a telltale sign of infection), her urine culture revealed an infection with E. coli. Formally known as Escherichia coli, it's a bacterium we're exposed to daily. However, when our immune systems are impaired—due to stress or illness—E. coli can multiply and cause infections. This includes urinary tract infections, a condition that drives 8.1 million visits to the doctor every year and which, as I assumed, Andrea was suffering from.

More prevalent among women than men, UTIs are frequently accompanied by the very symptoms she was experiencing, from a powerful, unrelenting urge to urinate to acute pain with urination. Dehydration—a common side effect of intense physical training—as well as the frequent sex Andrea and her new husband had enjoyed on their honeymoon and beyond, may have also contributed to her present urinary tract infection in that it can cause irritation to the urethra and vagina.

The good news? Her vaginal culture was normal, meaning she didn't have an overgrowth of yeast or bacteria there.

How I addressed the problem: For her acute infection—the UTI—I prescribed a combination of natural and Western medicine, utilizing "the best of both worlds." Urinary tract infections that have gone on for too long—usually greater than four days—are very difficult to treat with natural medicine alone, and sometimes an antibiotic is necessary to completely resolve the problem. (Most UTIs that I treat within that four-day window can be successfully treated with just natural medicines.)

Antibiotics: I gave her a prescription for an antibiotic that was shown to be sensitive to eradicating the bacteria found on her culture.

Botanicals: I prescribed several botanicals in the form of a tincture consisting of uva ursi (a diuretic), kava (an antispasmodic), goldenrod (an anti-inflammatory), and berberine (a natural antimicrobial). These herbs are known to support the extermination of a bladder infection.

Probiotics: I gave her a combination of lactobacilli and bifidobacter bacteria, taken orally, to replenish healthy flora in her intestines.

Marshmallow root tea: Drinking three cups a day to help rebuild and soothe the mucus membranes of her bladder and urethra.

Fruit extracts: I encouraged her to take one cranberry capsule a day to keep her urine acidic—thus preventing bacteria from thriving—and one teaspoon of D-mannose as well. A natural sugar found in pineapples and cranberries, D-mannose can further assist with the removal of bacteria from one's urethra and bladder by making the mucous membranes of the urethra more resistant to bacterial adhesion, thereby blocking bacteria from climbing up the urethra into the bladder.

One of Andrea's biggest complaints with the treatments she'd received for UTIs in the past was that she would often get them after sex. She would take antibiotics to solve the problem only to return to the health center a few weeks later with the same symptoms. To that end, we also took a look at her lifestyle. While her life was, as she described it, "wonderful," a surplus of stress—classically defined as anything that shakes up the nervous system and that can be negative (like a loss) or positive (like a new marriage)—may

weaken immune function and increase one's vulnerability to illness and infection.

I urged her to pair her demanding triathlon training with more relaxing "yin" exercises such as gentle yoga, stretching and walking, which have long been known to diminish stress and anxiety. I also advised her to increase her water intake to compensate for the fluid loss she likely experiences during training.

To decrease the possibility of tissue irritation, I urged her to use a natural lubricant with sex and to avoid using soap directly on her urethra (no matter how sweaty she may feel after training) as soap can alter the pH of a woman's vulvar tissue, create irritation and potentially allow unwanted bacteria to flourish.

I further encouraged her to wait at least 20 minutes before urinating after sex to allow her engorged tissues to resume their relaxed state. Urinating too soon after intimate relations can prevent bacteria from being adequately flushed from the urethra.

The patient's progress: Andrea resolved her acute UTI. Months later when I saw her for a different issue, she reported that she and her husband had returned to their healthy, happy life without any recurrence of UTI symptoms. Which, of course, was quite clear: She had that new-bride glow and boatloads of energy.

Does Your UTI Need an Antibiotic? What Older Adults Need to Know

The study "Antibiotic Management of Urinary Tract Infection in Elderly Patients in Primary Care and Its Association with Bloodstream Infections and All Cause Mortality: Population Based Cohort Study" was conducted by researchers at Imperial College London and published in *The BMJ*.

When is it appropriate to take an antibiotic? That's not an easy question to answer...even for doctors.

Antibiotics can kill the bacteria that cause a variety of illnesses, but overuse of these drugs can lead to antibiotic resistance—in which the bugs being targeted become stronger than the medicine.

As this thorny question continues to be investigated in the US and elsewhere, researchers in the UK have identified a scenario in which prompt antibiotic use appears to be life-saving. Their results have been published in *The BMJ*.

Study details: To better understand when antibiotics should be prescribed—and for whom—researchers from the Imperial College London crunched the data from 157,264 patients over age 65 who'd had a suspected or confirmed urinary tract infection (UTI). The patients were divided into three groups—those who had been given an immediate prescription for antibiotics…a delayed prescription (by up to seven days)…or no prescription at all.

Results: Compared with those who received an immediate antibiotic, adults who received a delayed prescription for the drug or no antibiotic at all were eight times more likely to develop sepsis, in which the body's response to an infection can lead to tissue damage, organ failure and even death.

Additionally, people who got a delayed antibiotic or no antibiotic had roughly twice the rate of hospital admissions (27%) compared with those who got immediate treatment with the medication (15%).

Among those at greatest danger: Older men—especially those over age 85.

UTIs are among the most frequently diagnosed bacterial infections in adults over age 65. These infections, often called "bladder infections," are frequently caused by E. coli bacteria and characterized by a relentless urge to urinate, burning pain and cloudy, pungent urine.

Caveat: The study authors noted that their results found an association but do not indicate that the delayed use (or no use) of antibiotics caused sepsis or death…and that the patients may have had other health conditions that contributed to their outcomes.

"Although antibiotic prescribing must be controlled to help combat the increasing problem of antibiotic resistance, our study suggests early use of antibiotics in elderly patients with UTIs is the safest approach," said Paul Aylin, MBChB, senior author of the research and professor of epidemiology and public health, Imperial College London.

Can a Yeast Infection Cause Incontinence?

Andrew Rubman, ND, medical director, Southbury Clinic for Traditional Medicines, Southbury, Connecticut. SouthburyClinic.com

After menopause, both vaginal yeast infections and bladder issues become more common. The two conditions aren't always connected—a weak pelvic floor can lead, all by itself, to overactive bladder (the urgent need to pee) and incontinence (leaking)—even if you rarely or never get vaginal yeast infections.

But what many women (and even some doctors) don't appreciate is that the two problems are often connected—chronic yeast infections can lead to bladder problems.

Here's how: Yeast can be a normal part of a person's internal flora—around 70% of people host yeast. Most people aren't bothered by it—but for others it can be a big deal, causing infections in a variety of areas of the body.

When yeast manages to invade the muscular wall of the bladder, it "niggles" at the tissue there to produce the sugar it needs to eat to survive. The inflammation and irritation that result will cause the bladder to become extra sensitive. The condition is called interstitial cystitis. And the result is exactly what you're describing—a need to pee more and an inability to hold as much urine.

The first step? Have your urine checked by your doctor to rule out a bacterial vaginal infection. If you do have chronic yeast infections contributing to urinary problems, the best way to get your bladder back to normal is to oust the yeast—think of it as getting squatters in a house you own to move on.

A Better Way to Fight Yeast

The idea is to change the environment of the bladder so that it's not as pleasant for the yeast to hang out there. One conventional way to do that is with a prescription anti-fungal medication such as or *ketoconazole* (Nizoral). But often drugs simply knock back the yeast without getting rid of it altogether. The yeast population starts to reproduce again and a few weeks later, bam…another urinary tract infection.

A longer-lasting solution is to use a combination of antioxidant vitamins, minerals and supplements to make your body a less comfy home for yeast. You'll need to work with a doctor to create a protocol that will be most effective for you—in other words, this isn't DIY advice. But it can be a successful way to deal with interstitial cystitis caused by yeast in the bladder. *Your doctor should guide you to some combination of…*

1. Vitamins A, C and E—especially C, which makes urine somewhat acidic. Yeast does not like an acidic environment.

2. Zinc. This mineral helps to enhance the junction strength between cells that line the bladder, making incursion by yeast more difficult.

3. Selenium, a trace mineral that helps improve immune function, which in turn helps the body identify yeast infections and fight them.

4. Goldenseal, a botanical remedy that has strong antimicrobial properties. When the extract from goldenseal is taken internally, it becomes highly concentrated in the urine, making it even more effective at fighting virtually all types of microbes, including yeast.

5. Cranberry extract. If you've ever been advised to chug cranberry juice to help treat a urinary tract infection, here's why. Yeast latches onto the lining of the urethra to climb up it, but cranberry contains substances called pro-anthocyanidins (PACs) that makes the walls of

the urinary tract slippery, and the yeast simply fall off. Although not all studies show that cranberry juice extract prevents UTIs by itself, cranberry juice extract—especially the freeze-dried form—contains concentrated PACs that have been shown to make incursions by microbes such as yeast more difficult.

This Herb Combo Helps Urinary Incontinence

Andrew Rubman, ND, founder and medical director, Southbury Clinic for Traditional Medicines, Southbury, Connecticut. He is author of the Bottom Line blog "Nature Doc's Patient Diary." Study titled, "Urox Containing Concentrated Extracts of Crataeva nurvala Stem Bark, Equisetum arvense Stem and Lindera aggregata Root, in the Treatment of Symptoms of Overactive Bladder and Urinary Incontinence: A Phase 2, Randomized, Double-Blind Placebo Controlled Trial," led by researchers at University of Queensland, Australia, published in *BMC Complementary and Alternative Medicine.*

U rinary incontinence puts a damper on your whole life. Drugs don't always help…plus, they have daunting side effects. (Constipation, memory loss, reduced libido anyone?)

Promising news: A new study found that urinary incontinence can be reduced—maybe eliminated—without drugs. How? With a combo of three well-known herbs that have been used for centuries in traditional medicine.

Australian researchers tested an herbal blend called Urox that is a combination of three herbs—Crataeva nurvala (common name, varuna), Equisetum arvense (horsetail) and Lindera aggregata (Japanese evergreen spicebush). The herbs have been used separately to treat urinary symptoms in traditional medicines for centuries and have long-established safety profiles.

For the study, 150 men and women who had urinary incontinence were given either a daily capsule containing 420 milligrams (mg) of Urox…or a daily placebo capsule that looked identical. Both groups took the capsules for eight weeks.

Results: The group that took Urox reported significant improvement. *On average...*

Those in the Urox group needed to urinate four fewer times during the day and two fewer times during the night than they had before the study. Meanwhile, there was very little difference (less than one fewer time on average for both day and night) in the need to urinate among those in the placebo group.

The Urox group had about two fewer episodes of urgency and two fewer episodes of incontinence per day compared with less than one fewer episode of either for the placebo group.

Even better: For 60% of participants in the Urox group, urinary symptoms returned to normal—meaning they no longer had symptoms of urinary incontinence—while this result was seen in only 11% of the placebo group. No significant side effects were reported for either group, although a small number of participants in both groups experienced transient diarrhea or urinary tract infections.

Naturopathic doctor Andrew Rubman, ND, commented that each of these herbs also is effective alone...

• **Horsetail** has been a common remedy for incontinence and bed-wetting in Europe since Shakespeare's time. The plant contains silica, which is anti-inflammatory and acts as an astringent in the bladder to "tone" the bladder wall, which helps restore normal bladder function.

• **Varuna** is an Indian Ayurvedic medicine that increases tone and coordination in bladder muscle. It helps the bladder empty more completely.

• **Japanese evergreen spicebush** is a Traditional Chinese Medicine (TCM) remedy for frequent urination and incontinence. According to TCM, incontinence and frequent urination are caused by "cold energy," and this herb moves warm energy ("chi") into the bladder to disperse the cold energy. But whatever the scientific reason, the remedy often works.

Urox is manufactured in Australia but is available in the US online for about $40 for a one-month supply. It should be noted that this study of Urox was funded by the maker of Urox, but Dr. Rubman points out that the study appears to have been conducted according to acceptable research standards, the researchers shared all their data and the study was published in a peer-reviewed medical journal.

Blood in My Urine!

Christopher Kelly, MD, a physician at Columbia University Medical Center in New York City, and coauthor of *Am I Dying?! A Complete Guide to Your Symptoms—and What to Do Next.*

It can be scary to see blood in the toilet bowl, but stay calm and consider these points...

• **Relax if you have recently eaten beets.** Some people have a genetic tendency to absorb beet pigment from the intestine. Even a small amount of beet salad or borscht can give urine a pinkish tint.

Caution: If you've eaten beets your whole life and only recently noticed urine-color changes, see your doctor.

• **Make an appointment if you see blood in the urine after intense exercise.** This is relatively common among serious athletes (such as marathon runners) but is unlikely to occur in casual exercisers. Dark urine (brown rather than red) that's accompanied by muscle pain could indicate rhabdomyolysis, the breakdown of muscle tissue. Blood in the urine also can be a sign of a urinary tract infection.

• **Get to an ER** (or see your doctor immediately) if you notice blood in the urine in any other situation, particularly if you're age 50 or older. It's the earliest symptom of bladder cancer. The vast majority of patients with bladder cancer will have visible blood—it might appear bright red, coffee-colored or yellowish—in the urine. Doctors assume that bloody urine in an older patient means cancer until they can prove otherwise.

A New Approach to Bladder Cancer Treatment: Watch and Wait

Study titled, "Conservative Management Following Clinical Complete Response to Neoadjuvant Chemotherapy for Muscle-Invasive Bladder Cancer: Contemporary Outcomes of a Multi-Institutional Cohort Study" by researchers at Columbia University Medical Center and Memorial Sloan Kettering Cancer Center and published in *The Journal of Urology*.

Treatment for muscle-invasive bladder cancer can be nearly as scary as the disease itself. It has typically included removing the bladder plus additional surgery to create another way to hold and excrete urine, within the body or with an external bag. Many patients with bladder cancer would dearly like an alternative to having their bladders removed—and now there may be one: A new study from Columbia University Medical Center and Memorial Sloan Kettering Cancer Center has pointed to a promising alternative.

What's Changed, What Hasn't

The first steps for treating bladder cancer are removing the tumor in a procedure called transurethral resection of bladder tumor or TURBT, followed by chemotherapy. Often these steps eradicate the cancer, yet the standard practice has been for doctors to suggest having the bladder removed in a separate operation, called radical cystectomy, after testing has been completed on the removed tumors and if the cancer was found to have extended into the muscle layer of the organ.

What the researchers wanted to learn was this: If a patient who had muscle-invasive cancer is cancer-free after TURBT and chemo, is it really necessary to then also remove the bladder? What would be the outcome if patients like this were monitored rather than automatically having their bladders removed?

To find out, researchers studied 148 patients who had had muscle-invasive bladder cancer but who had decided on monitoring (also called surveillance) rather than bladder removal after TURBT and chemo. These patients were followed for five years to see how many experienced a cancer recurrence. The average age of the patients was 62, and 80% were men. *Here's what happened over the five years…*

- **The survival rate related to the bladder cancer was 90%.**

- **64%** of the patients were still free of bladder cancer after five years.

- **18%** had a recurrence that ultimately required removing their bladders.

The researchers concluded that the high survival rate supports the option of surveillance for patients with no evidence of cancer after TURBT and chemotherapy.

Asking About Surveillance

If you have muscle-invasive bladder cancer and your oncologist suggests radical cystectomy, ask about the option of surveillance. It's not for everyone, but it might be an option for you if you're cancer-free after TURBT and chemotherapy. Talk about the risks and benefits of surveillance versus bladder removal. Consider getting a second opinion if your doctor won't discuss the option or isn't familiar with it.

This is what a surveillance program is likely to involve…

- **Every two to three months,** you will need an overall physical exam, an exam with a bladder scope (cytoscope) and urine testing to look for cancer cells.

- **Every four to six months,** you will need a CT scan or other imaging study of your bladder.

- **After five years,** if there are no signs of recurrence, these tests may be reduced to once a year.

Surveillance does require commitment on your part, but if appropriate, it can be a much easier adjustment than life without a bladder.

Strange Symptoms: Suddenly Spacey, Tired ...and Odd-Smelling

Andrew Rubman, ND, medical director, Southbury Clinic for Traditional Medicines, Southbury, Connecticut. SouthburyClinic.com

The patient: "Jeanette," a patient of mine for many decades, is a practicing Buddhist living in the Bay Area of California who meditates daily and enjoys eating a simple, clean diet. (She comes to visit with relatives in Connecticut, so I have seen her in the office as well as done distance consults.)

Why she came to see me: She called to tell me that she had been feeling "spacey" and tired. Her normal high energy and pleasant mood had been off for the better part of two weeks.

How I evaluated her: As she has always been a consistent creature of habit, I was sure there had been some change—in her environment, lifestyle, diet, etc.—that was affecting her. I asked about her digestion and then she related that her bowel movements had become quite light in color and she was experiencing unusual intestinal gas that was odd smelling. She then told me that the OMD (oriental medicine doctor) who had been treating her periodically with acupuncture for occasional insomnia had given her a package of Chinese herbs to make a tea out of. Jeanette's symptoms started within a few days of her taking this twice-daily tea.

How we addressed her problem: I advised Jeanette to immediately stop the tea and see her local MD that afternoon and ask to have a blood test to evaluate liver enzymes, kidney function and to rule out heart and brain involvement. The tests were ordered "stat" (meaning results requested immediately) and results reported to both the MD and me. Although kidney, heart and brain were not involved, Jeanette's liver enzymes were 15 to 20 times above healthy reference levels. With Jeanette's agreement, her MD and I worked to monitor my regimen to help her clear her system of the unfortunate contamination from the otherwise-innocuous tea. (Although uncommon now, contaminated herbal products coming out of mainland China had been a problem in the past in the Bay Area.)

The patient's progress: Jeanette's MD and I monitored her liver enzyme levels over the next two months with blood draws every two weeks. As we expected, her levels dropped to within reference levels in a manner consistent with recovery from oral poisoning affecting the liver. She has been fine now for the past four months. Part of my responsibility as a physician is to report adverse reactions to medication, whether available by prescription or over-the-counter. Both health authorities in Connecticut and California were alerted to investigate the incident.

Beware High Doses of Fat-Soluble Vitamins

Avoid high levels of fat-soluble vitamins, such as A, D and E. Your body stores excess amounts of these vitamins, mainly in the liver, and that can cause health issues. Vitamin A can bring on headaches, nausea, dizziness and more serious effects. Vitamin D can cause heart arrhythmias and kidney stones. Vitamin E can cause hemorrhages and even hemorrhagic stroke. Fat-soluble vitamins are more dangerous than water-soluble ones, which the body simply excretes if it does not need them. But it is never a good idea to overdo vitamin supplementation. Stick to the Recommended Dietary Allowances (RDA) unless your doctor advises otherwise.

HealthLetter.MayoClinic.com

A New Way to Manage Metastatic Liver Cancer

Xiling Shen, PhD, associate professor in the department of biomedical engineering at Duke University in Durham, North Carolina. His lab specializes in cancer and stem cell regeneration in the gastrointestinal tract.

When you're battling cancer, you want to do everything possible to improve your prognosis. Exciting research published in the journal *Cell Metabolism* found that making a simple change in your diet can have a significant impact on your health.

Most people who die from cancer don't die from their primary cancer, which can often be surgically removed, but from cancer cells that have metastasized to another part of the body. The liver is one place cancer cells like to go and grow. In fact, metastatic liver cancer is more common than primary liver cancer.

The study found that colon cancer cells that migrate to the liver learn to feast on fructose, the sugar that's extremely common in the American diet not so much because it's found naturally in fruit, but because it's added in great quanitities to processed foods.

Why is that so potentially significant for cancer patients? The liver is a major place in the body that stores and breaks down excessive fructose. So the theory is that reducing the amount of fructose eaten could deter the growth of these cancer cells. And if cancer hasn't yet spread to the liver, reducing the amount of fructose eaten might reduce the risk of liver metastasis taking hold.

The enzyme that the liver uses to break down fructose is called ALDOB, and colon cancer cells that find their way to the liver adapt to produce the same enzyme. The metabolized fructose fuels their growth in the liver, which is like a candy store to these cancer cells, said Xiling Shen, PhD, one of the study's researchers.

Blocking ALDOB could be a new way to manage liver metastasis, and Dr. Shen's team is working on a drug to do just that. But in the meantime, it makes sense for people with liver metastasis to cut back on fructose consumption, Shen said.

Because of all the added sugars in packaged and processed foods, the average American eats four to five times more fructose today than a century ago when our main source was the fructose found naturally in fruit. It sounds counterintuitive, but experts say that unless you're gorging on it, fruit doesn't contribute significantly to the problem (and fruit contains antioxidants and an array of other healthful nutrients). *Here are the foods you unquestionably want to avoid...*

• **All types of refined sugar,** such as white, brown and powdered sugars and packaged foods with high amounts of it like sweetened breakfast cereals.

• **Corn syrup and high-fructose corn syrup**—the primary sweeteners used in candy, sodas, sweetened juices and commercial baked goods.

• **Agave,** honey, molasses, sorghum, maple and pancake syrup.

This study looked at metastasis of colon cancer, but several other cancers also often travel to the liver, including lung, breast, pancreatic and stomach cancers and melanoma. It's reasonable to assume that other cancer cells would also take advantage of any fructose in the liver and grow quickly, said Shen.

Better Liver Cancer Test

G. Amit Singal, MD, associate professor of internal medicine and clinical sciences, UT Southwestern Medical Center, Dallas.

When doctors combined a blood test that detects levels of a substance called alpha fetoprotein—a protein that increases in the presence of liver cancer—with abdominal ultrasound (the standard screening method), detection of early-stage liver cancer increased from 45% with ultrasound alone to 63%. Both tests are readily available and should be covered by insurance.

Chapter 11

PAIN AND AUTOIMMUNE DISEASE

Headache Sufferers: Are You Misdiagnosing Your Pain?

When a headache comes on, sometimes you can just pop a pill and the pain goes away—end of story. But not all headaches quit that easily. If you've had a few that made you nauseated and foggy-brained, you might automatically assume that you have migraines. If you're congested, you might assume sinus headache. But the truth is that it's easy to misdiagnose the type of headache you're having. This guide will better help you interpret what you're feeling so you can take the right action.

The Garden-Variety Headache

A tension-type headache (TTH) is the most common headache, and more so among women than men. Typically, the pain is mild to moderate, feels like a tightness or vicelike sensation and affects your whole head—not just one side. This type of headache can last from 30 minutes to, quite surprisingly, a week. You might experience one only occasionally… or chronically—on 15 or more days a month!

While it's possible to experience nausea on occasion with a TTH, this type of headache typically doesn't interfere with ordinary activities—you can still go about your day, work, eat and even exercise. Still, easing the stress that often starts the chain reaction resulting in a headache can help you overcome it. And if you do need a pain reliever, acetaminophen or an over-the-counter nonsteroidal anti-inflammatory drug (NSAID) should do the job.

Migraine: The Headache Misnomer

A migraine isn't just a headache—it's a disabling neurological disorder with a strong genetic component, and it interferes with your daily routine and your ability to concentrate. By definition, a migraine must last from four to 72 hours and have two of the following four pain characteristics—throbbing pain, moderate-to-severe intensity, pain on one side of the head and/or pain that gets worse with routine physical activity. It also must have at least one of these features—

Nada Hindiyeh, MD, director of clinical research and clinical assistant professor of neurology and neurological sciences, Stanford University, Stanford, California, and principal investigator of many studies on migraine.

nausea (or vomiting) or sensitivity to light and sensitivity to sound.

So, for example, if you have a moderate headache that gets worse when you take a walk and find that it hurts to be in a brightly lit room, you meet the migraine criteria. About 25% to 30% of migraine sufferers also experience aura, a type of visual disturbance that precedes the actual pain.

The brains of people genetically predisposed to migraine are highly sensitive to stimuli. When you add in a trigger, such as a particular food, stress or a change in the weather, it seems to push the brain over the edge, leading to a migraine. Food triggers are very individual and include aged cheese, red wine, sugary processed foods, MSG and chocolate, among others. Dehydration or a change in barometric pressure, such as in the cabin of a jet, can set off a migraine. For women, the drop in estrogen right at the start of menstruation is a common trigger. (Three times as many women as men get migraines.)

Note: About two-thirds of women whose migraines are related to their menstrual cycle see an improvement after menopause, but it's also not unusual for a woman to get her first migraine after menopause.

Keeping a headache diary to track episodes and symptoms can help you pinpoint specific triggers to avoid. However, that alone may not be enough to prevent migraines.

There are abortive medications to reduce a current migraine and preventive ones to reduce headache frequency and severity. Depending on how often you get migraines and how disabling they are, you may need both. Until recently, drugs prescribed to prevent migraines had all been medications developed to treat other conditions. Then in 2018, the first migraine-specific drugs were introduced. They target a protein called calcitonin gene-related peptide (CGRP), which has been implicated in causing migraines.

But you can do a lot more than take medicine, starting with your posture. Next is engaging in regular, moderate aerobic exercise, such as a brisk 20-minute walk or cycling on a stationary bike. A healthy, protein-based diet that keeps your blood sugar steady, a regular schedule for eating and sleeping (going to bed and rising at set times) and stress-reduction techniques, such as meditation and biofeedback, all can help. Daily supplements, including magnesium, vitamin B-2 and CoQ10, have also been shown to reduce the frequency and severity of migraines.

Painful Yet Rare Headaches

Trigeminal autonomic cephalgias (TACs) represent a small group of distinct headaches. Best known among them are cluster headaches, so named because they come in clusters—say, three a day for two months—and then stop, often returning at the same time the following year. They cause excruciating pain, always on one side of the head, and can last anywhere from 15 minutes to three hours.

Notably, TAC headaches are accompanied by physical signs, such as tearing or red eye, facial flushing, a drooping eyelid or a feeling of fullness in the ear—in every case, on the same side of the head as the headache. Specific signs are key to identifying TAC headaches and distinguishing them from migraines. Each type of TAC has somewhat different symptoms, frequency, pain severity, underlying causes and treatment, and imaging tests usually are needed to make the right diagnosis.

The Headache That Isn't

Yes, it's possible to get a headache when you have a sinus infection or other sinus-related condition, but most people who think they have sinus headaches actually have migraines. If you get successfully treated for a sinus condition and find that your headaches don't improve, see a headache specialist.

The Headache from Headache Medication

If you take pain relief medications for too many days in a row, you can get a rebound headache (also called "medication overuse" headache). The risk is that a rebound headache can lead to chronic headaches. Keep track of the amount of pain relievers you take, and limit your use to 10 days a month.

The Headache That's a Medical Emergency

A headache that comes on very suddenly, feels like the worst pain you have ever had and is different from the headaches that you typically get should send you to the ER immediately, especially if you're over age 50. It could be an extremely dangerous condition, such as a stroke, other blood vessel problems such as an aneurysm causing a hemorrhage or a brain tumor. Other warning signs are neurological symptoms that are different from your normal headaches, such as weakness or numbness on one side of your body or slurred speech.

Bottom line: If head pain is interfering with your life, talk to your doctor. Once the underlying cause of the pain is found, you can start the appropriate steps to make it stop or at least keep it under control.

Safer, Faster Migraine Drug on the Horizon

Research presented by Sheena Aurora, MD, medical fellow and global launch leader, Eli Lilly and Company, Indianapolis, at the American Headache Society annual meeting, July 2018, San Francisco.

Yes, there are medications for migraine. Unfortunately, they don't always completely relieve the symptoms…can take a long time to work…and cause side effects, including serious ones such as high blood pressure and increased risk for heart attack. Now a new drug—and the first in a new class of migraine drug in nearly 20 years—that promises safer, faster relief for this debilitating condition may soon be available.

Triptans have long been the go-to drug for acute treatment of migraine symptoms once they start. These drugs—such as *sumatriptan* (Imitrex), *zolmitriptan* (Zomig) and oth-

ers—work by helping serotonin bind to sites in the brain called 5-HT receptors. Serotonin constricts blood vessels, and constricting blood vessels in the brain helps relieve migraine pain. Unfortunately, triptans constrict other blood vessels outside the brain, too, including heart vessels, which can cause chest pain, high blood pressure…and lead to heart attack.

The new drug, *lasmiditan*, also binds to 5-HT receptors—but only to those in the brain that are involved in migraine attacks. So the drug does not affect the heart or blood pressure. Lasmiditan is also very fast and effective—providing complete relief in as short a time as one hour.

Two clinical trials compared taking lasmiditan with a placebo among close to 4,500 people (average age 42) who reported three to eight debilitating migraines per month. Some but not all the participants had migraine aura, and most in both studies also had some risk factors for heart disease—and one study included people with known heart disease, arrhythmias and/or high blood pressure. The studies were conducted by Eli Lilly, the company that makes the drug, and the results were presented at the annual meeting of the American Headache Society in San Francisco.

Results: For migraineurs who took 200 milligrams (mg) of lasmiditan within four hours of a migraine attack, 32% in one study and 39% in the other were pain free—compared with 15% and 21% who took the placebo. Photophobia (pain associated with light) was about 41% to 49% relieved, compared with 30% to 33% for placebo. And even though they may not have had complete pain relief, 60% to 65% reported some pain relief, compared with 40% in the placebo group. (The researchers did not compare lasmiditan with triptans.)

Best: Cardiovascular side effects were not reported, even among migraineurs with known heart problems and/or high blood pressure. The most common side effects were mild-to-moderate dizziness, tingling or numbness, sleepiness, fatigue and nausea.

Lasmiditan is not yet available to the public, but Eli Lilly applied for FDA approval in November 2018. Meanwhile, let your doctor know if you are interested in trying the drug so that he/she can let you know as soon as it is available.

Mysterious Neck, Shoulder, Arm or Hand Problems?

Ying-Wei Lum, MD, MPH, assistant professor in the department of surgery, division of vascular surgery and endovascular therapy at Johns Hopkins University School of Medicine, Baltimore. He specializes in the treatment of thoracic outlet syndrome, peripheral artery disease and abdominal aortic aneurysms.

Thoracic outlet syndrome (TOS) is a little-known condition that's tricky to diagnose and treat.

This often painful and disabling disorder results from compression of nerves or blood vessels in the thoracic outlet, a narrow, bony, almost-triangular opening between the first rib at the top of the rib cage and the clavicle, or collarbone. It can cause a wide range of symptoms including neck, shoulder or arm pain…tingling or swelling in an arm, a hand or fingers…weakness in a shoulder, an arm or a hand…and/or impaired circulation in a hand.

Many other conditions (such as diabetes, carpal tunnel syndrome, Raynaud's disease, fibromyalgia or even a heart attack) can cause similar sensations, making it difficult to diagnose. But with the development of a clear set of criteria, vascular surgeons and other specialists can now identify TOS from a careful medical history, basic imaging tests and an in-office physical exam.

Too Close for Comfort

Two major blood vessels, the subclavian artery and vein, pass through the thoracic outlet. So does the brachial plexus, a bundle of nerves that travels to the shoulders, chest, arms and hands. The scalene muscles in the neck border the thoracic outlet.

Anything that crowds the blood vessels or nerves going through the thoracic outlet can cause TOS. This can include an extra rib that protrudes from the neck part of the spine (a cervical rib)…repetitive overhead motions—from activities such as swimming or house painting…and intense weight lifting, whiplash injuries or even weight gain. The symptoms usually affect only one side of the body but can sometimes affect both sides.

Nerves vs. Blood Vessels

Nerve-related TOS symptoms are different from those caused by pressure on an artery or vein…

•**Nerve pressure accounts for more than 90% of TOS cases.** These patients can have pain, numbness or tingling (or all three) that starts in the neck and radiates down to a hand. The discomfort may come and go but usually worsens when an arm is elevated. Patients will continue to have disabling symptoms without treatment.

•**Pressure on a vein or an artery can** restrict blood flow and cause swelling and discoloration of the fingers, hand or arm… or feelings of coldness in the hands. This type of pressure also can increase risk for blood clots in the shoulders or arms, which could potentially lead to a pulmonary embolism (a blood clot in the lungs).

A Diagnostic Challenge

If your doctor suspects TOS, you'll probably be given a chest X-ray to detect rib abnormalities, including the presence of a cervical rib. You'll also be given an ultrasound to help identify blood-vessel abnormalities and clots. But in many cases, doctors can't actually see what's causing the pressure, even with these imaging tests. A thorough medical history, along with an in-office physical exam, are among the best ways to diagnose TOS.

The doctor will take the patient through a variety of maneuvers. Patients with nerve-related TOS will usually notice an increase in pain/other symptoms when they rotate their head or tilt it from the ear to the shoulder. And raising the arms will usually cause an increase in symptoms within 30 to 60 seconds.

Also helpful: An injection of local anesthetic into one of the scalene muscles in the neck. In patients with nerve-related TOS, this will often stop pain almost immediately. The pain relief lasts only for about a day, so it's not a treatment—but it's a good diagnostic test.

A doctor also will look for physical signs like abnormal skin color and cool skin, which indicate severely restricted blood flow or a clot.

Next Steps

Surgery (see next column) is often advised for vascular-related TOS, while more conservative treatment can often be used to avoid (or delay surgery) for nerve-related TOS...

•**Stretches and/or physical therapy** can often help patients with nerve-related TOS. The movements stretch and strengthen muscles, restore normal posture and relieve compression of affected nerves.

Note: Be sure to get a physical therapist's consent before trying stretches on your own.

Sample stretch: Make an "OK" sign with your thumb and forefinger...turn your hand upside down...raise your elbow in the air...and place the circle over your eye. Your palm will be facing toward your face and your other three fingers will be touching your cheek. Hold the stretch for about 30 seconds. Other stretches can be found online (try YouTube) or from a physical therapist.

•**Massage and acupuncture** seem to help some patients with TOS caused by nerve pressure, and there's no downside to trying them, even though there's little evidence to prove these approaches work. But do get checked out by your doctor first to make sure you're not overlooking another problem.

•**Botox injections** in the scalene muscles will shrink these muscles and potentially open up the space in the thoracic outlet to relieve pressure. For about 10% of my patients, the injections provide long-term relief—sometimes for many years.

But more often, an injection gives relief for only two to four months and repeated injections are needed. Most patients aren't willing to keep getting injections, particularly because they tend to get less effective over time. If your symptoms have not improved after three or four attempts, the injections are probably not going to work for you.

•**Blood thinners** are an essential component of therapy when TOS presents with a blood clot in a vein. These patients are at risk for recurrent deep vein thrombosis (DVT) and pulmonary embolism if not treated with surgery (see below). Blood-thinning medications, such as *enoxaparin sodium* (Lovenox) or *rivaroxaban* (Xarelto), can be used until the clot is surgically removed.

If Surgery Is Needed...

In some cases, surgery is required to treat TOS.

For nerve-related symptoms, the goal of surgery is to remove the tissue—either bone or muscle—that's causing the pressure. For clot-related symptoms, surgery is a standard treatment. It's used to remove clots...reconstruct or replace damaged arteries...or remove bone/muscle that's pressing on the affected area.

These procedures typically require a one-to-three-night hospital stay, and patients should do physical therapy as part of their rehab.

Sudden Visual Disturbance

Nada Hindiyeh, MD, director of clinical research and clinical assistant professor of neurology and neurological sciences, Stanford University, California, and principal investigator of many studies on migraines.

It's relatively common for migraine sufferers to experience an aura an hour or so before head pain starts. It's also possible for them to experience an aura with no subsequent headache between 37% and 44% of the time. It happens more often after age 50. But up to 13% of people with no history of migraines have also experienced an aura alone.

If you think that you're experiencing a sudden aura, call your primary care doctor and describe your symptoms. He/she may want to see you to officially rule out a more serious underlying cause, such as retinal disease or a seizure.

Keep a journal to see if there's any pattern to your auras. If one lasts longer than normal, call your doctor. But if you get new symptoms, such as sudden loss of vision or weakness or numbness on one side of the body, call 911. These can be signs of a stroke.

Take safety measures at the first sign of an aura—for example, if you're driving, pull off the road. And because an aura can be stressful, practice your favorite relaxation method until it subsides.

Prevent Neck Pain

Clenching your teeth, perhaps unconsciously, can cause neck pain. To prevent it, repeat to yourself throughout the day, "Lips together, teeth apart."

Carol Krucoff, yoga therapist at Duke Integrative Medicine in Durham, North Carolina.

Could You Have Rheumatoid Arthritis and Not Know It?

Faizah Siddique, MD, assistant professor, department of rheumatology, Stritch School of Medicine, Loyola University, Chicago.

Are you frustrated because your joints are stiff, painful and swollen and you're tired all the time...yet your doctors can't tell you what's wrong? You may have a hard-to-diagnose form of rheumatoid arthritis. The longer it stays undiagnosed—and untreated—the greater your risk for permanent disability. You need to read this now.

Rheumatoid arthritis (RA) is an autoimmune disease. Antibodies produced by the body's immune system attack joint tissues, causing pain, swelling and stiffness in multiple joints. These antibodies, called rheumatoid factor (RF) and anti-CCP antibodies, are detectable in blood tests and help to diagnose RA.

However, up to 20% of people with RA have a form of the disease that doesn't show up in blood tests—seronegative rheumatoid arthritis. In the past, doctors thought that seronegative RA was a milder form of regular (seropositive) RA. It may be that patients with seronegative aren't producing enough antibodies to show up in current blood tests. Recent studies show that seronegative RA is just as serious as the regular kind...and for some patients can be hard to treat.

Getting Seronegative RA Diagnosed

To diagnose seronegative RA, imaging studies, such as X-ray and ultrasound, may be taken to look for joint changes. However, such changes may take time to develop. Blood tests, such as C-reactive protein (CRP) and erythrocyte sedimentation rate (ESR), also may be done to look for evidence of generalized inflammation. But without the confirmation of antibodies, diagnosing seronegative RA is mainly based on a physical exam and symptoms.

Unlike with osteoarthritis, which usually causes symptoms in a single joint, RA causes pain and stiffness in multiple joints all over the body—including hands, knees, elbows, hips, feet and ankles. Joints, especially knuckles but also throughout the body, are evaluated for swelling and stiffness...and then monitored over at least six weeks or longer for any progression of swelling and stiffness. *In addition, doctors check for...*

•**Morning stiffness** that lasts longer than 30 minutes after waking and gets better with movement.

•**Joint swelling** or redness throughout the body.

•**Unusual fatigue** that can't be explained by other causes.

Treatment and Prognosis

In most ways, seronegative RA acts just like regular RA and is treated the same. For mild cases, treatment may start with steroids to reduce inflammation and nonsteroidal anti-inflammatory drugs (NSAIDs) to reduce inflammation and pain. For more severe cases, drugs called disease-modifying antirheumatic drugs (DMARDs) may be used to try to halt or slow disease progression. Recently, new DMARDs called biologics have been found to be very effective for moderate-to-severe disease. To help reduce symptoms, doctors sometimes keep patients on steroids or NSAIDs while waiting for DMARDs or biologics to take effect, and then taper off the NSAIDs and/or steroids. The American College of Rheumatology guidelines support a "treat-to-target" strategy for medication, with the target being remission.

There are also nondrug approaches that can help ease RA symptoms, such as range-of-motion exercises, deep abdominal breathing and capsaicin creams.

Changing Diagnosis

Seronegative RA can change over time. Some patients will start to produce enough antibodies to become seropositive. Seronegative RA can also evolve into other seronegative diseases, such as psoriatic arthritis, spondyloarthritis, polymyalgia rheumatica or osteoarthritis. That is one reason why it's important to check with your doctor regularly if you have seronegative RA. If your diagnosis changes, your treatment may need to change.

And if you think you might have seronegative RA but confirmation is proving elusive, don't give up! Getting diagnosed and starting treatment as early as possible can prevent long-term disability. If your symptoms have lasted longer than six weeks without a diagnosis, ask your primary care doctor to refer you to a rheumatologist. This kind of specialist is best at diagnosing seronegative RA and at developing a treatment plan.

7 Natural Ways to Relieve the Pain of Rheumatoid Arthritis

Harris H. McIlwain, MD, a board-certified rheumatologist, founder of the McIlwain Medical Group in Tampa, and former chair of the Florida Osteoporosis Board. He is coauthor of *The NEW Arthritis Diet: A 5-Step Plan to Lose Weight, End Pain and Be Active Again!* and *The NEW Arthritis Diet Recipes: Recipes and Super Foods to Help You Lose Weight, End Pain and Be Active Again!*

If your rheumatoid arthritis (RA) pain has you reaching for medications more and more often, it's time to investigate natural ways to ease your symptoms.

Certain lifestyle habits can support the use of disease-modifying antirheumatic drugs (DMARDs) that you take to stop the disease's progression without increasing side effects and health risks. What's more, many bring overall health benefits, such as reduced risk for cancer and improved heart health.

Ease RA the Natural Way

•**Practice range-of-motion (ROM) exercises.** An active lifestyle is the single most effective way to keep joints bathed in soothing synovial fluid. It might be challenging—or even impossible during a flare—but done regularly, exercise can decrease pain and fatigue. RA responds particularly well to range-of-motion exercises.

These stretching moves, such as shoulder shrugs and circles, wall pushes and bending and straightening each leg while lying on your back, increase flexibility and keep your muscles strong. Work with a physical therapist to create a program tailored to your specific needs.

Bonus: Improved flexibility from ROM exercises translates into fewer falls, which are common among people with RA.

Tip: For extra pain relief, do as many of these exercises as possible while in a warm tub or shower or after applying heat directly to any painful joints with a hot, wet towel or heating pad for 15 minutes.

•**Rub on capsaicin.** Yes, the same compound that makes your mouth burn when you eat chili peppers can counteract the feeling of pain in your joints when applied to the skin surface. Capsaicin blocks substance P, a chemical responsible for transmitting pain signals to your brain. You'll likely feel a mild burning sensation that lessens over time. After a few days of thrice-daily applications to the affected joints, the capsaicin should begin curbing painful RA sensations. Once RA pain subsides, you may continue to apply capsaicin for maintenance or as needed, up to three times daily.

Good over-the-counter products: Zostrix and Capzasin. These are available as creams and gels and in different strengths—try a low-dose version first. If you don't get enough relief after a few days, step up to a higher concentration.

Caution: Use medical gloves when applying to avoid getting it directly on fingertips, and be sure not to get any near your eyes, nose, mouth or genitals. Also, don't combine capsaicin topicals with a heating pad—doing so can cause burns. Skip capsaicin if you have psoriasis, eczema or any other skin condition or rash, and stop using it if it causes a skin reaction, such as redness or swelling.

•**Work toward a healthy weight.** The more overweight you are, the more inflammatory chemicals are coursing through your body and the greater your risk for pain. One such chemical, C-reactive protein, is also associated with diabetes, heart disease and cancer. Extra weight is also harder on weight-bearing joints, such as hips, ankles and knees. Losing as little as 10 pounds can make a big difference in symptoms, especially when combined with an anti-inflammatory, plant-based diet—lots of legumes and produce. This one-two punch creates changes at the cellular level, decreasing inflammation and reducing pain, stiffness and disability.

•**Load up on fruit with deeply colored skins.** Purple grapes, blueberries, blackberries, raspberries and dark cherries all contain anthocyanins, pain-relieving plant compounds that are anti-inflammatory.

•**Consider cupping.** This centuries-old technique involves applying suction to the skin via glass cups filled with hot air (the treatment lasts five to 20 minutes). Despite the marks made, cupping doesn't hurt and seems to work well for localized RA pain. Exactly how cupping helps isn't known for sure, but one theory is that the suction may improve circulation and aid in tissue repair in the skin and muscles. For this reason, it may also help ease RA-related spasms and muscular pain. Seek out a certified acupuncturist, physical therapist or licensed massage therapist with training in the technique.

•**Calm the mind to calm the body.** Stress is a well-recognized pain trigger. It doesn't cause pain, per se, but the way your mind and body respond to stress can increase your interpretation of and response to pain.

Stress-relieving techniques include deep abdominal breathing, which oxygenates the blood, triggering the release of morphine-like pain-relieving chemicals called endorphins. Tai chi, a series of slow, graceful movements practiced while standing, increases balance, flexibility and strength while easing emotional stress. Beginners can call their local arthritis foundation for a nearby class recommendation. Music therapy, visualization and meditation also can help. Just be sure to choose a method that works for you. Set aside 10 to 15 minutes a day to practice it.

•**Slash caffeine.** RA fatigue can be more limiting than the pain itself, but consuming caffeine for energy can backfire. The stimulant mimics the body's natural stress response and, especially at higher amounts, might cause a short-term rise in heart rate and blood pressure and set up an inflammatory cascade that can ultimately lead to more pain. And while caffeine is sometimes added to pain medications, which can temporarily improve energy, caffeine also can heighten the side effects of pain medications, including anxiety and trembling.

Helpful: Green and black tea have beneficial antioxidant and anti-inflammatory effects but less caffeine than coffee.

Try holistic sleep strategies for fatigue, such as a warm bath before bed, keeping your bedroom cool and dark, and avoiding evening exercise. Tip: Make sure your mattress is firm—a soft mattress puts extra stress on your joints.

It may take a week or two of practicing these therapies to notice a difference, but many RA patients ultimately discover a significant degree of relief.

Walking: A Drug-Free Rx for Arthritis

Susan Besser, MD, primary care physician, Mercy Personal Physicians in Baltimore, Maryland.

Study titled "Effectiveness of a Scaled-Up Arthritis Self-Management Program in Oregon: Walk With Ease," led by researchers at Oregon State University, published in *American Journal of Public Health*.

Painful, stiff joints make it hard to get moving, but moving is exactly what you need for pain relief when you have arthritis. What many people don't realize is that the world's simplest exercise—walking—is an amazingly powerful arthritis pain-buster. But the trick is, you need to know exactly how and when to walk, and what to do before and after, to get the full benefit. Taking these steps will also help you get over the fear that any movement will be painful, which keeps many people glued to a comfy chair.

Getting on a smart walking program can help with inflammatory conditions such as rheumatoid arthritis and psoriatic arthritis and "wear and tear" osteoarthritis.

Walking is so beneficial that it's considered a natural medication for arthritis. It makes your muscles stronger, which takes pressure off your joints…and boosts the health of your cartilage, your joints' shock absorbers, by in-

creasing circulation and bringing nutrients and oxygen to the area. And while walking specifically targets the joints in your lower body, the feel-good endorphins released during exercise should make you feel better from head to toe.

As a calorie-burning exercise, walking can also help with weight loss—and every pound of overweight puts added pressure on your joints. Weigh less, and you have less pain.

Here's what to do…

How long to walk: Your goal is to walk for 30 to 60 minutes at a time, but if you can handle only five minutes to start, that's OK—start there and go a little longer every day.

How often to walk: Remember, walking is medicine for arthritis—so aim to take this medicine every day! If you're new to walking, begin with two or three days a week and build up from there.

How fast to walk: Walk fast enough to increase your heart rate while still being able to have a conversation. The key is to push yourself but not to the point that you're tiring too quickly or adding to your joint pain.

Of course, if you have any additional mobility issues or other chronic conditions, ask your doctor whether you should refine these guidelines.

You can follow a plan on your own, no gym membership needed. But you might find needed motivation through a walking group with friends or with a formal program such as Walk with Ease from the Arthritis Foundation. This six-week course, held in cities across the country, shows you how to manage arthritis as well as begin a walking routine. Researchers at Oregon State University surveyed 598 sedentary people with arthritis who participated in the program and found that those who completed it reported significantly less pain and fatigue. Not near a group? You purchase a self-guide book ($12) with all the information from their website and start reaping the benefits.

To make your walks more comfortable, warm up for a few minutes with easy walking in place, then stretch. Stretch again after walking—you should be able to increase your range of motion as these muscles will be quite warm.

Whenever your joints feel sore, use a shorter stride. This puts less pressure on them.

Maintain good posture, with your core engaged and your upper body relaxed.

Don't let pride or even forgetfulness keep you from wearing a brace if your doctor has recommended one. The support it offers will help stabilize the joint, make walking easier, and potentially prevent a fall.

Note: If starting out walking on land is simply too painful for you, get in a pool, said Susan Besser, MD, a primary care physician with Mercy Personal Physicians in Baltimore, Maryland. Walking in water is gentler on your joints yet adds some resistance, giving you an even better workout.

Your Wrist Pain May Not Be Carpal Tunnel Syndrome

Robert E. Markison, MD, hand surgeon and clinical professor of surgery at the University of California, San Francisco. MarkisonMD.com

Jane Bear-Lehman, PhD, OTR/L, FAOTA, FNAP, clinician and researcher in hand and occupational therapy.

Ann Porretto-Loehrke, DPT, CHT, COMT, CMTPT, therapy comanager at the Hand to Shoulder Center of Wisconsin in Appleton and instructor of continuing education courses on the hand, wrist, elbow and shoulder to therapists around the country.

Soft Tissue Injuries, Chapter 8: "Forearm, Hand and Wrist," by Stephen Southern and John Sloan.

D on't take wrist pain lightly! Our lives have become increasingly technology-centric, and this puts the vulnerable wrist joint at great risk for repetitive strain injury (RSI). Even nontech activities like riding a bike, playing a musical instrument, knitting or gardening and other hobbies can make your wrist hurt all the time—and many people don't realize just how debilitating wrist pain can be. They don't take their symptoms seriously early on, when they could do something about them—and then the condition could become permanent.

Another mistake: Assuming that any chronic wrist pain is carpal tunnel syndrome and treating it that way. It's often not—and in that case, treatment for carpal tunnel won't help you and can make matters worse. *Here's how to know what's going on with your wrist…*

Understanding Wrist Pain

Carpal tunnel syndrome is only one type of issue that can affect the wrist. It is (or should be) a very specific diagnosis involving compression of the median nerve at the wrist (the nerve itself starts in the neck and travels all the way down the arm to the fingers—its branches feed through the thumb, index and middle fingers and half of the ring finger). If you have carpal tunnel syndrome, you might experience not only pain in the thumb and index, middle and ring fingers as well as the hand but also numbness and tingling in your fingers, and symptoms might persist all day and even wake you up at night.

But other ailments could be causing your wrist pain. For instance, pain on the thumb side of the wrist, especially when you make a fist, twist or grasp an object forcefully, could mean de Quervain's tenosynovitis, an inflammation of the tendons that straighten the thumb and move the thumb away from the palm. Another possibility is ulnar tunnel syndrome, sometimes called Guyon's canal syndrome, which happens when the ulnar nerve (running from the neck down into the hand) is compressed at the wrist. This syndrome affects half the ring finger and the pinky, can make them numb and tingly, and can result in weakness in your hand grip or finger pinch.

When to See a Doctor

If you have numbness, tingling, swelling, weakness and/or pain in your hand or wrist that either persists for longer than a month or that repeatedly comes and goes, don't assume it's carpal tunnel syndrome…don't assume you can treat it with a drugstore splint or other device marketed for carpal tunnel syndrome…but instead, get yourself to a doctor for a real diagnosis. If you don't, you may miss the opportunity for a full recovery.

See a hand surgeon, a physician who has specialized training in the evaluation and treatment of hand, wrist and arm conditions. But don't be afraid that he or she will automatically recommend surgery. Hand surgeons are hand doctors first, and they don't perform surgery on everyone they see—far from it. Occupational medicine doctors or physiatrists can also diagnose RSI.

When surgery isn't necessary, healing will most likely involve working with an occupational or physical therapist, such as a certified hand therapist (CHT). You want a health-care professional with intricate knowledge of hand anatomy and hand conditions and your type of injury in particular. (These therapists can also help you postoperatively.) To determine the exact hand-therapy program you need, the therapist will do a thorough examination and perform tests appropriate for your situation.

What about the original cause of the injury? Your doctor and hand-therapy specialist will discuss with you which kind of movements provoke symptoms, how to limit these motions, how to reduce the pain…and then stay as symptom-free as possible. You can find a certified hand therapist through the American Society of Hand Therapists (ASHT.org).

Be Your Own Best Healer

What you do on your own, not just in therapy sessions, is also an important part of your recovery, and nutrition, including supplementation, can play a big role in success. *Robert E. Markison, MD, a hand surgeon and clinical professor of surgery at the University of California, San Francisco, often recommends these nutrients to his patients…*

•**Liquid vitamin D3,** which is more easily absorbed by the body than D3 in capsule form, to maintain musculoskeletal health. A periodic blood test can help you maintain your blood vitamin-D level between 50 and 80 ng/mL.

•**Vitamins B6 and B12, preferably from food.** These vitamins actively support central and peripheral nerve system function. Supplemental vitamin B6 can cause neuropathy (nerve pain) if you take amounts over the safe upper limit of 100 mg per day (the recommended daily allowance is only 1.3 mg), but high intake of this vitamin from food has not been shown to have adverse effects. Foods with generous amounts of B6 include chickpeas, chicken breast, yellowfin tuna and bananas. The recommended daily allowance of vitamin B12 is 2.4 µg. Foods high in B12 include beef liver, fish, meat, poultry, eggs and milk. Your doctor can monitor your levels of both vitamins with a blood test. For B6, the healthy range is between 5 and 50 µg/L, and for B-12, it's between 200 and 900 ng/mL. Dr. Markinson suggests aiming for at least the middle of the ranges.

•**Stay well-hydrated.** Microcirculation carries nutrients and oxygen to the cells and takes away waste. Regularly drinking water also ensures that you get up periodically to use the bathroom—sometimes that's the only break from computing that people get.

These ergonomic pointers can help, too…

•**As much as possible,** use a voice-recognition program, not a keyboard or touch screen, for computer work. For texting, use voice-to-text, not your thumbs.

•**When you must type at your computer,** use a split-and-tilt keyboard. It allows you to adjust the keyboard to fit your body, rather than having to contort yourself to a molded plastic keyboard. Also, use a light touch—don't pound on the keyboard.

•**If you use a mouse,** alternate it between your left and right hands to balance out the workload.

•**Sit tall and avoid a forward-head posture.** Relax your shoulders and keep your arms near your torso.

•**Keep your hands warm to improve circulation,** important for avoiding RSI.

A note about pain relief medication: Discuss options with your care providers before taking anything so that you don't mask symptoms and jump back into activities before you've truly healed.

When Your Thumb Hurts...

Leon S. Benson, MD, a hand surgeon at the Illinois Bone & Joint Institute, professor of clinical orthopaedic surgery at The University of Chicago Pritzker School of Medicine, and spokesperson for the American Academy of Orthopaedic Surgeons.

I t is extremely common for osteoarthritis to develop at the base of the thumb—where the thumb and wrist join together.

Osteoarthritis develops when there's a wearing away of the cartilage that buffers and protects the area where two bones come together. It is similar to wearing the rubber off a tire after many miles of use. This "wear and tear" arthritis can result from the aging process, overuse or injury. Currently, there is no way to prevent cartilage damage from worsening, other than to not use the joint that's involved. Obviously, not using your hand is certainly an impractical—if not impossible—task.

There are, however, some simple ways to relieve thumb arthritis pain. Using a splint to rest the thumb for a few hours a day can be very helpful. It is usually possible to use a mouse and keyboard even when wearing such a splint. To ensure that you get a splint that is customized for the shape of your hand, it's smart to see a certified hand therapist, an occupational therapist or physical therapist who specializes in treating the hand and upper extremity. Insurance often pays at least part of the cost of splint fabrication. To find a hand therapist in your area, check the on-line directory found on the website for the American Society of Hand Therapists.

Sometimes heat or cold (like an ice pack) can help ease the pain. Hand exercises can also help relieve any pain and stiffness in your thumb. However, they should be pursued carefully, because too much exercise can worsen the pain from arthritis.

Anti-inflammatory medication, such *ibuprofen* (Motrin), can significantly help ease arthritis pain. If the pain persists, a steroid injection into the thumb joint space may be even more effective. An injection can often give relief for six to 12 months, and as long as it is not administered too frequently (more than twice per year), is a very safe treatment. Topical medications are also available, such as anti-inflammatory creams, but they typically are less effective than oral medications or injections.

Although there are different devices that can be used in place of a computer mouse (like a trackball) or instead of the keyboard (like voice-recognition software), computer use itself is actually not the main cause of arthritis symptoms. People use their hands constantly for activities of daily living outside of the workplace, so computer use is neither a particularly bad activity for your hands nor is it done for a long enough duration to be a major cause or aggravation of arthritis pain.

If none of the above treatments are effective or last long enough, joint replacement is an option. Surgery for the most common type of thumb arthritis has been around for decades. It is performed in an outpatient setting, usually under twilight-type anesthesia, and allows most patients to resume normal use of their hand without pain. Post-operative immobilization in a splint or brace is often required for about four weeks, after which time many patients can use their affected hand with minimal limitations.

How to Sleep to Relieve Common Aches and Pains

Matthew O'Rourke, PT, DPT, CSCS, OMT, adjunct professor of physical therapy at Simmons University in Boston and a physical therapist in the outpatient clinic at Lahey Hospital & Medical Center in Burlington, Massachusetts.

W hether you like to curl up on your side or sprawl flat out on your stomach, you probably have a favorite sleeping position. But did you know that if you suffer from common aches and pains, this familiar position might be aggravating your pain?

Here's how to adapt your preferred sleeping style for pain relief and better sleep…

Neck Pain

Back-sleeping is often said to be the best position for neck pain. But back-sleeping can actually increase neck discomfort when using a pillow that's too thick (which causes the head to flex forward) or too thin (which causes the head to flex backward).

For back-sleepers: Be sure to use a pillow that keeps the neck in a neutral position, in line with the spine. When viewed from the side, the ear should be in line with the shoulders or slightly above them.

For side-sleepers: Add a thin pillow or rolled-up bath towel between the neck and the mattress in addition to your regular pillow to provide neck support and prevent the spine from bending to either side.

For stomach-sleepers: This position is the worst for neck pain because you'll need to turn your head to one side or the other, which puts strain on the neck. It's best to try another position, if possible.

Low-Back Pain

Many people say that their backs feel better when they sleep on their backs, particularly if they use a pillow or two to slightly elevate the knees. But side-sleeping often feels more natural.

For side-sleepers: Lie on one side in a "stacked" position, with your shoulders, knees and hips in up-and-down alignment and knees slightly bent.

Helpful: Place a pillow between your knees. This helps to prevent the top leg from rolling over the bottom, which can twist the spine.

For stomach-sleepers: This position can strain your lower back. However, if you find it difficult to try the positions above, place a pillow under your stomach to reduce excessive spinal extension.

Knee Pain

With knee pain, back-sleeping can be painful because the knees are extended all night…

but side-sleeping can cause irritation where the knees touch.

For back-sleepers: Try placing a pillow under the knees to prevent them from over-straightening.

Note: This position can be painful for some people.

For side-sleepers: Sleep with a pillow between your knees or use cloth knee pads (such as those that volleyball players wear), turning them sideways so that the area where the knees touch is well padded.

For stomach-sleepers: This position can put painful pressure on your knees. But if it's tough for you to switch to one of the above positions, put a pillow under your stomach to take some pressure off the knees.

Hip Pain

For back- or stomach-sleepers: People with arthritis-related hip pain often have more pain when sleeping on their back or stomach. It's best to try side-sleeping (see below). However, a small pillow under the knees (when lying on your back) or under the stomach (when lying on your stomach) may provide some relief.

For side-sleepers: Side-sleeping is usually best for arthritis-related hip pain.

Helpful: Keep your knees slightly bent and use a pillow (a body pillow works well) between the knees and thighs to keep the hip in a more neutral position. If lying on one side is more painful than the other, switch sides.

You Can Change How You Sleep

When you get into bed, start in the position in which you would like to sleep. Then spend about a minute visualizing yourself staying in this position for the night. If you wake up and are out of position, calmly go back to the position you are trying to change to. In most cases, good progress can be made in four to six weeks, but it's something you'll need to keep working on—it's easy to fall back into old habits.

The OTC Painkiller Trap

Leslie Kernisan, MD, MPH, clinical instructor, division of geriatrics, University of California, San Francisco. Board-certified in both geriatrics and internal medicine, she is founder of BetterHealthWhileAging. net, a website that provides practical information for older adults and family caregivers.

Many people assume that over-the-counter (OTC) drugs are less likely to cause dangerous side effects than their prescription counterparts. But that's not always true—especially when it comes to pain-relieving medications.

Nonsteroidal anti-inflammatory drugs (NSAIDs), a class of painkillers that includes *ibuprofen* (such as Advil and Motrin), *naproxen* (such as Aleve) and aspirin, causes more than 100,000 hospitalizations and 7,000 to 16,500 deaths each year.

Acetaminophen, the active ingredient in products such as Tylenol, Panadol and others, is generally safer than NSAIDs. But even this drug, the most popular painkiller worldwide, can cause liver damage and liver failure at too-high doses.

The problem: It's common for people who have chronic pain—whether it's from a bad back, persistent headaches or a bum knee—to take multiple doses daily and continue using the drug month after month, greatly increasing the dangers. This is particularly true for older adults, who metabolize drugs differently than younger people and are more likely to have health conditions (such as impaired kidney function) that increase the risks even more.

A Safer Choice

You've likely heard that acetaminophen isn't helpful for painful conditions that involve inflammation, such as arthritis and joint injuries. Studies generally find that NSAIDs are a bit more effective than acetaminophen for arthritis pain, which is one of the main reasons that older adults use OTC painkillers. Still, since acetaminophen is so much safer (when used at recommended doses) than NSAIDs, I almost always advise older adults to try acetaminophen first.

Important: Acetaminophen stops being safe when people exceed the recommended dose. This can happen when people think that they need a higher dose...or when they (often unknowingly) use other products that contain it.

Acetaminophen is an ingredient in dozens of OTC medications, including sleep aids (such as Tylenol PM) and cold and flu remedies (NyQuil and Theraflu). It's also used in some prescription painkillers (such as Vicodin). If you don't check ingredient labels, you could wind up taking far more than the recommended limit of 3,000 mg per day. (Aiming to take less than 2,000 mg per day is even safer.)

To prevent liver damage, people with a history of alcohol abuse—or those who drink alcohol frequently—definitely shouldn't take more than 2,000 mg daily. I advise patients who take daily doses of acetaminophen for long-term problems (such as arthritis) to ask their doctors if their liver enzymes should be checked—either occasionally or regularly.

Use Caution with NSAIDs

NSAIDs, such as ibuprofen and naproxen, are never my first choice because they frequently cause stomach/intestinal bleeding...increase blood pressure...and lead to kidney damage in those who already have impaired kidney function.

Sobering caution: In 2015, the FDA strengthened existing label warnings on nonaspirin NSAIDs to alert consumers about the increased risk for heart attack and stroke, which can occur even in the first weeks of using one of these drugs—especially when taken at higher doses...and in people with and without heart disease.

Caveat: Because some people get more relief from an NSAID than from acetaminophen, it's sometimes reasonable to accept the risks of using an NSAID for a short time, such as a few days to a week. But even then, I am cautious about recommending them for patients who take blood thinners (NSAIDs have a blood-thinning effect) or have impaired kidney function or other health problems.

My advice: It's probably OK for older adults to take an occasional NSAID if they feel acetaminophen doesn't provide enough relief...but these drugs are not safe for daily use. People with arthritis or other long-term conditions should talk to their doctors about nondrug ways to manage pain, such as weight loss, physical therapy, exercise and cognitive behavioral therapy—all of which have been proven to be effective.

What About Aspirin?

Doctors today almost never recommend aspirin as a pain reliever. Even at low doses (81 mg), it increases the risk for GI bleeding and for cerebral hemorrhage...and the risks for complications are higher among older adults and those with high blood pressure or other chronic diseases.

Aspirin is most likely to cause bleeding and other side effects when it's taken at doses of more than 100 mg daily for months or longer. But even low doses, as mentioned above, can be risky. Because of these risks, I try to discourage patients from taking aspirin as a pain reliever.

Exception: If you've had a heart attack or stroke, your doctor might advise you to take a daily aspirin (typically 81 mg) to prevent blood clots and a subsequent heart attack/stroke. The benefits of this so-called secondary prevention are believed to outweigh the risks.

However, experts no longer recommend aspirin for primary prevention (preventing a first heart attack/stroke) except for certain high-risk patients—for example, someone who has received a stent or has diabetes and another risk factor such as smoking or high blood pressure. Unless a person is at relatively high risk for a cardiovascular event, the risk of bleeding from a daily baby aspirin is generally higher than the chance of avoiding a heart attack or stroke due to this therapy.

The Topical Option

If you feel that you need an NSAID for pain relief, using a topical cream or gel reduces some of the risks. Topical NSAIDs used for musculoskeletal pain are effective, according to a Cochrane (a nonprofit group that evaluates medical treatments) review.

My advice: If your stomach can't handle oral NSAIDs—and acetaminophen doesn't seem to work—a topical drug (including OTC topical aspirin, such as Bengay, Aspercreme and other products with salicylate listed on the label) might be worth a try. Some people may also get relief from capsaicin cream.

What If You Really Need an Opioid?

Jane C. Ballantyne, MD, FRCA, professor of anesthesiology and pain medicine, University of Washington, Seattle. Dr. Ballantyne is coeditor of *Expert Decision Making on Opioid Treatments* and president of Physicians for Responsible Opioid Prescribing. SupportPROP.org.

Every day, more than 115 people in the US die after overdosing on opioids. And the efforts now being made to curtail addiction and stem the shockingly high death and overdose rates are all over the news.

Under-recognized problem: While there's no question that opioid addiction is a serious problem in this country, there are some circumstances where patients need these drugs.

Pain Specialists Are Wary

The majority of doctors, including primary care physicians, receive little training in the best ways to treat pain. Many of these doctors are now nervous about prescribing opioid medications due to increased government oversight (including voluntary opioid-prescribing guidelines issued by the CDC in 2016)...uncertainty, in general, about optimal dosing…and worries about the risk for addiction.

In a survey published in 2017 in *Practical Pain Management* that included more than 3,000 chronic pain patients, nearly 85% reported being in more pain than they were before stricter oversight recommendations were instituted.

Undertreated pain is a real concern when it prevents patients from engaging in normal activities and enjoying a good quality of life. This doesn't mean that doctors should dispense drugs more freely. Many people do better overall when they rely on drug-free methods of pain relief, including things like physical therapy, counseling or support groups. To find such a support group near you, ask your doctor.

Safer Opioid Use

Opioids are powerful drugs that need to be monitored. They aren't likely to cause problems when they're taken for a few days for acute pain (after surgery, for example), but long-term use can cause serious side effects, including osteoporosis, digestive problems (such as constipation) and opioid-induced endocrinopathy—decreases in testosterone and other hormones.

I provide long-term opioid prescriptions only for select groups of patients (discussed below). Patients with acute pain—after a back injury, for example—might need opioids, but should take them for as short a time as possible…and only if they can't get adequate pain relief from safer approaches, such as exercise, physical therapy and/or over-the-counter (OTC) acetaminophen (Tylenol) or a nonsteroidal anti-inflammatory drug (NSAID), such as *ibuprofen* (Motrin) or *naproxen* (Aleve). Prescription antidepressants or anticonvulsants also can reduce pain regardless of its cause.

With some exceptions, I advise patients never to start treatment with *hydrocodone* and *acetaminophen* (Vicodin), *oxycodone* (OxyContin) or other opioids and to try other pain-relief methods first.

Exceptions: Patients who are terminally ill can have a much higher quality of life when they take high doses of opioids—and not just because of pain relief. Someone with a terminal cancer, for example, might feel more at peace when taking the drugs. Similarly, patients with intractable diseases that impair their ability to function—such as spinal cord injuries, severe multiple sclerosis, etc.—might do better when they take the drugs.

But for those who can do without an opioid, lifestyle approaches, including cognitive behavioral therapy or physical activity, can sometimes relieve pain more than prescription or OTC drugs. Only take an opioid when other approaches don't work…and only take a dose that's high enough to relieve pain but low enough to allow you to function normally. *Also important…*

•**Set limits.** Some doctors continue to write opioid prescriptions too casually.

My advice: Don't take an opioid for short-term pain unless you have a very clear injury—after a car accident, for example. Even then, take the drug for a few days at most.

Also: The safest way to take opioid medications—both for acute and chronic pain—is to use them only as needed to control severe or sudden pain…not around the clock, unless it's absolutely necessary.

•**Attend a pain clinic.** Patients with complex pain do better when they work with pain specialists at an interdisciplinary clinic (available at most major medical centers), where the medical team typically includes doctors, nurses, psychologists and physical therapists. Opioid medications may be prescribed carefully in these settings, but the emphasis is on other safer, longer-lasting methods of pain relief.

•**Talk to your doctor about dosing.** It's common for patients taking opioids to develop tolerance—they gradually require more medication to get the same relief. This is not the same as addiction. However, the higher doses will increase the risk for side effects, including addiction. Do not change your medication or dose on your own. Get your doctor's advice.

• **Ask about longer-acting drugs.** Patients with acute pain after surgery or an injury often need a fast-acting drug, such as nasal or sublingual (under-the-tongue) fentanyl. But patients with chronic pain usually do better with longer-acting drugs, such as extended-release oxymorphone (Opana ER) or a buprenorphine patch (Butrans).

Long-acting drugs provide a steady level of medication to stabilize their effectiveness—with fewer "letdowns" that can lead some patients into inappropriate drug-seeking behavior. They're not a perfect solution because patients who take them may be given an additional prescription for a fast-acting drug to control "breakthrough" pain.

Addiction isn't likely to be a problem if you use these powerful medications only when needed and with the caveats described above.

Treat Pain Without Opioids

When 240 patients with moderate-to-severe back, hip or knee osteoarthritis pain were given either opioid medications, such as *oxycodone* (Oxycontin), or nonopioid pain medications, such as *acetaminophen* (Tylenol), *meloxicam* (Mobic) and/or *lidocaine* (Xylocaine), the nonopioid group reported significantly less intense pain and had fewer adverse side effects over the 12-month study period.

Erin Krebs, MD, associate professor of medicine, Minneapolis Veterans Affairs Health Care System.

More Coffee, Less Pain

Caffeine is associated with lower pain sensitivity, according to a new study of 62 men and women who underwent heat and pressure tests after reporting their caffeine consumption from coffee, tea, soda and chocolate over seven days. Each extra 100 mg of caffeine consumed per day (about one cup of

brewed coffee or two-and-a-half cups of tea) was linked to a reduction in pain severity that was deemed significant (the ability to withstand an additional 0.9°F increase in heat, a marker for pain tolerance).

Burel Goodin, PhD, associate professor of psychology, University of Alabama at Birmingham.

Better Care for Back Pain

Christine Goertz, DC, PhD, CEO, The Spine Institute for Quality, Davenport, Iowa.

Adding chiropractic care to traditional medical treatment, including pain relievers and physical therapy, reduced pain better than traditional treatment alone, according to a recent study. Chiropractic care included spinal manipulation plus hot/cold packs, exercise recommendations and other treatments. The chiropractic care participants were less likely to use prescription drugs and had significantly greater improvements in pain, disability and treatment satisfaction than those who received medical care alone. Specifically, 58% of those receiving chiropractic care reported at least a 30% improvement at six weeks, versus 32% of those in the medical care–only group.

Chiropractic care could offer a cost-effective and low-risk alternative to addictive opioids for those with low-back pain. Most insurance companies cover chiropractic treatment, however visit limits and high co-pays are common, so check first.

Back-Saving Chairs

Barbara Bergin, MD, orthopedic surgeon, Texas Orthopedics, Sports & Rehabilitation Associates, Austin, and author of the blog "Sit Like a Man." DrBarbaraBergin.com

By now, we all know how detrimental sitting is for our health. And of course, we all tend to slouch when sitting at the usual desk chair, and that can lead to back pain.

Standing desks can negate some risk, but standing all day can hurt, too.

The following three unusual chairs offer a sensible middle ground between standing and traditional sitting. All count as active sitting, meaning that they require you to engage far more muscles than with a normal chair—so you can strengthen your core, burn extra calories and maybe even alleviate or avoid back pain.

Each one will take some time to get used to, so plan to feel a bit awkward at first. A good way to adapt to any of these chairs is to sit in one for just an hour at a time for a few days and then gradually increase from there. *Here are the best kinds of "active" chairs...*

• **Saddle stool.** These stools look a bit like oversized bike seats or saddles on top of office chairs. When you sit in one, it causes your hips to open and feet to spread almost as if you were riding a horse. This can help stave off a host of painful back and hip problems as well as plantar fasciitis, all of which can come from sitting prim and proper with your knees and feet together. When you sit in a saddle stool, your feet will naturally fall at 11:00 and 1:00, with hips rotated outward, which helps reduce stress across the hips and knees. The backless nature of this stool can improve your own back strength by requiring you to keep your core muscles engaged as you sit. However, if you find this too tiring or uncomfortable, you can purchase a saddle stool with a back.

Example: Jobri Betterposture Ergonomic Saddle Chair, $199.95. SitHealthier.com

• **Wobble stool.** This stool looks a bit like a bar stool on a sturdy base. The seat will wobble from the natural little movements a body makes when sitting, and this motion keeps your abdomen, back and leg muscles moving as you compensate. All of that extra movement may counteract the negative health impacts of extended sitting.

Example: Uncaged Ergonomics Wobble Stool, $129. UncagedErgonomics.com

• **Recumbent chair.** A standard chair makes slumping easy, but a recumbent, or kneeling, chair features a seat that slants by about 20 to 30 degrees. This makes it easier to maintain good posture and avoid back pain. And because a recumbent chair takes pressure off the lower back and buttocks, it can help sciatic pain, too.

Example: Relaxus Recumbent Chair, $170. RelaxusOnline.com

Note: Recumbent/kneeling chairs can be hard on the knees, so anyone with arthritis, patellar tendinitis, kneecap pain or a meniscus tear should avoid them. People with leg swelling should steer clear as well, as these chairs may restrict your circulation. For most people, this isn't a problem, but getting up every hour or so for a short break will make using this type of chair for extended periods more comfortable.

Massage Yourself for Pain Relief and Other Benefits

Tiffany M. Field, PhD, director of the Touch Research Institute at University of Miami Miller School of Medicine, which focuses on the effects of massage therapy. She is author of *Touch*.

You may not be able to give yourself the giggles by tickling yourself, but you can tap into the proven health benefits of massage by letting your own fingers do the kneading. There are plenty of reasons to enjoy the oohs and aahs—massage can improve symptoms of health conditions ranging from chronic pain to depression to anxiety, high blood pressure and even painful autoimmune diseases.

With moderate-pressure massage, pressure receptors located directly under the skin are activated, starting a chain reaction that, among other benefits, decreases levels of the "stress hormone" cortisol. That's the source of many of the benefits. *How to tap into these benefits on your own...*

•**Grab a tennis ball.** If you're unsure of how much pressure to apply or if your fingers are stiff, a tennis ball is a perfect (and inexpensive) massage tool. Just hold the ball in one hand, and roll it up and down your legs, across your arms or over any place that needs some kneading. The movements can be circular or back-and-forth. As long as you are moving the skin in front of the ball as it rolls, you're getting benefit.

For a back massage, stand against a wall and put the tennis ball between the area you want to massage and the wall. Shift your weight from one leg to the other, or slide your back up and down along the wall to roll the ball.

For a foot massage, use your hands or place the ball on the floor and roll one foot over it at a time. Hold on to a table or counter for balance or try it sitting down.

•**Give yourself an extra hand.** Massage tools, available in fitness stores and online, are great for hard-to-reach areas.

Examples: Lie down on a cylinder-shaped foam roller, and roll back and forth over it to massage your entire upper body. If you prefer to sit up, try a curved massage stick or wooden massage-beads-on-a-rope.

Enhance the experience with an oil or lotion. You might find this more comfortable than a "dry" massage. Consider a lavender-scented product—lavender is scientifically proven to have a relaxing effect.

•**Get pro advice.** While you certainly don't need formal training to give yourself a massage, an instructional session with a certified massage therapist will be helpful. You'll learn new movements to keep the massages interesting and even prevent soreness. To find a massage therapist, contact your state's licensing board or go to the website of the American Massage Therapy Association (AMTAMassage.org) and click "find a massage therapist."

Hip Pain? Forget the Steroids and Do These Exercises Instead

Bill Vicenzino, PhD, professor in physiotherapy, chair in sports physiotherapy, director of sports injuries rehabilitation and prevention for health, School of Health and Rehabilitation Sciences, University of Queensland, Australia, and coauthor of the study "Education Plus Exercise Versus Corticosteroid Injection Use Versus a Wait and See Approach on Global Outcome and Pain from Gluteal Tendinopathy: Prospective, Single Blinded, Randomised Clinical Trial," published in *The BMJ*.

If hip pain has you wincing when going up stairs or when standing to put on your jeans, the problem could be weak tendons. Your doctor will probably recommend steroid shots. But that's only a short-term treatment—and you might not need it at all.

When weak tendons cause pain over the side of the hip at the widest bony point below your waist, it's called gluteal tendinopathy, and it can affect men and women of all ages.

Doctors typically treat this condition, called lateral hip pain, with steroid injections, but there's good news if you want to avoid the needle and the side effects that come with these drugs: Exercise is more effective at helping people with gluteal tendinopathy, according to a recent study at the University of Queensland in Australia. We spoke with Bill Vicenzino, PhD, professor in physiotherapy and director of sports injuries rehabilitation and prevention for health at the School of Health and Rehabilitation Sciences there and coauthor of the study, to find out what our readers can do to reduce hip pain and avoid steroids. *Here's what Dr. Vicenzino told us...*

Causes and Symptoms

This type of hip pain stems from a weakness in the tendons that connect some of the gluteal muscles of your butt to the hip bone. In severe cases, there are tears in the tendons.

You're more susceptible to hip tendon problems if...

- **You're a weekend warrior,** meaning you are inactive most of the time (maybe you work a desk job) and try to make up for it on the weekends with lots of exercise or by going on adventure vacations without getting in condition first.

- **You have poor posture** or stand with your weight on one hip.

- **You're a post-menopausal woman.** Hormone changes that occur during menopause may affect the tendons.

- **Being overweight** or sedentary can make it worse.

- **You're a runner.**

But hip pain tied to tendon trouble can hit even people who don't fit any of those descriptions.

Classic signs include tenderness or pain when you press on the bony protrusion on the side of your hip and pain that spreads from this area down your outer thighs…but not past your knee.

Pain may flare when you stand after sitting, sit with your legs crossed, or on the standing leg such as when putting on pants, Dr. Vicenzino said. The pain can be especially severe when walking at speed or up stairs or a slope. It may make it difficult to get to sleep or wake you up in the middle of the night if you were sleeping on your side.

Some pain involving the hip is not gluteal tendinopathy but can be mistaken for it. If your pain radiates all the way down your leg to your ankle and foot, if you feel pain in your groin, or if when sitting you feel stiffness and have trouble putting on shoes and socks, you probably have another condition, such as pain originating in the lower back or possibly osteoarthritis, Dr. Vicenzino said. Hip bursitis may also occur alongside gluteal tendinopathy, but the mechanical causes and treatments can be reasonably similar. So your first step is to be sure to get a proper diagnosis from your physician. Once you've been diagnosed with gluteal tendinopathy, the right healing can begin.

Exercises to the Rescue

You don't have to live with the hip pain of gluteal tendinopathy, nor are steroids the only (or best) way to get relief.

For the study done by Dr. Vicenzino and his colleagues, 204 men and women with gluteal tendinopathy were divided into three groups. One group received education about their condition and participated in an eight-week exercise program that focused on better body mechanics—the right way to move in everyday life—as well as exercises designed to strengthen certain muscles. The second group received a corticosteroid injection, a common treatment for the condition. The third group had one session with a physiotherapist during which they were given some general information about tendon problems, encouraged to keep moving within pain limits and to take a "wait and see" approach. Members of all three groups kept diaries of what they did and how they felt.

The bottom line: After both eight weeks and a year, people who exercised and learned how to move better in the exercise group reported greater improvement than the injection and control groups. (Note: At the end of the initial eight weeks, they were encouraged to continue with their program, but the researchers did not track whether they complied.)

Dr. Vicenzino recommends working with a physical therapist to develop a full program that addresses hip and gluteal muscles and can observe you while you do the exercises to see that you are doing them correctly. But you can make many of the exercises that the study participants used part of your daily routine.

Note: The participants began by doing less challenging exercises and gradually progressed to harder exercises as their movement control and pain improved, but never to the point of worsening their pain. At all times (including exercise) the participants were instructed to minimize hip drop/hang and knees crossing the midline, as a critical part of the education component.

The exercises target four specific goals…

Static abduction exercises gently activate the deep gluteal muscles at the side of the hips…

•**Lying abduction.** Lie on your back with a pillow under your knees. Buckle a belt around your thighs just above your knees, keeping your knees a little wider than your hips. Slowly move your legs apart to take up the slack in the belt, feeling a gentle tension at the 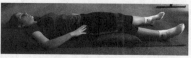 side of your hips and buttocks. Do 10-second holds for 10 repetitions twice a day.

•**Standing abduction.** Stand with your feet slightly wider than your hips. Think about slowly sliding your legs apart into an imaginary split and as you do this, allow a gentle tension along the sides of your hips and buttocks. (Your feet and legs don't move outwardly at all.) Hold the 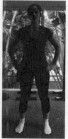 tension for five to 15 seconds and repeat three to five times…do this twice a day.

Bridging exercises strengthen the glutes and emphasize pelvic control.

•**Double leg bridge.** Lie on your back with your feet flat on the floor, and draw in your lower abdominal muscles. Pressing through your heels and tightening your gluteal muscles, lift your hips off the floor as high as is comfortable. Do not lift hips higher than a line from shoul- 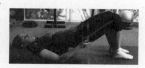 der to knees. Then slowly return your hips to the floor. Do 10 repetitions once a day.

•**Offset bridge.** Add this exercise after one week. Lie on your back with your feet flat on the floor. Bring one foot closer to your butt, and move your other foot further away. Press your hips into the bridge position primarily by pressing through the heel of the foot that is closest to you. Keep 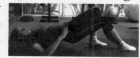 your pelvis horizontal. Do 10 repetitions once a day.

Functional retraining strengthens the glutes and thighs through the practice of good movement patterns…

•**Double leg squats.** Stand with good posture and bend at the hips and knees as if you're about to sit in a chair. Hold for three seconds, then return to a standing position for three seconds, pressing down through your heels to help you return to standing. Do 10 repetitions two times a day.

•**Offset squats.** Add this exercise after one week. Take one step 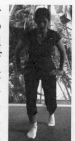 forward with your right foot and lean forward, placing the ball of the foot directly under your right hip. Squat as deeply as you comfortably can by bending the knee and taking your body weight onto the right side. Use your left leg to help you stay aligned and balanced. Both knees face forward and hips stay level. Take three to four seconds to get into the squat and three to four seconds to straighten up. Do five repetitions on each side every day.

•**Single leg standing.** Add this exercise after one week. Hold onto the back of a chair while standing 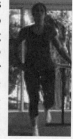 tall, and transfer your weight to one leg. Lift the foot of the other leg behind you and hold for five to 15 seconds, keeping your pelvis level. This may cause fatigue in the butt muscle, but it shouldn't cause pain on the side of your hip. Do five to 10 times on each side one to two times a day.

Weight-bearing abductor loading activates and strengthens the glutes and the tendons at the sides of your hip.

•**Sidestepping.** Keeping good posture with your knees facing straight ahead and feet hip dis- 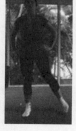 tance apart, take a controlled step out to the right side with your right leg, landing softly, then bring the foot back in to return to starting position (with feet hip distance apart). Switch sides and do the same move to the left with the left leg. Do 15 times with each leg once a day.

All these exercises condition key muscles in your hips and instill proper body alignment, enabling you to move with good posture and body mechanics to correct gluteal tendinopathy.

Remember if you are unable to perform these exercises without much pain or you do not improve, consult a physical therapist.

The High Risks of Low-Dose Steroids for Rheumatoid Arthritis

Study titled, "Association Between Glucocorticoid Exposure and Healthcare Expenditures for Potential Glucocorticoid-related Adverse Events in Patients with Rheumatoid Arthritis" by researchers at University of Pittsburgh, published in *The Journal of Rheumatology.*

Finding the best medication for your rheumatoid arthritis can take some time, and while you're waiting for it to work, other drugs can help, but it turns out that they also can lead to scary side effects.

We're talking about steroids—quick to relieve painful inflammation but with many side effects such as weight gain and high blood pressure. Doctors tend to prescribe them in low doses for the shortest amount of time that will bring relief. But a study published in *The Journal of Rheumatology* found that even low doses can be very risky for people with rheumatoid arthritis, some of whom are, surprisingly, taking them for too long.

Yes, steroids can block damaging inflammation from this disease, but they are not a long-term answer because, in addition to side effects, they don't change the course of rheumatoid arthritis. In contrast, a more recent class of drugs called "DMARDs" are a better ongoing treatment because they can actually slow or halt joint destruction.

You might sometimes also need a steroid to ease symptoms—such as when first starting a DMARD (because it can take weeks for it to take effect versus mere days for steroids) or when changing from one DMARD to another as you try to find the best one for your condition.

Know the Risks

For the study, researchers reviewed two years of medical records of 84,000 people with rheumatoid arthritis—they tallied the amount of steroids taken during the first one-year period and then looked at side effects during one year of follow-up.

They found that 48% of patients had taken oral steroids. Even though they were on a so-called low daily dose of 10 mg, many of them had taken this dose for relatively long periods—with terrible consequences. For example, patients who took steroids for between 80 and 180 days in the year had a higher risk for osteoporosis, fracture and infection than those who did not take steroids.

Even worse, those who took low dose steroids for a total of six months out of the year or more were at risk for an even longer list of complications that additionally included aseptic necrosis (bone loss from lack of blood supply), type 2 diabetes, heart attack or stroke.

The bottom line? If you have rheumatoid arthritis, it's important to get your pain and other symptoms under control, but you must also protect your overall health by making every effort to limit or avoid even low-dose steroids. *According to Johns Hopkins Medicine...*

• **Ask your rheumatologist** whether you can get started on a DMARD as early as possible after your rheumatoid arthritis diagnosis to preempt the need for steroids.

• **Try nonsteroidal anti-inflammatory drugs (NSAIDs) to reduce inflammation.** They are not as strong as steroids, but might be enough to ease symptoms until your DMARD kicks in.

• **If your doctor strongly recommends steroids,** ask for the lowest dose taken over the shortest amount of time that might work.

Steroid Injections for Arthritis Pain—Reasons to Think Twice

Beth Shubin Stein, MD, an orthopedic surgeon and member of the Sports Medicine and Shoulder Service at the Hospital for Special Surgery.

The studies titled, "Effect of Intra-articular Triamcinolone vs Saline on Knee Cartilage Volume and Pain in Patients with Knee Osteoarthritis: A Randomized Clinical Trial" led by researchers at Tufts Medical Center and published in *JAMA*. "Hip Steroid Injections Associated with Risky Bone Changes" led by researchers at Harvard Medical School and presented at the annual meeting of the Radiological Society of North America.

"Preoperative Hip Injections Increase the Rate of Periprosthetic Infection After Total Hip Arthroplasty" led by researchers at the Hospital for Special Surgery, published in *Journal of Arthroplasty*.

Steroids. Very few treatments will work as quickly. But know the downsides before you make the decision to try them.

For one thing, the effects of corticosteroid injections on arthritis pain are limited, meaning they aren't a long-term solution. While chances are good that your first injection will be very effective, bringing up to eight weeks of relief, each successive injection tends to be less effective than the time before. Subsequent injections may not help at all.

Beyond their limited effectiveness, growing research has uncovered of a variety of long-term risks from these injections.

One study by researchers at Tufts Medical Center published in *JAMA* found that patients with knee osteoarthritis who received corticosteroid shots over a period of two years lost significantly more cartilage than those who were given placebo injections…and there was ultimately no upside—they really felt no better.

For another study at Massachusetts General Hospital, radiologists who specialize in musculoskeletal diagnostic imaging compared follow-up X-rays of about 100 patients with osteoarthritis of the hip who had been given steroid injections for their pain to a placebo-injection group. They found that the bones of the patients in the steroid group deteriorated faster than those in the control group.

Another danger exists for those who get an injection too close to hip-replacement surgery. Researchers at Hospital for Special Surgery found that the injection increased the risk for post-surgery infection and other complications. The bottom line here? Wait at least three months after a cortisone injection before making the decision to go under the knife.

The most alarming risk factor has to do with spinal injections that use Depo-Medrol (methylprednisolone acetate), an off-label use of a steroid drug approved for muscle and joint injections. Although Pfizer, the drug manufacturer, warned the FDA about cases of blindness, paralysis, stroke and death resulting from injecting the drug into the spine, this information was not made public until a July 31, 2018, *New York Times* article noting nearly 2,500 serious adverse events related to Depo-Medrol, including more than 150 deaths between 2004 and 2018. Because of the reluctance of doctors to now prescribe opioids for pain, coupled with the fact that many doctors may not have heard about these reports, some are suggesting these injections as painkiller alternatives to their patients with back pain.

But the Pain Is Awful…

You do have other options to try short of what might be the ultimate decision to have a joint replacement, explains Beth Shubin Stein, MD, an orthopedic surgeon with the Hospital for Special Surgery in New York City. *What she recommends…*

• **Hyaluronic acid.** Hyaluronic acid can be injected into a joint to act as a shock absorber and lubricant. When you have osteoarthritis, your body's own supply of hyaluronic acid breaks down and your joints don't move as smoothly as they used to, causing pain. Typically, a series of injections are done over three to five weeks. Some patients have been able to delay knee replacements for up to three years with hyaluronic acid injections. There is a slight risk for an allergic reaction.

• **Platelet-rich plasma.** Platelets extracted from a patient's own blood are being used with more frequency these days. The idea is that growth factors found in your blood plasma could help you to regrow tissue. It also helps mitigate pain, though it's too soon to tell whether one, two or three injections are needed to get the benefits. If a patient finds that one helps, your doctor may repeat it a few times. A meta-analysis that included a total of 1,423 people and published in *Journal of Orthopaedic Surgery and Research* found that patients had less pain and better function with PRP than other treatments, including steroid shots, after a year of follow-up. The downside to PRP is that most insurance companies will not cover it, and a single injection can cost in the hundreds of dollars and up to $2,000, depending on your area of the country.

• **Stem cell injections.** Stem cells can be taken from your fat using liposuction. Another option is donor stem cells from amniotic fluid. The procedure takes about an hour in an outpatient setting. Like PRP, it might not be covered by your insurance and can be as costly. Also, it isn't yet widely available in the US. However, recent research published in *Stem Cells International* shows that it has promise, especially for osteoarthritis.

None of the existing treatments can regrow cartilage, and all have some drawbacks. With any type of injection, you may experience pain at the injection site, tissue damage or nerve injury, and there's always a slight chance of infection. But they can be helpful, at least in delaying knee- or hip-replacement surgery in many people.

Remember, too, that there are many conservative treatments that can help, such as losing weight, stretching, walking and other exercises, ice and nonsteroidal anti-inflammatory drugs (NSAIDs).

What Works for Knee Health

Increased fiber intake can reduce the chance of developing symptomatic knee osteoarthritis. People with the highest intake—21 grams daily from grains, legumes, nuts, fruits and vegetables—had a 30% lower chance of developing the condition over a four-year period, compared with those with lowest fiber intake. Weight loss may slow cartilage loss in the knee. Patients who lost 5% to 10% of body weight over four years had slower degeneration of their knee cartilage than those who stayed at a stable weight. Noisy knees, known as crepitus, may indicate development of arthritis pain in the near future. People with the most crepitus were most likely to develop symptomatic knee osteoarthritis within one to four years. A Mediterranean-style diet for people with knee osteoarthritis can reduce knee pain and bring a better overall quality of life. The diet focuses on olive oil, fruits, nuts, vegetables and whole grains.

Roundup of multiple research studies reported in University of California, *Berkeley Wellness Letter*.

Celebrex Is Safe for Your Heart

Chronic-pain drug *celecoxib* (Celebrex) is heart-safe after all—as safe as ibuprofen or naproxen. While it is similar to Vioxx—which was taken off the market in 2004—Celebrex doesn't have the same heart/stroke risks.

Why this matters: Celebrex is an appropriate nonopioid alternative for patients with chronic pain. The Food and Drug Administration is considering modifying safety warnings on the label.

Steven E. Nissen, MD, MACC, is chairman of the department of cardiovascular medicine at the Cleveland Clinic Main Campus, Ohio. His clinical research is the basis of the FDA's new evaluation.

Why It's Good to "Feel" Your Partner's Pain

Osteoarthritis patients whose spouses showed emotional support in daily interactions performed better on physical tasks over time than those with less responsive spouses. The osteoarthritis patients with supportive spouses did better on a series of tests, such as standing from a seated position without help, maintaining balance and walking—and people who perform better on these tasks are likely to live longer and maintain independence longer than those who perform worse.

Study of 152 patients diagnosed with knee osteoarthritis by researchers at The Ohio State University, Columbus, published in *Psychological Science*.

Ankle Replacements Are on the Rise

Ankle replacements are becoming more common. They can relieve the pain of ankle arthritis. Patients often live with the arthritis pain for decades until medication and rest no longer are enough to allow them to function. Now a device called the STAR (Scandinavian total ankle replacement system), available in the US since 2009, is increasingly being implanted surgically—in some 10,000 patients in 2017, twice as many as in 2011. The device has proved durable and long-lasting, although 25% of 761 recipients studied needed some sort of additional surgery within 15 years—usually to replace the device's plastic parts, which wear out faster than the metal ones. The replacement is not intended for all uses—recipients cannot run or jump—but it restores everyday function and relieves pain.

Cost: $19,000 to $30,000 or more, usually covered at least in part by insurance.

Roundup of experts on ankle replacement, reported in *The Wall Street Journal*.

Why Do My Legs Feel So Heavy at Night?

Janice F. Wiesman, MD, FAAN, clinical associate professor of neurology at New York University School of Medicine in New York City. She is author of *Peripheral Neuropathy: What It Is and What You Can Do to Feel Better.*

Waking up in the middle of the night to the feeling that the tops of your legs are so heavy...like dead weight...could be due to lumbar spinal stenosis (a narrowing of the lower spinal canal) or degenerative spine disease (changes to the spinal discs that are often related to aging). With both of these conditions, people typically experience low-back pain with tingling or shooting pain down one or both legs...and sometimes heaviness and aching in the legs.

With spinal stenosis, bony overgrowth slowly surrounds and compresses the nerves as they leave the spinal cord and run into the legs. I prefer physical therapy to treat this condition, while some doctors prescribe nonsteroidal anti-inflammatory drugs (NSAIDs), such as *naproxen* (Aleve), or the nerve pain medication *gabapentin* (Neurontin). If these approaches don't bring relief, minimally invasive surgery to open up the bony holes (called foramina) through which the nerve roots exit the spinal cord may be recommended. With degenerative spine disease, a protruded or herniated disc or spinal arthritis compresses one or a few nerves as they exit the spinal cord. Surgery is usually not required. Exercise to increase strength and flexibility and pain medication are often sufficient.

A muscle condition called inflammatory myopathy also could lead to heavy legs. People with this condition may have aching in the thighs and weakness when doing everyday tasks, such as getting up from a low chair or lifting the arms over the head, as well as trouble swallowing. Some patients may also have a rash on their face or other areas of the body. The cause of this condition is not known, but it is considered an autoimmune disorder. Inflammatory myopathy is usually treated with physical therapy, medication (sometimes including steroids to curb inflammation) and rest. A topical cream can be used to treat a rash or other skin problems.

Peripheral artery disease (PAD), a fairly common disorder in people over age 50, can cause a feeling of heaviness or aching in the thighs. With this condition, a buildup of fatty deposits in the arteries slows blood flow in the legs. Even though walking often triggers the pain associated with PAD, this form of exercise is usually the best possible treatment because, when done consistently, it brings more oxygen to the muscles, which improves circulation and helps curb the pain. Aspirin, blood-thinning medication and cholesterol-lowering drugs also may be recommended. If these therapies do not control the condition, the next step to consider is a minimally invasive procedure that involves placing a stent in the blocked artery.

If you're experiencing any of the above symptoms, visit your primary care physician, who can perform a thorough vascular and neurological examination. If any tests are abnormal, your doctor may want you to have a test known as an electromyography, in which small needles are inserted into the muscle to check the condition of your muscles and the nerve cells that control the muscles, and a nerve conduction study to check the functioning of your nerves.

Knee Arthritis Pain Helped by Whole-Body Massage

Knee arthritis pain is reduced by whole-body massage, says Adam Perlman, MD, MPH. Osteoarthritis limits movement and diminishes quality of life, but few treatments are effective for pain relief. A new study showed that weekly whole-body Swedish massage, which involves kneading, friction and vibration, significantly reduced knee pain and stiffness and improved function.

Adam Perlman, MD, MPH, is director of integrative health and well-being at the Mayo Clinic in Jacksonville, Florida, and lead author of a study published in Journal of General Internal Medicine.

Relieve Pain Without Drugs

If a loved one is in pain, hold his/her hand. Your brain waves will sync up—and pain will go down.

Study by researchers at University of Colorado, Boulder, published in Proceedings of the National Academy of Sciences.

Buzzing Foot?

Jerry Fleishman, MD, LAc, associate chair, department of medicine, and section chief, department of neurology, Medstar Franklin Square Medical Center, Baltimore.

Occasional twitches or feelings of buzzing in an arm, a leg, a hand or a foot are common and normal. They're called "fasciculations" and are most noticeable when you're resting. Moving the affected body part usually stops the buzzing feeling temporarily. Numbness and muscle cramps might accompany the buzzing.

Fasciculations are neuromuscular—your nerve cells (neurons) make your muscles move involuntarily. Possible triggers include a low level of calcium, magnesium or potassium… muscle strain…fatigue…alcohol…excess caffeine…and smoking. Certain medications, such as the antihistamine *diphenhydramine* (Benadryl), may also trigger fasciculations, as can anxiety and depression.

Muscle twitching that lasts for an extended time or recurs is called benign fasciculation syndrome (BFS), a neurological disorder marked by recurrent twitching of various muscles, usually in the calves and thighs, as well as burning, feelings of "pins and needles," tingling, buzzing, muscle fatigue and/or muscle pain.

There isn't a cure for BFS, but it's not a threat to one's general health, nor will it turn into a serious neuromuscular disease. BFS can be managed with diet, supplements and/or medications. Include bananas, oranges, avocados, leafy greens and mineral water in your diet to boost levels of potassium, magnesium and calcium...or take supplements of these minerals. BFS related to a muscle injury may just need time to heal. If these measures aren't enough, you may need a beta-blocker, an antiseizure drug, a muscle relaxant or an anti-inflammatory.

Hope for Fibromyalgia Sufferers

David Sherer, MD, a board-certified anesthesiologist who is president and CEO of Consolidated Medicine. He is coauthor of Dr. David Sherer's Hospital Survival Guide: 100+ Ways to Make Your Hospital Stay Safe and Comfortable. *His blog on BottomLineInc.com is titled "What Your Doctor Isn't Telling You."*

Fibromyalgia as a disease and diagnosis has been around for decades. But many doctors, even today, don't believe it exists. Characterized by any combination of muscle and joint aches, sleep disturbance, headaches, "brain fog," anxiety, depression, migraines and irritable bowels, this condition was often dismissed as a bogus diagnosis. There was never, until recently, any lab test or other medical study that could confirm its presence. For those who do believe it is real, it seems to afflict one out of 12 women and one out of 20 men. Children can even be affected.

The condition confounds patients and caregivers alike. Many patients fear being labelled hypochondriacs and doctors who don't know much about fibromyalgia and how to treat it have been frustrated when its signs and symptoms present themselves.

All that may be changing. Dr. Bruce Gillis, a California doctor and researcher, in conjunction with the University of Illinois/Chicago and the Harvard School of Public Health, has been examining the issue. He and his research team have designed a test specific for fibromyalgia, the fm/a test, which is said to measure certain chemicals (called cytokines) from white blood cells. The test sees if these chemicals are altered in their function in a specific way indicative of fibromyalgia.

Not all insurance companies will cover the cost of the test. Also, there have been critics who say that since Dr. Gillis has a financial stake in the company (he is CEO of EpicGenetics, the company selling the test), the test should be regarded with caution. You can learn more about the test at thefmtest.com.

Concurrent with the test has been the discovery that an old TB medication, BCG, has shown promise in treating patients with fibromyalgia. I would encourage anyone who is suspected of having the condition do the necessary research and ask your doctor if he/she is aware of this information (including clinical trials on BCG). For a disease that has been so mysterious and elusive these many years, perhaps there is a game-changing diagnostic test and treatment on the horizon.

Stress Can Give You an Autoimmune Disease

Angelos Halaris, MD, PhD, professor of psychiatry and behavioral neurosciences and medical director of adult psychiatry and researcher in psychoneuroimmunology at Loyola University Chicago Stritch School of Medicine. The study "Association of Stress-Related Disorders With Subsequent Autoimmune Disease" by researchers in Sweden and Iceland and published in JAMA.

We know the debilitating effects that stress can have on the mind and body in terms of anxiety and fatigue and even heart attack. But now we've learned that stress can also cause a very specific, serious and lifelong health condition—an autoimmune disease.

The connection is understandable when you think about it. Stress throws your body out of balance and sends your immune system into high gear—too high. To learn just how deeply stress can affect the immune system, researchers in Sweden and Iceland followed more than 100,000 patients diagnosed with a stress-related disorder, such as PTSD or acute stress reaction (which results from witnessing a traumatic event), for an average of 10 years to see how many developed autoimmune diseases, compared with other people who didn't have stress disorders.

What they found was alarming. People with stress disorders had, on average, a 36% higher risk of developing an autoimmune disease—a huge added risk. For people with PTSD, the risk was 46%, and they were more likely to develop multiple autoimmune diseases than people with other stress disorders.

The autoimmune diseases people developed included rheumatoid arthritis, psoriasis, diabetes, lupus, ulcerative colitis and multiple sclerosis and more than 30 others, all diseases that can be caused by an immune system on constant high alert.

Recognizing and Reducing Your Stress Level

Chronic stress is, simply put, toxic, said Angelos Halaris, MD, PhD, a psychiatrist and professor at the Loyola University Chicago Stritch School of Medicine, whose groundbreaking work in the new field of psychoneuroimmunology explores the association between autoimmune diseases and stress-related disorders. Like many toxins, stress causes both physical and psychological warning signs.

Dr. Halaris explained that stress activates substances in the body called cytokines—think of them as the firefighters for the immune system. Under extreme stress, cytokines invade the blood, spinal fluid and brain tissues, and while trying to restore balance, they can create collateral damage…such as an autoimmune disease. And once that happens, you can never be rid of the disease, be-

cause it permanently affects your body—you can manage it but never actually cure it.

Important: Even if you haven't been diagnosed with a stress-related disorder, to reduce your risk for an autoimmune disease, Dr. Halaris says to look out for signs that your body and mind are suffering from high stress, then take action to reduce it. *These are all indicators that your stress level is too high…*

•**Physical signs such as a pounding heart,** headache, sweating or flushing.

•**Changes in sleep,** especially insomnia and waking too early in the morning.

•**Overeating and food cravings.**

•**Mood swings.**

•**Irritability.**

•**Sudden outbursts of anger.**

•**Dependence on caffeine,** alcohol or drugs.

Dr. Halaris said the following stress-reduction tips have been the most helpful for his patients…

•**To improve sleep,** avoid stimulating your brain in the evening. Don't eat late at night or work late into the night.

•**Allow yourself at least 30 minutes of down time every day,** and whenever possible, use it to take a walk, a great stress reducer.

•**Practice more formal stress-reduction techniques** and get the wellness benefits of social interaction by joining a stress-reduction group or taking a yoga class.

•**Don't use food, alcohol, drugs or smoking to reduce stress**—that's just substituting one negative lifestyle habit for another.

What about medication to help deal with stress? The stress and autoimmune disease study found that antidepressants greatly reduced the risk for autoimmune disease in people with PTSD, though not in people with other stress disorders. Dr. Halaris said that the antidepressant Zoloft can be very effective for PTSD, but before taking any drug, be sure to be evaluated by a mental health professional—not only by your primary care doctor—to help determine the best course of action for you.

Chapter 12

PHYSICAL INJURY AND BONE HEALTH

How to Stay Injury-Free

During the past 30 years, exercise physiologist Tom Holland has completed more than 60 marathons, 25 triathlons and several ultramarathons stretching as far as 50 miles. Although the 50-year-old has asked a lot of his body, he has not endured a single significant injury since he separated his shoulder playing football in high school. Avoiding injury is vital to staying active and independent as we age—and even to avoiding physical therapy, which could easily cost $100 per session. *So we asked Holland to share his secrets for remaining injury-free despite being extremely active…*

• **I listen to my body.** I don't subscribe to the saying, "No pain, no gain." If I feel an unusual twinge or tweak while I'm exercising, I stop what I'm doing. If I felt something was really wrong in the middle of a marathon, I'd take myself out (thankfully, it has never happened). Pushing through pain is how small issues become major injuries.

That doesn't mean I get to skip my workout whenever something seems off. It just means that I switch my focus to a different part of my body. If the twinge was in my knee, for example, I do upper-body exercises that day instead.

• **I do a little of many things rather than a lot of one thing.** I love running. I could happily run every day. I'm less a fan of swimming and biking, but I took up triathlons anyway—because excessive focus on one activity puts great stress on certain body parts while leaving others underdeveloped, increasing the odds of injury.

A balanced fitness plan includes upper- and lower-body work and addresses all five components of fitness…

• **Cardiovascular endurance.** Activities that get the heart rate up and keep it up for at least several minutes, such as jogging, swimming and biking.

• **Muscle endurance.** Using a muscle continuously over an extended period, such as holding a plank position or ascending long staircases without pausing.

• **Muscle strength.** Such as lifting weights.

• **Body composition.** Making sure, through diet and exercise, that you develop and maintain a healthy balance of fat and muscle.

Tom Holland, exercise physiologist and certified strength and conditioning specialist based in Darien, Connecticut. He serves as chief fitness adviser for Nautilus, Inc., and is author of *The Five-Minute Exercise Plan.* TeamHolland.com

• **Flexibility.** Such as from stretching, yoga or Pilates.

You can incorporate all of the above without spending hours a day exercising—just don't do the same thing every day!

I begin *very* slowly with unfamiliar exercises and activities. The risk for injury is greatest when we try new things. We don't yet know the proper forms and techniques... and our bodies aren't yet used to performing the necessary actions.

The first few times I try something, I set aside my ego and keep the reps slow and the difficulty low. There have been times when I've lifted so little weight at the gym that people have asked me if something is wrong. Better that my pride gets hurt than my body.

I'm extremely cautious about group fitness classes. Fitness classes tend to be designed to be challenging for the strongest people in the class—which can leave novices at risk for injury as they struggle to keep up. Many instructors do not closely monitor participants' technique, either—they just shout encouragement from the front of the room. Even yoga can be dangerous for novices. I have a number of friends who sustained injuries in yoga class that could have been avoided with better oversight from the instructor.

Fitness classes can be socially fun and great motivators—I myself take some. But before trying any new class, I confirm that it's appropriate for someone at my level...and I ask the instructor to keep a close eye on my form. If I find that I can't keep up during the class, I don't try to—in fitness classes, ego gets people injured.

I'm always working on my balance. Falls cause injuries. Preventing falls requires maintaining your ability to keep your balance, which naturally declines with age from loss of muscle strength and joint flexibility and changes in the inner ear.

Incorporating balance exercises into your day is as simple as standing on one foot while you brush your teeth, put on your socks or ride an elevator.

For even better balance, add to your workouts an exercise called a *single-leg floor touch*. Stand with your feet hip-width apart. Lift your right foot off the floor, raising the leg behind you, and hinge forward at the waist until your torso is parallel with the floor. As you do so, lightly touch the floor with your right hand. (You should bend your left leg as you do this—this is not a stretching exercise.) 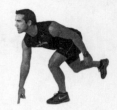 Balance for a few seconds in that position, return to start, then repeat for a total of 10 reps. If needed for balance, hold your left arm out to the side or grasp something sturdy. Then switch sides, and do 10 reps with your left leg raised and left hand touching the floor.

I don't do exercises that often cause injuries. I don't do straight-leg lifts—an exercise where you lie flat on your back and lift your fully extended legs. These put too much strain on the lower back. I don't do upright rows, where a barbell (or pair of dumbbells) is lifted repeatedly from waist height to collarbone height with the hands facing inward toward the body in an overhand grip. These put too much stress on the shoulders. And I don't do behind-the-neck lat pull-downs, where a bar attached to weights by a cable is pulled down until it is behind the neck. This also puts excessive stress on the shoulders. (Lat pull-downs are safe when the bar is pulled down to a position in front of the head.)

I do lateral training. The most common exercise equipment includes treadmills, ellipticals, stationary bikes and stair climbers. The most common outdoor exercises include jogging and biking. What do all of these have in common? They all feature forward-only or forward-and-back movement, not side to side. That's one reason why seemingly fit people often get hurt when they play basketball, tennis or touch football for the first time in a while—these sports require rapid side-to-side movement, which their exercise routines have not prepared them to do.

I include side-to-side, or "lateral," exercises in my workouts. A lateral elliptical machine, which many gyms now have, is one way to do this. You also can train laterally with simple lateral lunges—stand with your 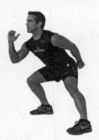 feet shoulder width apart... take a big side step to your right, leaving your left foot where it is...bend your right knee until your right thigh is almost parallel with the floor, keeping your left leg straight, your right knee approximately above your right foot, and both feet pointed forward. Return to standing without repositioning your left foot, then repeat to the left, and do 10 lunges on each side.

4 Ways to Build Better Balance

Carol Clements, MA, who has more than 45 years of experience as a personal trainer and teacher of many movemeant arts, techniques and methods. She is also author of *Better Balance for Life* and works privately with clients in New York City. CarolClements.com

B alance is a crucial but under-recognized element of good health. Unfortunately, loss of muscle strength and other factors cause us to become more wobbly as we age. So it's no surprise that one of every four adults age 65 and older in the US reports falling each year.

The good news is, balance is a skill that you can improve. *Here's how*...

Getting Started

Feeling insecure about your balance can lead to a fear of falling, which will inhibit your daily activities—and actually increase your risk of falling. Practicing your balance will help you gain more confidence and overcome any fear you may have.

Important: Balance problems can be caused by a variety of medical conditions. Some of the most common causes are abnormalities in the vestibular system (the inner ear)...weak muscles or unstable joints...less visual acuity...certain medications...alcohol... and various neurological disorders, including peripheral neuropathy—especially involving nerves of the feet. Your doctor can rule out any medical problems that may make balance practice unsafe or give you the go-ahead to begin the regimen described below.

4 Balance Boosters

To improve your balance, a good strategy is to fit a few targeted moves into your everyday activities. Within a matter of days, you'll begin to incorporate them into your daily routine—and without even breaking a sweat. *My favorite everyday balance boosters can be done while...*

•**Watching television.**

What to do: While sitting, take off your shoes and socks, prop one foot up on a coffee table or the couch, and interlace your fingers between your toes. Use your fingers to spread out all five toes so that they are not touching one another. Maintain this position for one minute. Relax. Repeat on your other foot. Then alternate flexing and pointing each foot 10 times. Finally, try to wiggle each toe one at a time. This may be difficult at first, but remember that you will improve with practice. These relaxed micro-movements of the foot are an important part of standing and balancing.

•**Brushing your teeth.**

What to do: Lightly place the fourth (ring) finger of your nonbrushing hand on the edge of the sink or vanity, so as you stand, you have that bit of support from your finger on the counter but are not holding on tightly. (Use this finger, since it is capable of only light touch to steady yourself.) Move one foot slightly behind you and off the floor. This exercise will force you to adjust your center of gravity and recruit more hip and core muscles to stabilize yourself. Alternate feet

To Check Your Balance, Start with This Self-Test

Balance is a critical element of our overall well-being. But it's not something you can take for granted. It can decline almost imperceptibly, and a dangerous fall can happen in a split second.

A frightening trend: Deaths from falls are on the rise in the US, according to a 2018 report from the Centers for Disease Control and Prevention. The number of people aged 65 and older who died as a result of a fall jumped from 18,334, in 2007 to 29,668 in 2016. While the reasons for this steep increase are not fully understood, good balance is undoubtedly among the best defenses against this serious danger. If you're concerned about your balance, be sure to discuss it with your doctor. There can be a variety of underling causes. If you think your balance is fine, give yourself the following quick self-test to see just how steady you really feel on your feet.

What to do: Stand upright, with your feet together, behind a sturdy chair. Cross you arms over your chest and slowly close your eyes. If necessary, place one hand on the seat back for support. Do you feel stable? Wobbly? Nervous? Notice how you react to this balance challenge. (By excluding sight, you rely on your body's use of sensory nerve endings and other body-orienting input that contributes to achieving balance.)

It's a good idea to tell your doctor about your results—and to repeat the self-test periodically to informally check your balance.

morning and night, optimally for as long as it takes you to brush your teeth. If you lose your balance at first, touch the nonstanding foot to the floor lightly to steady yourself and calmly resume balancing.

To up your game: Stand on one foot without touching the sink...then with your free arm extended overhead.

- **Talking on the phone.**

What to do: Stand up. With your feet hip-width apart and your knees directly over your ankles, imagine yourself squeezing a balloon between your shins. This squeezing motion, called adduction, will strengthen your adductor muscles of the inner thighs and hips to help keep you stable.

- **Walking down a hallway.**

What to do: Find a safe, clear hallway and walk down it backward at least once a day.

This exercise requires coordination of reversed foot mechanics and the transfer of weight in the less familiar backward direction. The first time you do this, look over your shoulder and count the number of steps it takes until you reach the end. After that, you can count out that number of steps in your head while keeping your gaze forward. If you feel unsteady, reach out to the wall on either side of you or have someone with you.

Gazing forward is easier on the neck, and you can't use sight to orient yourself in the familiar forward direction.

Most important: In addition to these exercises, find an enjoyable activity that keeps you on your feet. Whether it's dancing, playing table tennis, flying a kite or walking your dog, the more you move, the better your balance!

Best Exercise to Prevent Falls: Tai Chi

Study titled, "Effectiveness of a Therapeutic Tai Ji Quan Intervention vs a Multimodal Exercise Intervention to Prevent Falls Among Older Adults at High Risk of Falling," by researchers at Oregon Research Institute, Eugene, published in *JAMA Internal Medicine*.

It's a fact of life that the older you get, the greater the chances that you'll trip, stumble, lose your balance, miss a step or do something else that will cause you to fall. Of course, exercising can keep you fit so that taking a tumble is less likely. But if you really want to stay strong and steady—and on your feet—there's one kind of exercise that's best.

While plenty of research shows that exercise is effective at preventing falls among seniors, there is not much scientific consensus as to what kind of exercise is the safest and most effective. So researchers at Oregon Research Institute compared the fall-preventive effects of different kinds of exercise in 670 adults age 70 and older who had had a fall during the previous year or were at increased risk for falling because of impaired mobility.

The participants were randomly assigned to one of three exercise programs—stretching (the control)...a multimodal program of aerobic, strength and flexibility exercises...or a popular tai chi program for seniors called *Tai Ji Quan: Moving for Better Balance* (TJQMBB). Each group exercised for 60 minutes twice a week for 24 weeks.

Results: Compared with the multimodal exercise, TJQMBB reduced falls by 31%... and compared with the control (stretching), TJQMBB reduced falls by 58%. During the course of the study 733 falls were reported among 324 of the participants—363 falls in the stretching group...218 falls in the multimodal group...and 152 in the TJQMBB group. Also, fewer participants had falls in the TJQMBB group compared with the other groups—85 participants in the TJQMBB group reported falls, compared with 127 in the stretching group and 112 in the multimodal group.

There were no injuries related to any of the exercises and all the exercise programs were deemed equally safe. The researchers concluded that TJQMBB offers a significant reduction in fall risk for older people compared with traditional exercise programs.

Tai Ji Quan: Moving for Better Balance is based on the ancient Chinese martial art of tai chi and incorporates eight movements that have been modified into exercises that synchronize movement, balance and breathing. TJQMBB is being promoted for older adults by the National Council on Aging. You can find additional details about the program on its site. If you want to try TJQMBB, classes are offered at many YMCAs.

You Broke a Bone... How to Avoid Another

Susan Ott, MD, professor of medicine at the University of Washington School of Medicine in Seattle and a specialist in bone diseases.

You tripped and broke a bone when you landed on the floor. The pain is gone, your recovery is complete, but you're left with an unwanted vestige of the event—the fear of falling again...and suffering another break.

Giving up all activity and plopping yourself into a cushy chair is not an option. So we asked Susan Ott, MD, a specialist in bone diseases, for a step-by-step plan to help people who have broken bones and healed to actually get back to living. *Here's what Dr. Ott recommends...*

•**Get evaluated for osteoporosis.** This should be your first step if you don't already know your bone density status. Other diseases such as cancer or infections can weaken your bones, but if you're over 50 or a younger woman who already went through menopause, your break was likely osteoporosis-related. Depending on the severity of osteoporosis, a strong cough or even a sneeze can be enough to cause a fracture—so you don't want to be in the dark about it.

Typically, an osteoporotic fracture is one caused just by a simple fall from a standing height rather than by a trauma. Bones in the spine (vertebra), the hip and the wrist are the most bones most often affected, although fractures of the ankles and feet can also be early indications of osteoporosis. (Fractures of toes, hands and fingers don't count as osteoporotic fractures.)

The lower your bone density, the more careful you'll need to be. One out of five women who have a spine fracture will have another one the next year if they don't get treatment, warns Dr. Ott. Those with a hip, leg or arm fracture also have a high risk of more fractures. Medications for osteoporosis aren't perfect, but they can help prevent future fractures, Dr. Ott said. In clinical trials that have included thousands of women, those treated with placebo had about twice as many second fractures as those treated with osteoporosis medicines, even when they followed advice about exercise, nutrition and fall prevention. Unfortunately, only about 20% of women who are admitted to a hospital with a fracture receive any medical treatment for their osteoporosis. Sadly, osteoporosis is still often ignored. Many fractures could be prevented with more attention paid to treatment. Sometimes women don't want to take medication because they are worried about side effects, but once you have had a fracture the benefits are far greater than the side effects. After one fracture, the best way to prevent another fracture is to take a medicine and to work out a plan for activities you can do to help strengthen the bones, said Dr. Ott.

• **Create a bone-boosting exercise plan.** Bones really respond to exercise, and they also respond to a lack of exercise: If you sit or lie around much, your bones will become weaker. If you're up on your feet, bones get stronger. Different types of exercise can work together to also make your muscles stronger so you're better able to prevent a fall that could lead to another break.

• Weight-bearing exercise isn't just any exercise where you lift weight—it's specifically activities in which you move against gravity when you're upright, benefitting your whole frame. Walking is an example (and a good one). The purposeful stress placed on your bones in weight-bearing exercise causes them to draw in more nutrients and become denser. Do some form of weight-bearing exercise five times a week for at least 30 minutes each time. Besides walking, this can include tai chi, dancing and hiking. If you don't have arthritis or balance problems, climbing stairs is good, too, says Dr. Ott.

• Strength training will develop your muscles so that they can better support your bones. An international panel of experts found that strength training and balance training help prevent falls, resulting in fewer fractures. Do strength training with weights two to three times a week—and don't feel pressured to weight-train more often because it's actually essential to wait at least 48 hours between sessions to allow muscles to recover. Two sets of at least one exercise per muscle group is recommended. The guidelines also suggest getting instruction on proper form, using free weights rather than machines if you're at high risk of a spinal fracture because the forward bending and twisting puts too much strain on your bones, and starting with low weights, especially if you're new to strength training.

• **Balance training can take many forms.** Tai chi with its combination of gentle movements and mindfulness is very effective for balance as well as weight-bearing exercise. One study found that practicing tai chi for at least four weeks not only led to fewer falls, but also reduced the participants' fear of falling. Yoga is another great choice for improving balance and flexibility.

While exercising is critical to bone health, knowing what not to do will also help you avoid another break. If your fracture was due to osteoporosis, skip high-impact exercises, such as jumping and running because they put too much pressure on weak bones. Also, avoid activities that require twisting or bending at the waist such as sit-ups, toe touches and golfing, which pressure the spine and can cause (another) fracture.

• **Don't let fear paralyze you.** After you've broken a bone, it will probably take some time for you to regain your self-confidence. That's understandable—don't beat yourself up about it—but be alert to the risk of staying afraid and tentative for too long a time. If you don't get emotionally as well as physically stronger from exercise, consider working with a physical therapist who can refine your workout program to make you feel more secure when exercising. If the problem is literally in your head, a few sessions with a mental health professional might help. Cognitive behavioral therapy in particular helped older adults who had a fear of falling overcome that fear.

Practical Steps to Avoid A Second Break

• **Eliminate or reduce home hazards.** If you haven't done so yet, go room-by-room and clear the floor where you walk of all tripping hazards ranging from loose throw rugs to electrical cords to furniture or planters with legs that jut out (and, of course, any stacks of books and such if you are prone to clutter!). Area rugs should have skid-proof backing or be placed on non-slip rug pads. Install grab bars in the tub and shower—never rely on a towel rack to help you stop a fall. Don't ever leave packages or other items sitting in hallways or at the bottom of stairs—it's too easy to forget they're there.

• **Improve home lighting.** Have you been making do with dimly lit rooms? Now is the time to upgrade to brighter bulbs and additional light fixtures where needed. Be sure there's a light switch at every room's entrance so you can turn lights on before you walk in. Keep a flashlight and extra batteries in your night table in case your power goes out. Stay up to date with vision checks. Wearing eyeglasses with an outdated prescription increases tripping and bumping risk significantly, Dr. Ott said.

• **Wear appropriately soled shoes indoors and out.** At home, low-heeled shoes rather than socks or even slippers will give you better footing. Outside, choose rubber-soled shoes and boots.

• **Don't smoke cigarettes.** Not only are they harmful to your heart, lungs, and blood vessels, they also reduce strength of the bones.

• **Eat your calcium.** Getting this vital nutrient from food is better than relying on supplements, Dr. Ott said. Put yogurt, cottage cheese and dark green leafy vegetables (other than spinach—your body doesn't absorb much of its calcium, she said) on the menu. You can get calcium's partner, vitamin D, from 10 to 15 minutes of sun exposure two to three times per week, but depending on where you live, that's not always possible

and some people need to avoid the sun. It's safe to take a D supplement of 1,000 IU daily, Dr. Ott said.

Note: Alcohol interferes with your body's ability to absorb calcium. And if you're even a bit tipsy, you're more likely to fall. Limit alcohol to one drink a day or less.

• **Know how to fall.** It's best to fall forward in a ball or backward on your butt. Tumbling sideways or straight down increases your risk of a broken hip. With falling forward, you may break wrist or arm, but those are not as severe as a hip fracture. If you're at high risk for a fracture, consider underwear or pants with padding at the hips, available online at sites such as AliMed.com, which will absorb some of the trauma to your bones in case of a fall (research on their effectiveness is mixed, but some research found that they aren't more effective simply because people don't wear them).

• **Review medication side effects with your doctor.** A number of drugs for very common conditions ranging from high blood pressure to insomnia to allergies can interfere with your balance. Ask about other medication options.

Better Bunion Surgery— Less Pain, Big Gain

Rebecca Cerrato, MD, a board-certified orthopedic surgeon, The Institute for Foot and Ankle Reconstruction at Mercy Medical Center in Baltimore.

Have you been putting off bunion surgery because of the daunting months-long, painful recovery? (Besides the fact that even if you go through all that, you might be unhappy with the results.) A new bunion-correction procedure might change your mind. It is much less painful, has a shorter recovery...and could have you wearing stilettos in just eight weeks!

Hallux valgus—the medical term for bunion—afflicts about one-quarter of adults under 65, and about 35 % of people older than that, with women outnumbering men more than two to one. A bunion is a deformity of the big toe joint. The big toe becomes misaligned, bending toward the toe next to it and causing a bony protrusion to develop on the outside of the foot at the base of the big toe. The misalignment and bump typically worsen over time—interfering with the fit and comfort of shoes, especially those with narrow, pointy toes…and swelling and causing pain. Icing the bump, taking anti-inflammatory drugs such as ibuprofen or naproxen, and wearing flat, wide-toed shoes won't correct the deformity but can relieve or reduce the pain. When that isn't enough, surgery is the next step.

The Old Way

Traditional bunion-correction surgery typically involves an incision on the side of the foot that is wide enough to allow the surgeon to use a saw to perform bone cuts to both realign the toe and to remove the bony bump. The surgeon then realigns the big toe, often using pins (usually later removed) or screws (usually kept in permanently) to hold the bones in place while they heal.

The problem with this procedure is that the surgeon usually has to perform the cuts within the toe joint itself, which can reduce its ability to move and bend freely even after healing is complete. So while the bunion may be eliminated—as well as most, if not all, of the pain—often range of motion in the toe is significantly reduced.

Recovery for traditional bunion surgery also is long and painful—usually involving a splint, crutches, staying off the affected foot as much as possible for several months, plus keeping it elevated most of the day for the first several weeks.

Of course, if bunion pain has been interfering with quality of life anyway, this kind of recovery may seem worth it. *But now that there's a much better option, you may not have to…*

Minimally invasive bunion surgery (MIS), also called a percutaneous procedure, actually has been around since the 1970s. However, only recently have improved techniques and instruments made the procedure so successful and the outcome so predictable. MIS not only has a shorter, less painful recovery period than traditional bunion surgery, but because the procedure does not involve performing the bone cuts within the toe joint, the toe's range of motion is not compromised—so those stilettos are not out of the picture!

MIS—How It's Done

Surgery: The procedure is performed under anesthesia, and the anesthesia used varies from surgical center to center. Rather than the large incision of traditional bunion surgery, MIS involves only small keyhole incisions and a kind of X-ray machine that is used to help guide the surgeon. And instead of a saw moving back and forth, the surgeon cuts away the bump with a burr—an instrument similar to what dentists use—that allows for smaller, more precise cuts. After the bone is cut, it is shifted to correct the toe alignment and secured with screws.

Recovery: The patient goes directly into a postsurgical weight-bearing shoe that allows him/her to walk immediately after surgery. While patients tend to have much less pain after MIS than with the traditional procedure, typically a prescription pain medication may be needed for the first several days—usually less medication and for a shorter period of time than with traditional bunion surgery. At about two weeks, stitches and other surgical dressings are removed, and the post-surgical shoe is worn for another four to six weeks or so. After that, back to regular shoes!

If you have certain foot conditions, such as big toe arthritis or another foot condition that is contributing to your bunion, you may not be a candidate—but it's likely that condition would make you not a candidate for traditional bunion surgery, either. Otherwise, anyone who can have traditional bunion surgery qualifies to have MIS. Most insurance companies cover bunion-correction surgery.

Finding a surgeon near you who performs MIS may take some searching. The company

Wright Medical, developers of a minimally invasive bunion surgery procedure called PROstep, list surgeons who perform MIS on its website.

The Diet That Reduces Hip Fracture Risk

Teresa T. Fung, ScD, RD, CD/N, professor at the Harvard T. H. Chan School of Public Health and at Simmons University, both in Boston, and coauthor of the study "Association between Diet Quality Scores and Risk of Hip Fracture in Postmenopausal Women and Men Aged 50 Years and Older," published in *Journal of the Academy of Nutrition and Dietetics.*

You already know the importance of calcium and vitamins D and K for maintaining bone health, but it may be time to take a bigger-picture view of your diet.

Researchers at Simmons University and the Harvard School of Public Health analyzed 32 years of health and diet records from over 74,000 postmenopausal women, who participated in the expansive Nurses' Health Study, and nearly 37,000 men, age 50 and older, who participated in the Health Professionals Follow-Up Study. They created a retrospective study to see how a healthy diet could reduce the risk of hip fracture, a potentially devastating event.

The researchers assessed each participant's diet according to how closely it followed three healthy-eating plans—the Alternate Mediterranean diet (a stricter version of the standard), the DASH (or Dietary Approaches to Stop Hypertension) diet and the Alternate Healthy Eating Index-2010, originally developed in 2002 at Harvard in response to shortcomings in the government's nutritional guidelines and later updated. Then they looked at hip fracture risk in relation to how well or how poorly the three diets were followed and which diet conveyed the most benefits.

Study results: Not surprisingly, women whose diets most closely mirrored any of these healthy diets had fewer hip fractures than those whose diets mirrored them the least. While all three diets suggest getting most daily calories from plant foods—vegetables, fruit, whole grains, nuts and legumes—and limiting red and processed meats, sugar, salt and alcohol, there are subtle differences between them (more on that below), and the Alternate Healthy Eating Index-2010 was slightly more beneficial than the other diets. Women who followed it most closely had a 13% greater reduction in hip fractures than women who followed it least closely. Adhering closely to the Mediterranean diet, as good as it is for other reasons, didn't convey much risk reduction, while adhering closely to DASH hinted at some risk reduction, though numbers weren't significant.

Important: The benefits were much more apparent for women under age 75—so don't wait to start healthy eating, especially if you're already in menopause.

Because the percentage of men who had a hip fracture during the course of the study was very small, the researchers couldn't draw any firm conclusions for men, but did see a hint of a positive association between diet and avoiding hip fracture.

Another study limitation: Because of the low number of minority participants in both surveys, the researchers were only able to analyze the diets of Caucasian men and women, so the findings can't automatically be applied to other groups. But since all three diets have an assortment of benefits, including fighting off heart disease, diabetes and even neurological diseases, following one of them can't hurt and could help.

Drilling Down on the Alternate Healthy Eating Index

Because the "Index" is a set of guidelines rather than an exact diet to follow, it involves more planning, one reason why it may not be as popular as the DASH and Mediterranean diets. But it's not complicated. Every day, eat five or more servings of vegetables, four or more servings of fruit, five or six servings of whole grains and one serving of nuts. Get your protein—typically 5 ounces a day is all you need—from seafood, legumes and chicken—but be sure to eat at least 1,750 mg of omega-3 fatty acids from fatty fish a week—that's about one 4-ounce serving. Choose plant-based fats (oils) over animal-based fats (butter, lard). Limit dairy to one serving a day, avoid red meat and cut out processed meats. Also cut out all sugary beverages, from soda to fruit juices to high-sugar flavored coffees. Eat as little salt as possible and avoid alcohol or limit it to one drink a day for women, two for men.

If you find that the Alternate Healthy Eating Index diet is too complex, one of the others might better suit your needs and your tastes—and you'll be more inclined to stick with a diet if you like it. For instance, the Alternate Healthy Eating Index-2010 recommends eating only whole grains and polyunsaturated fats whereas DASH doesn't have specific guidelines for omega-3s and polyunsaturated fat and allows for some refined grains as well moderate amounts of low-fat dairy. The Mediterranean diet is known for its red wine allowance and abundance of fish.

Natural First-Aid After a Fall

Andrew Rubman, ND, medical director, Southbury Clinic for Traditional Medicines, Southbury, Connecticut. SouthburyClinic.com

The patient: "Sophie," now 84, is a well-functioning, active senior who has been a patient for almost 30 years.

Why she contacted me: Sophie called my office after she had slipped and fallen on the ice in her bank's parking lot, banging her head and cutting her hand. Even though the bank manager was insistent that he call an ambulance for her, she would have "none of that" and told him that her doctor (meaning me) would come and evaluate her.

How I evaluated her: I spoke with her to determine the mechanism of injury and assess her cognitive state. I brought her into my vehicle and conducted a focal physical exam.

We decided to adopt a "watchful waiting" approach to her head injury, which appeared to be limited to facial bruising. I explained to her that if she were to be picked up by an ambulance, because of her age she would be processed in a hospital emergency department, referred to an in-house neurologist, sent for a CT scan, and probably held overnight for routine blood work and observation.

Based on my neurological assessment and lack of concerning signs, I didn't feel that an immediate neurology consult was appropriate. I knew that I would spend the next three hours observing her and could better confirm my decision after that time had passed.

How we addressed her problem: She traumatized one of her hands when she fell and required a compression dressing to control bleeding, so we drove to one of the imaging centers I use and to have X-rays done on the spot. (I love having a facility where I am recognized and can come in with a patient, or send someone over, and receive immediate attention.) Within 30 minutes, I was back in my office with Sophie and chatting with the radiologist, who confirmed my suspicions from my limited physical exam that there were no fractures.

In that the damage to her hand, although extremely painful, was relatively superficial—there was no laceration or involvement of vital structures deep in the skin involving finger movement or circulation—I replaced the initial compression dressing, anointed with Neosporin, and provided her with Yunnan Paiyao, an herbal supplement from Traditional Chinese Medicine developed for trauma and excessive menses, to control the remaining bleeding.

I saw Sophie the next day and inspected the wound, then squeezed fresh aloe vera gel into the area and replaced the dressing. I also conducted another more thorough neurological evaluation, which was entirely negative.

The patient's progress: I explained to Sophie that it would be wise for us to speak daily for three or four days to continue to exclude the possibility of a slow brain bleed, which initial CTs often miss but is always a concern with those over 60. But in my clinical opinion, she hadn't needed the ambulance, emergency department, specialist, overnight stay or anything else that the local hospital would, by protocol, have provided in their abundance of caution. Such treatment would have merely led to a $10,000 bill that Medicare would have paid most of and legally indemnified the hospital against negligence. (Sophie was quick to chime in, "So who pays for Medicare really? We all do.")

After a few weeks, Sophie returned to her exercise classes and her weekly lunches "with the girls." The bruising on her face was almost gone. When I asked her how she explained her bruised cheek and black eye to her friends, she told me that she just says she "had been in a bar fight over a handsome gentleman!"

Gastric Bypass Alert

In a recent study of nearly 39,000 bypass patients, this weight-loss surgery increased their risk for fracture by 30% compared with a matched group who didn't undergo the surgery.

Theory: Increased fractures may be due to falls or weaker bones from malabsorption of calcium and vitamin D caused by the surgery.

If you had gastric bypass surgery: Ask your doctor to evaluate your fracture risk with, for example, the FRAX risk calculator and bone density testing.

Mattias Lorentzon, MD, professor and head of geriatric medicine, Institute of Medicine, Sahlgrenska Academy, Mölndal, Sweden.

Your Bones Are in Danger

Neil Binkley, MD, professor in the divisions of geriatrics and endocrinology at University of Wisconsin (UW) School of Medicine and Public Health, Madison. He is director of the UW Osteoporosis Clinical Research Program and associate director of the UW Institute on Aging. Aging.wisc.edu

We've been told that the best way to prevent fractures is to prevent or treat osteoporosis—diet, exercise and, if needed, medications. But that approach has not been successful.

For people with osteoporosis, medications do prevent many spinal fractures—but fewer than half of hip and other fractures, according to a major study published in *The New England Journal of Medicine*. And many people who fall and break bones don't even have osteoporosis.

Example: An overweight or obese person may have good bone density (from carrying that extra weight) but still get fractures. Unless he/she has the muscle strength to carry that extra weight, mobility issues—such as difficulty getting up off the toilet or climbing stairs—can lead to falls that cause fractures. Rather than hip fractures due to weakened bones, they tend to get ankle or lower-leg fractures.

In the end, it's preventing fractures—from any cause—that really matters. Many of us think that if we break a bone, our friendly orthopedic surgeon will put it back together and life will go on as usual. But after age 50—and especially after age 65—a fractured bone can threaten independence and quality of life. And that's what we fear most about aging—losing independence…not being able to drive…and winding up in a nursing home. The classic example is a hip fracture, which often sends people to nursing homes and is linked to a shorter life span. But breaking an ankle, an arm or even a wrist can make daily life harder at home…and make it tougher to be mobile.

To find out what is really needed to prevent fractures, we spoke with geriatrician and endocrinologist Neil Binkley, MD. He started with a simple question—"What causes most fractures in older people?"

The answer: Falling.

Here's how to prevent falls—and the fractures that could end your independence…

•**Eat for muscle strength, not just bones.** Getting enough calcium and vitamin D—standard elements of osteoporosis prevention—still is important. But pay close attention to calories and protein, too. These are essential to maintaining muscle strength—and that's as important as strong bones in preventing fractures. After all, when our muscle strength declines, we fall. And when we fall on weak bones, guess what? They break.

Protein needs are based on your body weight. To calculate your individual needs, multiply your body weight by 0.45. For a 150-pound woman, that's 67 grams a day…for a 185-pound man, 83 grams. To get a sense of what that looks like, a three-ounce serving of tuna or salmon contains about 22 grams of protein and an egg contains six grams, on average. Aim to include good sources of protein—seafood, lean meat, poultry, eggs, nuts, seeds, soy and legumes such as beans and peas—at every meal.

For some older people, a waning appetite also can mean that they just don't eat enough calories. If you're not eating enough, a registered dietitian can help find practical ways to help you get enough protein and calories each day.

•**Get strong—and balanced.** Now that you're nourishing muscles, make them work. Exercise helps keep your bones and muscles strong, so it's vital for lowering your fracture risk. The best exercise is the one that you'll actually do, whether it's walking, biking, swimming or team sports. Beyond general fitness, exercises that improve core strength and balance are key to fall prevention. *Suggestions*…

•Join a tai chi class. This ancient Chinese set of gentle, slow-moving exercises strengthens lower limbs and improves balance. Several studies have found that practicing tai chi regularly significantly reduces fall risk in older adults.

•Yoga may help, too. It can strengthen bones, and while it is less well-studied for fall prevention, it has been shown to improve balance and mobility in older people.

•**Take fall-prevention classes.** One popular, evidence-based program is Stepping On, a seven-week, two-hours-per-week workshop, first developed in Australia, that now is offered in 20 US states. It is geared to healthy adults over age 65. One study, published in *Journal of the American Geriatrics Society*, reported that people who participated in Stepping On had 31% fewer falls over the next 14 months, compared with a similar group of people who didn't go through the program. To find programs like this in your area, check with the National Council on Aging's Fall Prevention website (NCOA.org/healthy-aging/falls-prevention).

•**Consider physical therapy.** If you've fallen and have been injured—even if you didn't break a bone—you're waving a red flag that a fracture could be in your future. A physical therapist can do a formal strength-and-balance assessment…show you exercises to strengthen muscles, bones, walking posture and balance…and help you find classes in your community.

•**Make your home safer.** A key part of fall prevention is taking a look at what you can do to make it less likely that you'll trip and fall…

•Do you have night-lights in your home? Consider putting a night-light in your bathroom for those middle-of-the-night trips.

•Are there throw rugs that you might slip on? Get rid of them!

•Is there clutter on the floor or stairs that you could stumble on? Declutter!

•Do you need to get on a chair or step stool to reach things on high shelves? Put everyday items on lower shelves that are easy to reach.

• Is it hard to get in and out of your bathtub without slipping? Consider installing grab bars or replacing your tub with a walk-in shower.

Some of your safety changes may need to be in your own behavior—such as drinking less alcohol. That's a fall risk that many older people don't consider.

And don't forget to get your vision checked regularly. If you can't see it, you can trip on it.

• **Review your medications.** Some medications (prescription or over-the-counter) or medication interactions can cause dizziness, light-headedness or low blood pressure, which can increase the risk of falling. Key medications to be aware of include antihistamines, sleep aids, pain pills, antidepressants and antianxiety medications. In addition, some medications, such as glucocorticoids (steroids taken for inflammatory and autoimmune conditions) contribute to bone loss. If you are taking medications that increase your fall risk, talk to your doctor to see if you can reduce the dose, find an alternative—or modify how you take it, such as only at bedtime.

It's not that strong bones aren't important—they're a key part of a fracture-prevention plan...but only one part. If your doctor has prescribed a diet, exercise program or medication for you to prevent or treat osteoporosis, continue following those instructions. Osteoporosis medications often are prescribed based on an individual's estimated risk for fracture. For individuals at high fracture risk, the benefits of reducing that risk far outweigh the risk of side effects. But just taking medications is not enough.

Now you know what else you need to do to protect yourself.

This Exercise Prevents Falls

One of the simplest and most effective exercises—and one that you can do almost anywhere—is the Chair Rise. *Do this daily to strengthen the muscles in your thighs and buttocks, which can help keep you steady on your feet and prevent falls...*

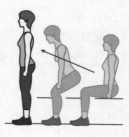

• **Sit toward the front of a sturdy chair,** with your knees bent and feet flat on the floor, shoulder-width apart.

• **Rest your hands lightly on the seat on either side of you,** keeping your back and neck straight and chest slightly forward.

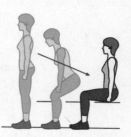

• **Breathe in slowly.** Lean forward and exhale as you stand up—feel your weight on the front of your feet.

• **Pause for a full breath in and out.**

• **Breathe in as you slowly sit down.** Try not to collapse down into the chair. Rather, control your lowering as much as possible.

• **Breathe out.**

Repeat for a total of 10 to 15 stand/sits. Rest and breathe for a minute, then do another set of 10 to 15. You may need to work up to this level over several days or a few weeks. The goal is to get to the point where you can complete two sets without using your hands at all.

Best Foods for Bones and Joints

Best foods for bone and joint strength. Calcium-fortified cereals—choose one that is high in fiber and low in sugar...salmon, an excellent source of vitamin D...dark leafy greens and vegetables, including spinach, kale, Swiss chard and bok choy, are high in vitamin K, which keeps bones healthy...yogurt...milk alternatives such as almond, soy, cashew or hemp milk, which are almost always fortified with both calcium and vitamin D.

Kathryn Weatherford, RD, LDN, registered dietitian, Beth Israel Deaconess Medical Center, Boston.

Feeling Anxious? Watch Your Bones

Study titled, "Anxiety Levels predict Fracture Risk in Postmenopausal Women Assessed for Osteoporosis," Antonio Catalano, MD, PhD, et al., University Hospital of Messina, Italy, published in *Menopause: The Journal of the North American Menopause Society*.

You already know that keeping your bones strong and healthy means taking care of yourself physically. Now new research has found that your mental health can affect the health of your bones, and in a big way. If you tend to have anxiety, it can even lead to fractures. Here's why…and what to do about it.

The Mind-Bone Connection

It was already known that certain psychiatric disorders, including depression, were associated with fracture risk. But how anxiety might affect bone health hasn't been well studied. So researchers at the University Hospital of Messina in Italy led a study that investigated the role of anxiety in postmenopausal women, a group that is already, of course, at increased risk for bone problems because of hormonal changes from menopause. The women studied, about 200 of them, had not been diagnosed with anxiety and were not taking osteoporosis medications at the start of the study. They answered questionnaires that assessed their overall levels of anxiety and were given bone mineral density tests.

Results: Women who had higher anxiety scores had lower bone density in the lower vertebrae and in the femoral neck, the part of the thigh bone just below the ball of the hip joint. In fact, based on their bone-density scores, women who reported the highest levels of anxiety had a 22% greater probability of having a major fracture over the next 10 years (24.94% vs. 20.44%)—and a 34% greater likelihood of a hip fracture (9.26% vs. 6.91%—compared with women with the lowest anxiety scores. (Women with higher anxiety scores were also slightly more likely to have already had a fracture, compared with women with the lowest anxiety scores—but the difference was not considered statistically significant.)

The researchers postulated several ways anxiety could affect bone health…

• **Inflammation.** People with high anxiety levels are likely to have high levels of systemic inflammation, which leads to bone loss and is a contributor to osteoporosis.

• **Cortisol.** People with anxiety tend to have higher levels of the stress hormone cortisol, which also contributes to bone loss.

• **Oxidative stress.** Anxiety may cause more oxidative stress, which means that the body has a harder time fighting free radicals, molecules that can harm cells. Research has found that oxidative stress may be related to osteoporosis in postmenopausal women.

• **Falls.** Research links anxiety with an increased likelihood of falls.

• **Medications.** While this study did not include women who were taking medications for mental health disorders, antidepressants are known to reduce bone density—and people with anxiety often take antidepressants.

What to do: Understand that anxiety may be one of the factors that can harm your bone health—and besides the smart bone-health measures you already know about, such as getting enough calcium and vitamin D, strength training and aerobic exercise, do whatever you need to do to reduce stress and curtail your anxiety.

When to Be Concerned About a Bruise

Eric H. Kraut, MD, hematologist, professor of internal medicine, The Ohio State University, director of benign hematology, Hemostasis Thrombosis Treatment Center, The Ohio State University Wexner Medical Center, both in Columbus.

Whether you closed a drawer on your thumb or knocked your knee into a table leg, a bruise is a sign that small blood vessels under the skin have broken and leaked blood.

About half of all people are considered "easy bruisers." Bruises show up at the slightest bump or even when you can't remember injuring yourself. Conditions that can make you an easy bruiser include taking medications such as blood thinners, aspirin and ibuprofen…being deficient in certain vitamins, such as vitamin C or vitamin K…taking supplements, including fish oil, gingko biloba…spending a lot of time in the sun…and even consuming large amounts of garlic or alcohol.

Different people have different healing times when it comes to bruises. Some people's bruises disappear within two or three weeks, while others' linger longer. Age can be a factor. Bruises tend to last longer for people older than 65 because of changes in the skin.

Tip: As with swelling, you can speed the healing of a bruise by elevating the area above the heart, icing it for about 15 minutes every hour for the first 24 hours, and resting the injured area.

It might take longer for a bruise under a nail to heal and may have to do with growth with the nail. Most likely your current bruise isn't something to worry about, especially if it's moving up the nail, albeit slowly, as the nail grows out. Still, there are certain signs that any bruise, regardless of location, warrants a trip to the doctor.

When to See a Doctor

• **You have swelling and pain.** If you had an injury and there's swelling and pain at the bruise site, you could have a sprain or a fracture that needs evaluation and treatment.

• **You have other signs of a bleeding disorder.** You'll experience more bruising and other types of bleeding if you have a disorder that impacts your blood's ability to clot. Besides easy bruising, other signs to look for including having frequent nosebleeds, bleeding excessively after getting a cut or having dental work done, having heavy menstrual periods or bleeding at unusual spots, such as around your joints.

• **You have symptoms of anemia.** Anemia, a problem with red blood cells, deprives the body of oxygen. If you may have abnormal bleeding and bruising, you may have anemia. Other symptoms of anemia include shortness of breath, dizziness, a faster heartbeat, cold hands and feet, weakness, chest pain, pale skin and headaches.

• **You have a large bruise on your torso.** Small bruises or bruises on your arms or legs don't usually point to an underlying issue. A large bruise on your chest, back or stomach, especially if you haven't fallen and don't know what caused it, should be examined. This could be a sign of abnormalities in clotting due to low or abnormal platelets in your blood and or an inherited bleeding disorder. This should be evaluated by a physician since blood tests may explain the problem.

• **There's a sudden change in your bruising pattern.** A good rule of thumb is to pay attention to what's common for you. If you suddenly experience more bruising for no known reason, get checked out by your doctor.

Best Treatments for Ankle Arthritis

Judith F. Baumhauer, MD, MPH, professor and associate chair of the department of orthopedics at University of Rochester School of Medicine, New York. Her research has been published in *The New England Journal of Medicine, Foot & Ankle International* and other leading medical journals. She is the recipient of the American Orthopaedic Foot & Ankle Society's Roger A. Mann Award for outstanding clinical study in 2017.

Remember that sprained ankle you suffered years ago? Or maybe it was an ankle fracture that left you hobbling around for weeks. Whatever the specific problem, be forewarned that ankle injuries can come back to haunt you—years or even decades later. *Here's how…*

Self-Care for Arthritis

The ankle is vulnerable to the same types of arthritis that affect other joints. Post-traumatic arthritis is the most common form in the ankle, followed by age-related osteoarthritis and rheumatoid arthritis. For these forms of ankle arthritis, you might be able to manage discomfort with simple remedies.

But self-care is tricky. You can't "go easy" on the ankles in the same way that you would with certain other joints. People use their ankles all day, every day. *My advice for people with ankle arthritis…*

• **Choose activities that minimize ankle wear and tear.** To stay active and keep the muscles supporting the ankle strong, try biking, swimming, walking, rowing, elliptical workouts or other low-impact, weight-bearing exercises that don't cause relentless pounding.

• **Keep your weight down.** People with ankle arthritis tend to gain weight because they find it too painful to walk or exercise much…and the extra pounds accelerate joint damage by increasing the weight load on the ankles.

Helpful: Losing even five pounds can reduce the ankle load by 20 pounds, which may be enough to minimize symptoms.

• **Exercise the ankles.** Ankle-specific exercises will build up the muscles surrounding the joint, keep the joint from getting stiff and reduce the bone-on-bone friction that occurs with arthritis.

Example: Several times a day, flex your foot upward (dorsiflexion) as far as it will go…hold for a few seconds…then flex it downward (plantarflexion). You can find dozens of ankle exercises on the Internet.

• **Wear shock-absorbing shoes.** Also known as "stability sneakers," they have a densely cushioned heel/sole that absorbs shocks when you walk, exercise, etc.

Not Ready for Surgery

In addition to the steps above, some simple therapies can help slow the progression of arthritis. For example, it may help to wear an over-the-counter ankle brace that gives support and stability…apply cold packs when the ankle is hurting…and/or take as-needed doses of a nonsteroidal anti-inflammatory drug (NSAID), such as *ibuprofen* (Motrin) or *naproxen* (Aleve).* If you're lucky, these and other self-care therapies—including physical therapy—may be the only treatments you'll ever need.

Very helpful: A cortisone injection. Cortisone (sometimes combined with lidocaine) is a strong anti-inflammatory that can reduce or eliminate pain within a day. The shot is good for patients who are having moderate daily pain—and might be helpful for an upcoming vacation, for example, or when the pain is unusually severe. This shot won't stop the arthritis but can get you through a rough patch. In some cases, hyaluronic acid injections may be used but may not be covered by insurance.

When Surgery Is Needed

Even with the approaches described earlier, many people will eventually develop "end-stage" arthritis that does not improve and interferes with their daily activities. Once ankle arthritis progresses to that extent, it's serious business.

Until about 10 years ago, most patients with end-stage ankle arthritis were advised to have a procedure called ankle arthrodesis, commonly known as ankle fusion because affected bones are fused together to reduce pain and inflammation. Now, patients (based on their age and other factors) have a second option—a total ankle replacement.

Because long-term comprehensive studies haven't yet been done, there's still debate about which approach is better. Both procedures are effective…and both have downsides that patients need to know about. *Specifically…*

*Discuss the use of NSAIDs with your physician—they can cause side effects such as stomach upset, ulcers and high blood pressure.

• **With ankle fusion, the affected bones are locked together (with screws alone or plates and screws) and eventually fuse into a solid mass of bone.** This eliminates the rubbing/friction that causes the pain and disability of ankle arthritis. Most patients will walk in a shoe (without a cast) in eight to 12 weeks. And unlike ankle replacement (discussed below), the procedure is permanent. You're unlikely to require an additional procedure unless it doesn't fuse.

Downside: Bone fusion eliminates ankle mobility. You might walk haltingly when you go up hills or down a flight of stairs. And because the ankle is locked in place, other structures in the foot assume more of the burden of daily movements—and could become more susceptible to arthritis.

Ankle fusion might not be the best choice if you have a highly active lifestyle that involves, for example, strenuous hiking, tennis, etc., and want your ankle to move "naturally"…or if you have other arthritic areas of your foot that couldn't take on more responsibility when the ankle is locked up.

• **With a total ankle replacement, the arthritic surfaces are replaced**—as also occurs with a knee or hip replacement—with an artificial joint. Surgeons advise patients that the implants might last for eight to 12 years. A recent study found that 73% were still working after 15 years.

The advantage of total ankle replacement is that the ankle will flex. Patients retain a greater degree of motion and experience less stress on surrounding joints.

Downside: The risk for additional procedures to repair/replace a damaged implant.

My take: I might recommend joint replacement for someone who's over age 60 and in good health but has other arthritis in the foot…or a person who is active with sports, such as tennis, that involve jumping and cutting. However, the choice between fusion and replacement is highly individualized.

Important: See a surgeon who's experienced in both procedures to get an unbiased opinion about the pros and cons of each. To find such a surgeon near you, consult the American Orthopaedic Foot & Ankle Society, AOFAS.org.

Insurance typically covers these procedures, but be sure to ask.

How to Make Yoga Safe for Everybody

Carol Krucoff, C-IAYT, E-RYT, a yoga therapist and codirector of the Integrative Yoga for Seniors Professional Training at Duke Integrative Medicine, Durham, North Carolina. She is coauthor of, most recently, *Relax into Yoga for Seniors: A Six-Week Program for Strength, Balance, Flexibility and Pain Relief.* HealingMoves.com

I'd love to try yoga, but… It's a common lament of people with arthritis, osteoporosis or other chronic health problems. But yoga doesn't have to be off-limits if you have one of these conditions.

With a few precautions and a tailored approach, yoga is a wonderfully effective, research-backed method of improving strength, balance and flexibility…easing pain…and relieving the anxiety and depression that are often associated with chronic health complaints.

For anyone with one or more painful and/or limiting chronic conditions, the relaxation breathing and mindfulness that are central to yoga also can be exceptionally helpful.

Note: Older adults and people with health challenges should look for a class called "Gentle Yoga" or one geared to their needs, such as "Yoga Over 50" or "Yoga for Creaky Bodies." *Follow these steps to ensure that you stay safe if you have…*

Arthritis

Decades ago, people with osteoarthritis and rheumatoid arthritis were advised to rest and "save their joints." Now we know that inactivity can actually cause stiff joints. Yoga relieves pain and stiffness, improves range of motion and sleep, and boosts energy levels and overall mood. *If you have arthritis, be sure to…*

•**Avoid putting excessive pressure on arthritic joints.** Arthritis in your left knee? Keep the toes of your right foot on the ground in single-leg balance poses like Tree Pose. If you have arthritis in both knees, you can relieve the load on your joints by lightly touching a wall or chair.

•**Understand the meaning of different types of pain.** Sharp, immediate pain—especially in a joint—is a sign to ease up. If you have dull pain in your muscles the day after a yoga session, that's likely delayed-onset muscle soreness after using your muscles in new ways—a sign that you're getting stronger! It generally goes away in a few days.

•**Don't overstretch.** This is especially true for people with rheumatoid arthritis, which can render joints loose and unstable.

To tell whether it's a good or risky stretch: Check your breath. If your breath is compromised in any way, back off.

•**Avoid chin-to-chest poses that place pressure on your head.** Poses, such as Plow, place undue pressure on vulnerable cervical spine joints.

•**Turn certain poses around to "take a load" off.** If a pose is bothering an affected joint, try turning it upside down or sideways, taking weight off the joint and letting gravity do the work for you. Child's Pose, for example, can be done while lying on your back in bed.

Caution: Hot, red and/or swollen joints indicate active inflammation. Stick with rest or gentle range-of-motion activities for that joint. Talk with your health-care provider about appropriate treatment.

Osteoporosis

Yoga is an effective way to improve strength, balance and flexibility in people with osteoporosis. And because yoga improves your balance and strengthens bone, it may help lower your risk of falling and breaking a bone. *If you have osteoporosis, be sure to…*

•**Avoid rounding your spine when sitting or standing, since this position in-** **creases the risk for vertebral fracture.** In yoga poses—and in daily life—keep your spine long and hinge forward at your hips, rather than bending at your waist.

•**Don't twist your spine to its end range of rotation.** Instructors may encourage their students to twist as far as possible, using their hands to move even deeper into the twist. This is called end-range rotation and can increase fracture risk in people with osteoporosis. Keep any twists in the midrange, as you would when turning to look over your shoulder while driving. Move slowly, don't round your back and keep your spine elongated.

•**Avoid loading body weight on your neck and/or shoulders** as occurs during such poses as Shoulder Stand and Plow.

•**Keep your head on the ground during supine (face-up) poses.** Lifting your head when lying on the ground creates the forward-flexing, "abdominal crunch" action that can be dangerous because it places excess pressure on vertebral bodies and can lead to compression fractures. Yoga poses that can create this "crunch" are not necessarily supine—they include Standing Forward Bend and Seated Forward Bend. To perform these poses safely, hinge at the hips and keep your spine in neutral (don't round your back).

Stay Safe in the Cold!

Shoveling snow: Keep the shovel close to your body, and favor your leg and rear-end muscles for shoveling rather than those of your arms and back. Be sure to emphasize balance while shoveling.

Even better: Use someone else's strength to your advantage—hire the teenager next door who may be eager to earn some extra cash.

Walking on icy paths: Move one foot forward slowly, be sure you are stable, then put weight on the foot. Now do the same with the other foot.

AARP the Magazine.

Can Osteoporosis Cause a Backache?

David G. Borenstein, MD, clinical professor of medicine, division of rheumatology, The George Washington University Medical Center, Washington, DC. He is managing editor of *The Spine Community* website and author of *Heal Your Back: Your Complete Prescription for Preventing, Treating and Eliminating Back Pain.*

I'm 55 and recently started having back problems. My mom had osteoporosis starting in her 50s. Could my back pain be due to osteoporosis?

While there are many possible causes of back pain, you may want to get your spine checked for tiny fractures. About one out of every five postmenopausal women has these vertebral spine fractures—and most don't know it. Thin bones in the back can fracture suddenly during a routine activity, such as opening a window, bending over or even sneezing. In some cases, there is no pain at all, but in others there's a sharp pain in the back that doesn't go away. These fractures are a sign of osteoporosis and can eventually reduce your mobility and your quality of life.

Given your mother's history of early osteoporosis, you may be a candidate for a bone density scan that includes an assessment of your spine. Typically, based on screening guidelines from the American College of Obstetricians and Gynecologists, a bone density test known as DEXA (or DXA) is recommended only for women aged 65 and older. But some women should be screened earlier if they have significant risk factors for osteoporosis such as early menopause...a chronic health condition such as celiac disease (which interferes with absorption of calcium) or (as in your case) a family history of early osteoporosis. When you get a DEXA test, your doctor can use the same machine to give you a vertebral fracture assessment (VFA). Good indications for including the VFA are that you've gotten significantly shorter with age (more than one-and-a-half inches since your tallest height), have a stooped posture,

have had a previous fracture (of any type) or have...unexplained back pain.

So, yes, get it checked out. But don't assume this is why your back hurts. There can be many reasons for back pain in a 55-year-old woman! It could be caused by a muscle injury or weakness, for example, or by degenerating discs between vertebrae. Osteoarthritis can also develop in the joints of the spine and cause pain. And a narrowing of the spinal canal can result in a painful condition called spinal stenosis.

To get to the bottom of your back pain, see an internist or a rheumatologist, a doctor who specializes in arthritis and other disorders of the bones, joints and muscles. In addition to the DEXA test, the doctor may use an imaging test, such as magnetic resonance imaging (MRI) or computed tomography (CT), to find the cause of your back pain. Treatment will depend on the cause.

If your DEXA test does indicate thinning bones, your treatment will typically include calcium and vitamin D supplements and weight-bearing exercise like walking for 30 minutes five days a week. Your doctor can also prescribe medications that can slow bone loss. In some cases, especially if these drugs aren't successful, biologic therapy—genetically engineered drugs such as *denosumab* (Prolia, Xgeva)—may be used.

Relieve the Pain of Whiplash for Good

Mitchell Yass, DPT, a specialist in diagnosing and resolving the cause of pain and creator of the Yass Method for treating chronic pain. He is the author of *Overpower Pain: The Strength Training Program That Stops Pain Without Drugs or Surgery* and *The Pain Cure Rx: The Yass Method for Diagnosing and Resolving Chronic Pain.* MitchellYass.com

You get into a car accident and end up with neck pain. You seek medical care and you are told it is whiplash. You may get chiropractic care, physical therapy and/or take medications all under the diagnosis of whiplash. It may or may not help. Why? Because there is a problem with this diagnosis: Whiplash is merely, mechanism of injury. It describes the fact that upon impact, your head was jerked forward and back. That is all it means. It doesn't attempt to define the tissue in distress that is eliciting your pain. It is not a diagnosis.

Think about it…if you tripped and fell and bruised your knee, you wouldn't say that your wound was a trip, right?

So…What Does Happen with Whiplash?

The most-common tissue that is affected by the quick, jerky motions of whiplash is muscle. Muscle has a certain tone to it. If it is forced to stretch excessively in a quick manner, the tone in the muscle will try to prohibit the stretching. This can lead the muscle to strain and pain.

In the neck region, the muscles that support the head attach from the skull and top of the cervical spine to the shoulder blades. If these muscles are quickly stretched, they could strain and elicit pain at the neck and between the shoulder blades. This type of muscular deficit does not show up on diagnostic tests, so conventional practitioners won't treat it. It will continue to elicit pain… and could lead to chronic pain.

A pre-existing muscle imbalance can make a whiplash-related injury worse. Many people have developed a forward-shoulder posture. This is where the person has a rounded upper back and his/her head hangs forward excessively in front of the spine. This altered posture results from a muscle imbalance between the pecs (chest muscles), anterior deltoids (shoulder) and biceps versus the muscles between the shoulder blades, posterior deltoids and triceps.

The muscles in the front of the body have a tendency to shorten because they are stronger. Once they shorten, they pull the shoulders forward causing the shoulder blades to move outward away from the spine. This overstretches the muscles between the shoulder blades, including the muscles that support the head. and they become susceptible to straining. The mechanism of whiplash causes the quick stretch that leads these muscles to finally strain and emit pain.

If the improper posture and muscle imbalance that lead to this were corrected before the whiplash, a lot of the resultant pain would be tamped down. In fact, some people would not experience any pain in the event of whiplash.

When I have treated patients with a diagnosis of whiplash, I focused on correcting the muscle imbalance that leads to the improper posture. And this, indeed, resolves the pain at the neck and between the shoulder blades.

If *you* present with forward shoulder posture with a forward-leaning head, I urge you to address the issue now and potentially save yourself a lot of pain down the line.

Exercises to Relieve (or Prevent) the Pain from Whiplash

You need to strengthen the *rhomboids/ midtrapezius* (muscles in the upper back between the shoulder blades), *lower trapezius* ("trap"), *posterior deltoids* (muscles in the back of the shoulders), *rotator cuff* (muscles that stabilize the shoulders) and *triceps* (muscles in the backs of the upper arms).

For each exercise, perform three sets of 10 repetitions with a minute rest in between each set. Perform the series three times a week with a day of rest between. Resistance should be progressed to eventually get the muscles strong enough to perform all functional tasks without straining and eliciting symptoms.

1. Lat Pulldown (interscapular muscles: midtraps and rhomboids).

Tie a knot in the center of a resistance band and secure it in place at the top of a closed door. Sit in a sturdy chair facing the door and lean back with an angle at the hip of about 30 degrees. Reach up for the ends of the band so that the start position begins with the arms nearly straight and the elbows

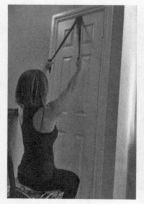
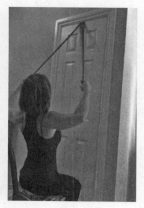

START · FINISH

just unlocked. Pull the band down, keeping your arms wide and bringing the elbows just below shoulder height and slightly behind the line of the shoulders. At this point, you should feel the shoulder blades squeeze together (the elbows will barely reach behind the line of the shoulders if performing this exercise correctly). Then return to the start position.

Important: If the elbows start to drop so they are lower than the shoulders, you are using the incorrect muscles to perform the exercise.

2. Lower Trap Exercise (lower trapezius muscle).

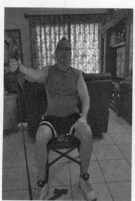
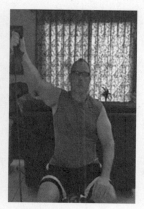

START · FINISH

Sit in a sturdy chair with a back and lean back slightly—about 10 degrees. This posture will prevent the resistance from pulling you forward. Step on one end of the resistance band to secure it and hold the other end in your working hand. Start with your arm half-

way between pointing straight forward and pointing straight to the side, with your hand at shoulder height and your elbow just unlocked. Begin to raise the resistance until the arm reaches about 130 to 140 degrees (about the height of the ear). Then return to the start position at shoulder height.

3. Posterior Deltoid Exercise.

Stand with your feet more than shoulder width apart, knees slightly bent, and your butt pushed behind you. Your weight should be mostly on your heels. Step evenly on the band and hold the ends in front of your thighs with your palms facing in and your elbows unlocked. Begin to move the resistance out to your sides from the shoulders like a pendulum. Go out until you feel the shoulder blades start to move inward (about 60 degrees), and then return to the beginning position.

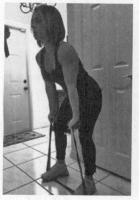
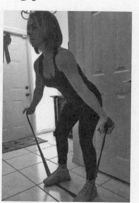

START · FINISH

4. External Rotation Exercise (rotator cuff).

You can do this exercise using a dumbbell or resistance band. With the elbow supported at the end of a surface so that the elbow is just below shoulder height, the elbow should be maintained at a 90-degree angle through the whole motion. The elbow of the arm performing the exercise should be in a line with both shoulders (if the elbow is in front of this line, the rotator cuff will have difficulty performing the exercise). The start position is with the forearm facing about 20 degrees below parallel. The resistance is pulled upward until the forearm is facing about 20 de-

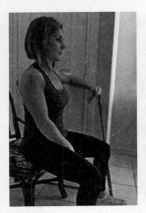
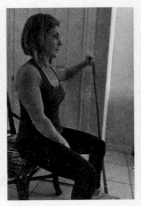
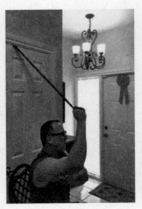
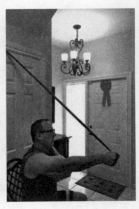

START   FINISH   START   FINISH

grees above parallel. Then return to the start position.

Careful: This is an exercise where people want to go through too much range of motion. If excessive range of motion is performed, there is a chance of straining the rotator cuff.

5. One-Arm Triceps Extensions Exercise.

This exercise is done sitting in a chair. If you are using a resistance band, secure one end at the top of a closed door and sit with your back to the door. If you are using a hand weight, hold it over your head, with your arm straight up and your elbow close to

your head. Bend your elbow and lower the weight just behind your neck, then raise it back up. Repeat with the other arm.

I have treated patients who had pain for years after a car accident and they continued to say the cause of their pain was whiplash. If you continue with this thought process the odds of resolving your pain diminishes because you are focused on the mechanism that led to your pain. Unless you identify the tissue in distress eliciting the pain and treat that tissue, it will continue to elicit pain indefinitely. Remember: Whiplash is not diagnosis; it is a mechanism.

Chapter 13

PREGNANCIES AND REPRODUCTION ISSUES

Timing Pregnancy: When to Have Another Baby

You've always dreamed of having kids and can't wait to get started (or get pregnant again). But there's an important piece to consider when contemplating family planning: The length of time between pregnancies.

A new study looked at 148,544 pregnancies of women who had more than one baby. Researchers found that an interval of 18 months between giving birth and getting pregnant again was ideal for both baby's and mom's health. There is still some benefit for waiting at least 12 months. This was true for women of all ages, but even more so for women over age 35.

For baby: Getting pregnant again within six months increased the risk for preterm delivery among all women in the study—the risk was 5.3% for women ages 20 to 34 and 5% for women over 35 vs. 3.2% and 3.6%, respectively, for those who waited 18 months. Babies who are born too early face a host of health problems including lung issues, poor feeding and slow weight gain.

For mom: For women 20 to 34, the risk for serious complications, such as organ failure

or the need for blood transfusions, or death was only slightly changed—0.23% after six months vs. 0.25% after 18 months. But for women over 35 who got pregnant six months after a previous birth, that risk was 0.62% compared with 0.26% among those who waited 18 months.

Younger women may find it easier to wait longer between pregnancies. They likely don't feel the biological clock ticking as loudly as women over 35 who face issues including having a hard time getting pregnant and growing concerns over birth defects. These factors often lead women over 35 to more closely space pregnancies. After all, waiting even 12 months between babies means, at best, four and a half years to have three children, and that's if conception goes like clockwork—it's entirely possible that it won't, and that longer intervals would result in not being able to have as many children as desired. So, what's the answer?

Stephanie Teal, MD, MPH, professor and division chief of ob/gyn-family planning at University of Colorado School of Medicine in Aurora and coauthor of "Balancing the Risks and Desires for Pregnancy in Older Mothers," invited commentary to study titled "Association of Short Interpregnancy Interval with Pregnancy Outcomes According to Maternal Age" by researchers at University of British Columbia, Canada. Both were published in *JAMA Internal Medicine.*

If the ideal waiting period isn't ideal for your circumstances, take these steps to protect your health and your baby's…

●**Work very closely with your doctors.** See your primary care doctor for a full checkup before getting pregnant again. This is important for all women, but especially those 35 and over because health risks rise with advancing age. Make sure that your blood sugar, blood pressure, cholesterol and weight are in a healthy range or are being properly managed. Testing may also include a mammogram if you are 40 or older. Estrogen levels rise during pregnancy, and this can feed a breast cancer and make it grow faster. You should also be up to date on your vaccinations including your yearly flu shot. Vaccines can help keep your immune system in tip-top shape, so it can better protect you and your baby.

●**Work hard to lose any excess weight.** It's definitely difficult to lose pregnancy weight, and shorter intervals between pregnancies make it even harder. But when you're overweight, your risk for diabetes, high blood pressure, high cholesterol and fatal blood clots is higher. Being at your ideal weight when you become pregnant again helps to lower all of these risks and makes for a safer, healthier pregnancy.

●**Use protection.** Many closely spaced pregnancies are actually unintended. Regardless of your age, use contraception if you don't want to get pregnant…yet.

●**Don't panic.** While the study did show higher risks with shorter intervals between pregnancies, the absolute risks are still low. Most pregnancies result in a healthy baby and mom.

What Makes a Pregnancy High-Risk and How to Protect Yourself

Kimberlee McKay, MD, an obstetrician/gynecologist in Sioux Falls, South Dakota, and coauthor of "What Can We Do About Maternal Mortality—And How to Do It Quickly," published in *The New England Journal of Medicine*.

With modern medicine, it's almost unthinkable that women still die in childbirth in the US. But the fact is our rate of maternal deaths is higher than that of other industrialized nations and, what's worse, it's rising. The latest numbers show that 24 women die for every live 100,000 births—a 26% increase since 2000. Considering there are four million babies born every year, that's 1,000 women. The problem is the greatest in rural communities where many local hospitals have shuttered, leaving women without access to the care they need. But pregnancy-related deaths can and do happen anywhere.

What puts a woman at risk?

●**Preexisting medical conditions** such as high blood pressure, chronic kidney disease, HIV, lupus and thyroid disease raise the risk for serious pregnancy complications, including a life-threatening form of high blood pressure called preeclampsia, hemorrhaging and fetal embolisms (pregnancy-related particles that get into the bloodstream and can block arteries to your heart).

●**Diabetes, both types 1 and 2, as well as gestational diabetes** (the type that first develops during pregnancy) can cause the baby to grow larger than normal, making delivery more difficult.

●**Being overweight.** Obesity in itself increases risk of having diabetes and high blood pressure. When BMI is high, the risk of C-section and hemorrhage increases as well.

• **Being 35 or older.** As we age, we're more likely to develop conditions such as high blood pressure and diabetes. Women who get pregnant after the age of 35 seem to develop gestational diabetes at a higher rate than younger women...and women who become pregnant after age 40 are at higher risk for preeclampsia. All of these things combined can increase the risk for the most common causes of severe maternal morbidity including hemorrhage, blood clots and hypertensive urgency (extreme high blood pressure).

• **Carrying twins**—or more, which increases the chances of an early delivery. Twins can essentially outgrow the uterus and cause a woman to go into labor early. Also, after delivery, the uterus does not stop its bleeding as effectively as it does after having a single baby.

What should you do? Beyond following a healthy lifestyle, the key to having a safe pregnancy and delivery with any of these conditions is having a skilled obstetrics team in place to closely monitor you and baby. *Here's how...*

Choose an ob/gyn who specializes in high-risk pregnancies. The doctor you've been seeing for gynecology care may not be the best obstetrician if you have any preexisting conditions. Ask for a referral to a doctor who is certified as a perinatologist, a maternal-fetal medicine specialist. A perinatologist has two to three years of additional training in medical complications that can arise during pregnancy. You can also use the search option on the Society for Maternal Fetal Medicine site to find a specialist near you.

Maternal-fetal medicine specialists work with all obstetric providers, including physician assistants, nurse practitioners and traditional ob/gyns to provide care for you and your baby.

Note: Do not consider a home birth or birthing center for a high-risk pregnancy.

You're mostly likely to find a perinatologist at urban medical centers, which might require you to travel to get this care. Depending on your situation and the specialist's geographic availability, a perinatologist may work alongside your existing ob/gyn, see you intermittently and then be at the delivery...as long as he/she has delivery privileges at a hospital in your area. If not, you'll need to decide if, logistically, you'll be able to travel to his hospital (and find out if your insurance will cover it) when baby comes.

What can you do if you don't have access to a perinatologist? Have a candid conversation with your existing ob/gyn to discuss his experience with the most serious and most common threats to a pregnant woman's health. Ask how he will monitor you and the baby and make sure neither is in distress. If his experience with high-risk pregnancies is limited, ask if there's a colleague you can be referred to. Also, find out if the hospital you're scheduled to deliver at has a neonatal intensive care unit (NICU) for your baby should it be needed. Though you may be the one who needs intensive care, hospitals that have NICUs are likely to have high levels of care for mom as well.

What care can you expect? If you're high risk, you may need to be seen as much as twice a week throughout your pregnancy. You likely will need more blood tests and ultrasounds than normal and possibly other specialist visits, such as a cardiologist or nephrologist (kidney specialist), depending on your unique needs. Telemedicine initiatives in some rural communities are making this easier for women who don't have local access to certain specialists.

If your experts aren't all in the same health network, be your own advocate and ask that all workups are shared with all other members of your care team. While there are initiatives under way from leading health organizations to improve maternal health, it's important to advocate for yourself until that happens.

Marijuana Warning for Pregnant Women

Kelly Young-Wolff, PhD, MPH, Kaiser Permanente Division of Research, Oakland, California. She is lead author of the study titled, "Association of Nausea and Vomiting in Pregnancy with Prenatal Marijuana Use," published in *JAMA Internal Medicine*. Clinical report titled, "Marijuana Use During Pregnancy and Breast-feeding: Implications for Neonatal and Childhood Outcomes," from the American Academy of Pediatrics, published in *Pediatrics*.

The number of pregnant women using marijuana, especially if they have morning sickness, is growing—possibly influenced by a perception that it's safe now that it's been legalized in many states. In fact, a recent study by Kaiser Permanente of Northern California found that among pregnant women with mild nausea and vomiting, 8.4% were using marijuana in the first trimester...and among those with severe nausea and vomiting, 11.3% were using marijuana in the first trimester.

The danger: There is no proof that prenatal marijuana use doesn't affect the developing baby...while evidence is mounting of serious harms. Tetrahydrocannabinol (THC), the psychoactive ingredient in marijuana, crosses the placenta. How THC affects a developing baby is not completely understood—more research is needed on the health effects of prenatal marijuana use. That's why there is no medically approved use for marijuana during pregnancy (or breastfeeding)—in fact, guidelines recommend against such use.

It can be hard to tease out the effects of marijuana from other lifestyle factors common among women who use marijuana—such as cigarette smoking and use of alcohol or other drugs. Nor is anyone going to set up a controlled study in which some pregnant women are given marijuana. So researchers have to rely primarily on retrospective studies. But the compelling evidence from these, including a recent clinical report from the American Academy of Pediatrics, suggests that using marijuana during pregnancy is as-sociated with lower birth weight and neuro-developmental and behavioral problems in childhood.

It is also known that THC passes through to breast milk. Unfortunately, there is not much known about what effect this has on the nursing baby because there have been very few studies. One survey done in Colorado, where marijuana is legal, found that 18% of women who have ever used marijuana also used it while breastfeeding.

Another factor: The potency of THC in marijuana is increasing, and the potential harms may be greater now than in the past. Also, today's marijuana crops are more likely to be grown with pesticides, herbicides, rodent killers and fertilizers, adding other possible toxins to the mix.

Bottom line: Women experiencing morning sickness should ask their doctors for ways to reduce nausea that are known to be safe for their babies.

Ease Endometriosis Pain...Naturally

Andrew Rubman, ND, founder and medical director, Southbury Clinic for Traditional Medicines, Southbury, Connecticut, and author of the Bottom Line blog "Nature Doc's Patient Diary." SouthburyClinic.com

Endometriosis can be extremely painful, so the enthusiasm for the newly FDA-approved drug to treat the pain, Orilissa, is understandable. However, the drug comes with a serious potential side effect.

Alternative: A natural protocol that reduces the pain and inflammation of endometriosis (when tissue from inside the uterus grows outside the uterus)—but doesn't compromise the rest of your health.

Orilissa—its chemical name is *elagolix*—is a pill that is taken once or twice a day and has just been approved for moderate-to-severe endometriosis pain. Studies show that it reduces endometriosis menstrual pain, pain between periods and pain during sexual intercourse. However, it can be taken for only two to six months, depending on the dose, because it creates a risk for irreversible bone loss.

Why would a pain drug cause bone loss? Orilissa works by blocking the effect of gonadotropin-releasing hormone, which stimulates the ovaries to produce estrogen and progesterone. Since the inflammation and pain of endometriosis are triggered by estrogen, blocking its production results in less pain. However, estrogen is also important for bone health—which is why extended use of the drug can cause bone loss. Other side effects of low estrogen include night sweats, hot flashes and mood problems such as anxiety and depression.

The good news is that inflammation can be reduced naturally without the side effects of medications, says Andrew Rubman, ND, naturopathic doctor and medical director of the Southbury Clinic for Traditional Medicines in Southbury, Connecticut. This is especially important for women who are trying to get pregnant...who already are pregnant (Orilissa cannot be taken during pregnancy)...or whose pain is not severe enough to require medication. Natural inflammation reducers also won't interfere with medication if it becomes necessary.

Diet changes that can reduce the pain of endometriosis...

• **Eat an egg every day.** Eggs have cholesterol, the source material for the steroidal hormone cortisol, a hormone that helps control inflammation. (You may think of cortisol as an inflammation producer, but that's because as levels of cortisol increase, another hormone called cortisone, which needs to stay in balance with cortisol, decreases—encouraging inflammation.)

Best: Boil the egg or poach it in water because frying the cholesterol produces oxides, which are inflammatory. And don't worry about creating any heart issues by adding this bit of cholesterol to your diet because inflammation is the trigger that makes cholesterol form plaques on artery walls.

• **Eat wild-caught cold-water fish such as salmon and sardines,** rich sources of anti-inflammatory omega-3 fatty acids. You can also get omega-3s from fish oil supplements. A typical recommended daily dose is 1,000 mg of combined eicosapentaenoic acid (EPA) and docosahexaenoic acid (DHA). (Interestingly, Dr. Rubman reports that his patients who move to Florida and stop eating fish from cold water start having more inflammation issues.)

• **Get some seeds into your diet,** especially the inflammation-fighters chia and flaxseeds. Both also are high in omega-3 fatty acids.

• **Get plenty of antioxidants from brightly colored fruits and vegetables,** especially dark blue and purple berries...beets...and green, leafy vegetables. Also include cruciferous vegetables such as broccoli, cabbage and kale.

• **Three supplements that can help the liver bind and remove inflammatory compounds are vitamin B, dandelion root extract and methylsulfonylmethane (MSM).** These are generally safe for most people, but check with your doctor if you are being treated for a medical condition or have allergies (such as to ragweed in the case of dandelion supplements). Dosages should be prescribed by your doctor based on the severity of your endometriosis. Typical daily amounts: 50 mg vitamin-B complex, taken twice a day...2 grams (g) to 6 g of MSM, divided into two or three doses...about 30 drops (1 milliliter) dandelion root extract once a day.

Exercising regularly to reduce body fat and limiting intake of caffeine and alcohol also help keep estrogen levels lower.

If natural therapies and drugs fail to relieve your pain, endometrial tissue outside the uterus may be surgically removed. Women who have this surgery often find that their bodies respond better to anti-inflammatory foods and supplements afterward.

The Endometriosis/ Cancer Connection: What You Need to Know

Oskari Heikinheimo, MD, PhD, professor in the Department of Obstetrics and Gynecology, Helsinki University Hospital, physician in chief at Helsinki University Hospital and coauthor of the study titled "Risk of Gynecologic Cancer According to the Type of Endometriosis," published in *Obstetrics and Gynecology*.

You already know the basics about endometriosis. Tissue that's usually found inside the uterus grows outside of it, causing pain for most women with the condition and fertility problems for many. *But you may not know that there are three different types of endometriosis based on the location of the growth…*

Peritoneal endometriosis: The most common type. Growths develop anywhere in the pelvic cavity.

Deep infiltrating endometriosis: The rarest type. Growths develop within the pelvic cavity but also extend deep into tissues.

Ovarian endometriosis: Just as it sounds, growths develop within the ovaries.

The study: Researchers in Finland analyzed the hospital records of women who had had surgery to treat their endometriosis to look for associations between the three types of the disease and various types of cancers of the reproductive organs.

The good news: None of the types of endometriosis raised the risk for endometrial cancer or other uterine cancers, cervical cancer or genital cancer. Surprisingly, there was a decrease in the risk for squamous cell cervical cancer among women with endometriosis, though it's unclear why.

The not-so-good news: Women with ovarian endometriosis had a higher risk for ovarian cancer than the average woman, particularly for two rare types of cancer—clear cell ovarian cancer and endometrioid ovarian cancer. The number of women with ovarian endometriosis who got ovarian cancer was relatively small at 2%, but that risk was higher than earlier studies had found and higher than the 1.3% risk for ovarian cancer among women in general. These women also had a higher-than-usual risk for borderline ovarian tumors, growths that begin along the outer edges of the ovaries, meaningful because these are thought to be starting points for ovarian cancer due to endometriosis.

What This Means for You

The study authors said that even though the absolute risk for ovarian cancer remained relatively small, knowing about this risk could help women make decisions about treatment of ovarian endometriosis—in particular, whether to opt for ovarian conservation (keeping the ovaries) vs. removing the ovaries. (Once the ovaries are removed, the risk for ovarian cancer drops substantially.)

Bottom line: Each woman with endometriosis should talk with her doctor about the type she has…any resulting effect on her risk for ovarian cancer…and her treatment options based on this risk. Also consider getting a second opinion from an oncologist who specializes in gynecologic cancers to make the most informed decision.

Eat Fish to Get Pregnant Faster

Audrey J. Gaskins, ScD, research associate, Harvard T.H. Chan School of Public Health and instructor of medicine, Harvard Medical School and Brigham and Women's Hospital, all in Boston. She is the lead author of "Seafood Intake, Sexual Activity, and Time to Pregnancy" published in *The Journal of Clinical Endocrinology & Metabolism*.

Trying to get pregnant? Here's some news that could boost your chances. Couples who eat more seafood have more sex and get pregnant more quickly, a recent study has found.

Background: Many people avoid seafood these days—especially when trying to have a baby—because they're concerned that the mercury in fish is harmful. But seafood is a good source of protein and contains other important nutrients such as heart-healthy omega-3s. Now researchers have discovered that eating the right type of seafood is safe and is actually linked to faster conception in couples who enjoy fish regularly.

Recent research: The study, published in the May 23, 2018, issue of the *Endocrine Society's Journal of Clinical Endocrinology & Metabolism*, included 501 couples (women were ages 18 to 44) who were trying to conceive. The researchers, from Harvard University and the National Institute of Child Health and Human Development, asked participants to record their seafood intake and sexual activity in a journal every day for up to a year (or until pregnancy was confirmed).

Study results: Of the couples in which at least one partner ate seafood less than twice a week, 79% were pregnant at the end of the year…but a whopping 92% of the couples in which both partners consumed seafood two or more times per week were pregnant. The fish-feasting couples also reported having more sex, which one might suspect led to the more impressive conception stats.

However, the additional sexual activity did not completely explain the link between eating seafood and faster conception. The researchers suggest that other factors, such as seafood's potential effects on semen quality, ovulation and/or embryo quality, could also have played a role. They theorize that seafood's omega-3 fatty acids, which have been linked to other reproductive benefits, may be a contributing factor. It's unclear, however, whether fish oil supplements would confer the same beneficial effects. More research is needed.

Best choices: The US Food and Drug Administration (FDA) and the Environmental Protection Agency (EPA) categorize fish and shellfish into "best choices"…"good choices"…and "fish to avoid." The agencies recommend that men and women eat two to three servings of a variety of best-choice fish per week. (A typical serving size is four ounces of fish, measured before cooking.)

Good news: Ninety percent of the fish we eat in this country—including catfish…cod…flounder…oysters…pollock…salmon (wild and Alaskan, canned or fresh)…shrimp…tilapia…sardines…and tuna (canned light)—falls into the "best choice" category.

All types of fish contain at least trace amounts of mercury, which can harm the brain and nervous system if consumed in excess amounts over time. There are seven fish, however, that have higher mercury levels and should be avoided, according to the FDA and EPA. These are tilefish from the Gulf of Mexico…shark…swordfish…orange roughy…bigeye tuna…marlin…and king mackerel.

Bottom line: A healthy diet for both partners, not just the women, is important when you're trying to start a family…and incorporating more seafood into your diet may hasten conception. It may even increase the frequency of sexual activity, which is definitely worth a trip to the local fish market!

After a C-Section: What You Need to Know Before Another Pregnancy

Ilan E. Timor-Tritsch, MD, professor, department of obstetrics and gynecology, NYU Langone Health, New York City, and lead author of study titled "A New Minimally Invasive Treatment for Cesarean Scar Pregnancy and Cervical Pregnancy" published in *Obstetrics*.
Report titled, "Cesarean Scar Pregnancy, Incidence, and Recurrence: Five-Year Experience at a Single Tertiary Care Referral Center" by researchers at Yale-New Haven Hospital, Connecticut, published in *Obstetrics & Gynecology*.
Study titled, "Cesarean Scar Pregnancy—a New Challenge for Obstetricians" by researchers at Regional Polyclinical Hospital, Poland, published in *Journal of Ultrasonography*.

Nearly all ectopic pregnancies—pregnancies in which the fertilized egg implants itself somewhere other than healthy tissue within the uterus—occur in a fallopian tube. But in women who've had a cesarean section, it's possible for a future pregnancy to implant and develop in the scar tissue of the uterus where the C-section was done. This rare type of pregnancy is called a cesarean scar pregnancy, and it can be extremely dangerous. At times they are mistakenly referred to as "cesarean scar ectopic pregnancy." However unlike the real ectopic pregnancies, this type of pregnancy may result in a newborn.

Estimated to occur in about one in every 2,000 pregnancies, the number of cesarean scar pregnancies has been steadily increasing over time, along with the number of cesarean deliveries themselves.

It's not possible to predict who this will happen to. More than half of women who have a cesarean scar pregnancy had just one prior C-section. For reasons that aren't clear, women who undergo IVF after a C-delivery are at a higher risk than women who conceive naturally.

Most cesarean scar pregnancies are discovered between five and 10 weeks into a pregnancy. You may not have any symptoms early on. The first sign may be vaginal bleeding, which could easily be mistaken for a miscarriage, so it's important to make sure that your provider knows to screen you for a cesarean scar pregnancy. Rarely, women also have abdominal pain. Both pain and bleeding can worsen over time.

And time is not on your side. Early diagnosis is essential because a cesarean scar pregnancy can become life-threatening in a matter of weeks. Risks include the uterus rupturing and severe hemorrhaging, or dangerously excessive bleeding.

Some positive news: Transvaginal ultrasound has made diagnosing cesarean scar pregnancies easier and more accurate because it can detect where in the uterus the pregnancy is developing.

Once a diagnosis is made, many patients will be able to choose between two courses. The first is to continue the pregnancy with the understanding that complications could arise at any time, leading to a premature delivery and the possibility of an eventual hysterectomy, depending on how affected the uterus is.

The second option is ending the pregnancy. This may be done surgically in an operating room by aspiration or resection of the pregnancy, and requires general anesthesia and a short hospital sty. It also can be achieved by minimally invasive means such as a local injection into the embryo of methotrexate (the same drug used to treat rheumatoid arthritis and some forms of cancer) or other drugs. A less invasive procedure was recently developed by experts in the department of obstetrics and gynecology at the New York University School of Medicine. It involves placing a special catheter (usually used in labor and delivery rooms to induce labor) with two balloons into the uterus and, under continuous ultrasound guidance, filling them with fluid to exert pressure against the embryo and stop the pregnancy. This method, tested in about 50 cases, has been shown to be more effective and safer than other methods. It is usually performed in an office setting, may only require sedation and does not necessarily need hospitalization.

Sometimes a combination of approaches is needed to ensure that the embryo is fully removed and, in turn, to prevent complications that could require a hysterectomy—that's how serious a cesearean scar pregnancy is. What's most important after being diagnosed with a cesarean scar pregnancy is to ask for an ob-gyn experienced in treating this type of pregnancy. Specialists working at a large medical center will likely see them more often than doctors at a small practice.

Being treated as quickly as possible gives you the greatest chance of preserving your uterus and your fertility. Most women will have a normal pregnancy after a cesarean scar pregnancy, but you'll want to have an ultrasound as early as possible to make sure the new pregnancy is developing in the right spot.

8 Ways Pregnancy Has Changed Since You Had a Baby

Kathy Hartke, MD, an obstetrician/gynecologist in Brookfield, Wisconsin. She is past chair of the Wisconsin Section of the American College of Obstetricians and Gynecologists as well as its current legislative cochair. She also serves on the board of the WI Association of Perinatal Care. She has seven grandchildren.

I f your daughter, granddaughter or daughter-in-law (or niece!) is expecting, you may be tempted to give all sorts of "helpful" advice. *Here's a tip…*

Most of it will be dead wrong.

What medical science now knows about pregnancy and labor has changed enormously since you had a baby. *Here are the latest evidence-based "best practices" for having a baby—so that you can be a truly helpful advice giver…*

You may think: Bed rest prevents preterm labor.

But the truth is: Bed rest does most pregnant women no good—and even may be harmful. Doctors used to order women who were at risk of delivering prematurely to take to bed day and night. The goal was to prolong the pregnancy. But then studies showed that bed rest didn't actually accomplish that or, indeed, improve outcomes in any way. Plus it comes with dangerous side effects, including an increased risk for blood clots. Today doctors recommend bed rest only in rare medical circumstances—and often in a modified form that allows for walking around.

You may think: Epidurals slow down labor and lead to C-sections.

But the truth is: Epidurals are safe. Epidurals—regional anesthesia or "nerve blocks" used to dull pain during labor—have been around for decades. But they fell out of favor in the 1980s and early 1990s because they often reduced a woman's ability to push or feel anything below the waist, thereby increasing her chances of needing a cesarean section.

Update: New epidural drugs are more effective, easy to calibrate and safe for both baby and mother. They don't slow labor and don't lead to more C-sections. A woman can safely get an epidural during the earliest stages of labor so that she can experience less pain right away.

You may think: Once a C-section, always a C-section.

But the truth is: Doctors now encourage most women to try for vaginal birth after cesarean (VBAC), especially if they want to have more kids later. Doctors used to be reluctant to have a woman give birth vaginally after she had delivered a child via cesarean— they believed that the risk for a rupture at the site of the uterine incision, leading to excessive bleeding and possible brain damage to the baby, was too high. That's no longer the case. Successful VBAC, which occurs between 60% and 80% of the time, means less risk for hemorrhage, infection and blood clots, shorter recovery and a reduced chance of complications in future pregnancies. But a failed VBAC can lead to complications, so it needs to be done in a facility capable of emergency delivery via C-section.

You may think: A woman who exercises during pregnancy should take it slow and stop exercising if her heart rate gets high.

But the truth is: Pregnant women should work out! If you exercised during your own pregnancy, you were probably told to not let your heart rate go too high—and to bring it down if it did. Now doctors are encouraging moms-to-be to swim laps, lift weights, take fitness classes—even compete in 5K runs. Being sedentary is as harmful for expectant women as it is for anyone else, and it's not good for the fetus either, so moms-to-be should exercise at a moderately intense pace for at least 20 to 30 minutes, four to five times a week. But while they don't have to watch their heart rates, they should stay away from activities where there could be trauma to the abdomen such as skydiving, horseback riding and martial arts. Scuba diving also is off limits because the fetus may be harmed during decompression.

You may think: Just eat! It's OK to gain 25 pounds or more.

But the truth is: It depends on how much the pregnant woman weighed before. Weight-gain guidelines are tailored now to a woman's prepregnancy weight. While 25 pounds still is the guideline for women who were normal weight before they got pregnant, those who were overweight or obese should gain less.

Example: A woman with a body mass index (BMI) of 30—that's 180 pounds for a five-foot, five-inch-tall woman, which is considered obese—will be advised to keep her weight gain to between 11 and 20 pounds.

You may think: Never eat sushi when you're pregnant.

But the truth is: It's no more likely to be unsafe than many other foods if you know your restaurant. For years, sushi was off the menu for expectant women because of the chance of parasites from undercooked or raw fish. But in the US (as in most developed countries), the fish common in sushi, such as salmon, flounder and tuna, almost never have parasites, according to *Obstetrics and Gynecology*. Pregnant women are encouraged to avoid raw and undercooked fish in general, but sushi that is prepared in a clean, reputable establishment is unlikely to pose a risk. Pregnant women should eat two or three servings of fish a week, but avoid fish high in mercury such as swordfish, shark and marlin. Canned light tuna is OK.

Bonus advice: Caffeine is safe for most pregnant women up to 300 milligrams a day, about the amount in two or three cups of coffee.

You may think: If a woman's labor isn't progressing rapidly, it's time for medical intervention.

But the truth is: Most of the time, it's best to let labor progress at its own rate. Physicians have come to view childbirth the way

midwives always have—if they're patient, it usually will progress naturally, and every woman progresses at her own rate. During the latent (early) phase of labor, if the fetal heart tracing is normal, mothers may be sent home until contractions get stronger. Hydrotherapy, massage, self-hypnosis training, walking and changing positions may provide pain relief for mild contractions. Active labor officially begins when a woman has dilated to six centimeters, but new research shows that this can take from just a few hours to eight, 10 or more—and that's fine. Today if an expectant mom dilates to four centimeters—and stays that way for two hours—doctors will give her more time rather than rush to do a C-section. Labor and delivery tend to be patient-led these days. If her pregnancy is considered low-risk, she doesn't need to be hooked up constantly to fetal monitors or IVs…told to push as soon as she's fully dilated (in most cases, she can wait until she feels the need to push)…or have her water broken artificially. Most women will go into labor within 12 hours of water breaking, but there still are some circumstances in which it makes medical sense to induce labor.

You may think: Babies deserve a cozy place to sleep.

But the truth is: Bare cribs are best. Before you splurge on a gift of crib décor, be advised that bumper pads, pillows, quilts, sheepskins and stuffed animals for the crib are considered unsafe. To reduce the risk for sudden infant death syndrome (SIDS), babies must sleep on a firm mattress covered with a tight-fitting sheet—and nothing else. It's still OK to swaddle a newborn or put him/her in a sleep sack (on his back, of course), but there shouldn't be anything soft or loose in the crib. After one year, these precautions aren't necessary.

Now that you know the facts, you can be a source of wisdom as the mom-to-be in your family prepares for the big event. To stay up to date, visit the website of the American College of Obstetricians and Gynecologists (ACOG.org) and click on the "For Patients" section.

When Someone You Love Is Struggling to Conceive

Jonathan Scher, MD, an obstetrician/gynecologist and fertility specialist in New York City and coauthor of *Preventing Miscarriage: The Good News.*

There is no struggle like that of trying to have a child, and it can be hard to know the right thing to say—or not say—when a loved one is going through this tumultuous process.

To someone trying to have a baby, it seems like everyone else is pregnant and sailing through her pregnancy. She zeroes in on belly bumps, strollers and happy parents frolicking wherever she goes, which can make her feel sadder, angrier and even hopeless.

Some women may have trouble conceiving, while others may have difficulty carrying a pregnancy to term…or experience both. And for those who opt for fertility treatments, getting hormone shots and other drugs may cause mood swings, nausea and other side effects on top of the roller coaster of emotions already coloring her days. Each cycle offers renewed hope…which can be dashed in an instant when a pregnancy test has just a single line or a developing fetus does not have a heartbeat.

So, what can you do as you watch your loved one go through this emotional and physical roller coaster? *There is no one set script, but there are things to say and, more important, not say, to support anyone who is trying to have a child…*

•**Let her know you're available…on her terms.** Say something such as, "I know you're going through a lot and if you ever want to talk about it, that's great, and if not, that's perfectly fine, too." But remember to be available, not judgmental if you don't personally agree with what she shares with you.

•**Be positive.** There's a lot that can now be done even if gold-standard fertility treatments such as in vitro fertilization and intra-uterine insemination haven't worked. Gently suggest getting another opinion if she's frustrated. Sometimes the man's genes are too similar to the woman's genetic make-up, so her immune system rejects the embryo. This will happen over and over again unless the immune system is tweaked. Newer fertility treatments can target her immune system so that it allows the fertilized egg to implant and grow.

•**Share your struggles…if asked.** Many people don't talk about their fertility issues or miscarriages, but if your friend/daughter opens up to you, sharing any personal struggles can help her feel less alone.

But don't offer unsolicited anecdotes. Most of the time couples are doing everything right, yet one in five may experience "unexplained infertility," meaning that everything is normal on the fertility work-up, but the woman still can't conceive. Telling her about another friend, coworker or sister-in-law who struggled for years and finally got pregnant with twins may only make your friend feel more isolated rather than give her renewed hope.

•**Never presume there's a pregnancy.** On girls' night out, your friend, who usually joins you in a glass of rosé, orders a club soda instead. Your antenna immediately goes up because you know she has been trying to conceive for several months and you want to coax her into sharing the big news. Don't. There are many reasons that someone may abstain from drinking alcohol. Pregnancy is but one of them. Also, many people are, or become, superstitious about disclosing a pregnancy early on. Give your friend time and space to share any news.

Take No Chances with the Flu

Everyone who gets the flu picks it up from someone else, which is why mass vaccination is so crucial—it creates community immunity in addition to protecting individuals. During flu season 2017-2018, 80,000 people in the US died from flu—the highest death toll from the flu in 40 years. In addition to people at high risk—the elderly and those with compromised immune systems—pregnant women need to be especially attentive to getting a shot. It protects a woman during pregnancy and her newborn baby for several months after birth. But fewer than half of pregnant women got a shot last flu season.

Daniel Jernigan, MD, director, influenza division, National Center for Immunization and Respiratory Diseases, Centers for Disease Control and Prevention, Atlanta.

First-Ever Postpartum Depression Drug Gives Relief Fast

Samantha Meltzer-Brody, MD, director, perinatal psychiatry program, University of North Carolina at Chapel Hill. "FDA Approves First Treatment for Postpartum Depression," FDA News Release.

New babies truly are little bundles of joy. Sadly, though, for many women, childbirth comes with debilitating depression. Antidepressants don't always help…or can take weeks or months to work—putting both mother and baby at serious risk.

Good news: A new drug promises almost immediate relief from even the most severe postpartum depression.

The US Food and Drug Administration (FDA) recently approved the first-ever drug that specifically treats postpartum depression. A single intravenous dose of the drug, *brexanolone* (Zulresso), provides relief as quickly as within 48 hours. There is no need for additional doses…and it doesn't interfere with other antidepressants the patient may be taking. It is even safe to resume nursing within a few days after receiving the drug.

While brexanolone is an important breakthrough, there are considerations that may be drawbacks for some women. The drug is administered over a 60-hour period, requiring a two-and-a-half day stay at a hospital or other medical center while being monitored for headaches, nausea, sleepiness, dizziness and/or fainting—temporary side effects noted in clinical trials of the drug. The drug also is not cheap—possibly as much as $34,000, not including hospital or medical facility costs. Whether or how much of treatment costs will be covered by insurance is not yet clear.

Note: A pill that will work similarly to brexanolone is in clinical trials. If successful, the pills could potentially improve both availability and cost.

Even taking potential drawbacks into consideration, for the millions of women who suffer each year from postpartum depression, brexanolone could be a welcome light at the end of their dark tunnel. Postpartum depression is a serious condition, affecting one out of seven women who give birth. Severe postpartum depression can be life-threatening. But even milder forms interfere with the care, bonding and nurturing between mother and child that is so essential for healthy child development.

Chapter 14

RESPIRATORY HEALTH AND ALLERGIES

Think You've Been Exposed to "Toxic Mold"? Here's What to Do

You've just learned that a building where you spent a lot of time is contaminated by mold. It's being removed...but should you do anything else to protect your health?

You may have heard of "sick building syndrome"—illnesses, especially upper-respiratory problems, attributed to airborne contaminants, including "toxic mold." Whether mold really is at the root of the symptoms is controversial and remains unproved. *However, according to the Institute of Medicine (IOM), evidence links indoor mold exposure to...*

• **Upper-respiratory-tract symptoms** (coughing, wheezing) in otherwise healthy people.

• **Asthma symptoms** in people with asthma.

• **Hypersensitivity pneumonitis,** a lung disease where lungs of people prone to the condition become inflamed when airborne pollutants, including molds, are inhaled.

Plus, other research suggests that early exposure to indoor mold may be linked to development of asthma in children, especially if they are genetically at risk.

Realistically, you can't completely avoid mold. Scientists estimate that it's been around for 500 million years and forms 25% of Earth's biomass. Nor would you want all mold eliminated—think cheese (especially blue, Roquefort, Gorgonzola), beer, wine, cider, vinegar...and penicillin.

How Mold Takes Hold

While many kinds of mold can grow inside buildings, the most common culprit is Stachybotrys atra, also called Stachybotrys chartarum or black mold. S. atra is greenish black and thrives where there is a continuous supply of moisture (a water leak, condensation, humidity) and nutrients (cellulose-based building materials such as ceiling tiles, wood, wood products...paint, insulation, drywall, carpet, upholstery, etc.). Mold also can grow inside building vents and air-conditioning systems. (*Note:* Legionnaires' pneumonia is caused by the bacterium Legionella pneumophila—not mold.)

S. atra is not itself toxic, but it can produce toxins, as can other molds, called mycotoxins.

Andrew L. Rubman, ND, naturopathic doctor, founder and medical director, Southbury Clinic for Traditional Medicines, Southbury, Connecticut, and author of the Bottom Line blog "Nature Doc's Patient Diary." SouthburyClinic.com

But even when mycotoxins are not present, inhaled spores can cause an allergic reaction…an immune system reaction…or nonallergic irritation of lungs and nasal passages.

People with allergies, asthma or other respiratory conditions such as chronic obstructive pulmonary disease (COPD) are most likely to have a reaction or a worsening of the symptoms of their condition when they inhale mold spores. In otherwise healthy people, typical symptoms include stuffy nose, itchy eyes and wheezing—which usually clear up quickly once the exposure stops.

Mycotoxins, on the other hand, can be nasty. Some mycotoxins are powerful enough to kill bacteria (penicillin, for instance, is a mycotoxin)…and mycotoxins have been weaponized for chemical warfare. Mycotoxins from common indoor molds are not as deadly but still can cause acute and chronic illness.

Acute symptoms from mycotoxin exposure typically include headache, fatigue, disorientation, dizziness and vomiting. Most of the time, these symptoms clear up when exposure is stopped. However, long-term exposure can cause some people to develop more severe symptoms that affect the nervous system, mood, memory and concentration.

"Detoxing" After Mold Exposure

There are no medications to treat mold toxicity, but you can help your body recover from the effects of exposure to mold by strengthening your immune system.

Obviously, you first need to make sure that you're no longer being exposed to the mold that you suspect is causing your problems. This may be easier to do if the source is your own house than if it's an office building, school, college dorm or some other public building over which you have less say in whether it gets remediated.

But once you've dealt with the source of mold exposure—or while you're waiting for that to happen—take steps to keep your immune system as healthy as possible. Start by making sure you're following basic healthy lifestyle recommendations—stay well-hydrat-

ed (drink at least six glasses of water daily)…eat plenty of fresh fruits, including colorful berries, and vegetables…avoid foods that promote inflammation, such as added sugar and fried, refined and processed foods…get enough sleep (ideally, about eight hours a night)…and enough exercise.

Then consider adding the following supplements…

- **Vitamin C.**
- **Vitamin B-12.**
- **Selenium,** a trace mineral that increases an important immune system protein called immunoglobulin A (IgA).

All three are available as supplements and are in most multivitamins, but it's best to consult a naturopathic doctor for appropriate dosages for you. Nasal irrigation with a neti pot and a nasal wash, such as Alkalol, also can help reduce respiratory symptoms.

If you have symptoms that you suspect may be related to mold exposure, besides following these steps you may need a specialized diagnosis and/or treatment. Not all medical doctors (MDs) are familiar with diagnosing and treating illnesses stemming from exposure to indoor mold. You may need to consult a naturopathic physician (ND). Check the site of The American Association of Naturopathic Physicians to find one near you who can either treat you himself/herself or refer you to a naturopathic environmental medicine specialist.

Cleaning Your House Can Harm Your Lungs

Philip J. Landrigan, MD, dean for global health and professor in the departments of pediatrics and environmental medicine and public health, Icahn School of Medicine at Mount Sinai in New York City.

You might expect people who clean houses or offices for a living to develop lung problems from harsh cleaning products. But it happens even to people who regularly clean just their own homes.

So finds a new study published in *American Journal of Respiratory and Critical Care Medicine* that followed more than 6,200 adults for 20 years. Compared with people who didn't clean their own homes, those who did so at least weekly scored significantly lower on a measure of overall lung function. In this one measure, the decline was similar to that found in people who have been smoking cigarettes for years.

To learn more, we spoke with environmental expert Philip J. Landrigan, MD, of the Icahn School of Medicine at Mount Sinai in New York City. *His advice to keep your lungs from being harmed...*

• **Use your nose.** Ammonia and bleach are known irritants that can, over time, impair lung function even when inhaled in low concentrations. You can tell just by opening a product and giving it a sniff that it is irritating—avoid those products.

• **Buy safe.** Choose gentler products. While labels are no guarantee—they're not regulated—look for products that use terms such as "gentle," "nontoxic" and "ecofriendly."

• **Make your own.** For total control over what you breathe in when you clean your house, use ingredients such as distilled white vinegar or borax to make your own safe cleaning products.

Example: Mix three-quarters cup of vinegar with three-quarters cup of water in a spray bottle to clean windows and mirrors.

No matter how long a person has been using irritant chemicals, there are health benefits that come from stopping their use. Some will be immediate...others take months or years...but all the results are positive.

Lung Disease Link to Dementia

Compared to those with healthy lungs, people with obstructive lung disease, such as chronic obstructive pulmonary disease (COPD) and asthma, had a 33% higher risk of developing dementia, according to a 23-year study of 14,000 men and women.

Theory: The low blood oxygen levels resulting from these conditions lead to inflammation, stress and damage to the brain's blood vessels.

Pamela L. Lutsey, PhD, MPH, associate professor, Division of Epidemiology & Community Health, University of Minnesota, Minneapolis.

Triple Therapy for COPD: Greater Benefits But Also Greater Risk

Study titled, "Triple Therapy in the Management of Chronic Obstructive Pulmonary Disease: Systematic Review and Meta-analysis" by researchers at Guangdong Medical University in China and published in *BMJ*.

Few feelings are as frightening as the inability to breathe, something experienced by most people with COPD, chronic obstructive pulmonary disease. The focus of COPD care is medication-based treatment to avoid breath-robbing flare-ups called "exacerbations," usually using one or two inhaled drugs. But what if that's just not enough? The answer, triple therapy, can help, but it can come at a health cost, as new research shows.

Background: Patients diagnosed with COPD are often started on single inhaler, usually a long-acting beta 2 adrenoceptor agonist (LABA) or a long-acting muscarinic receptor antagonist (LAMA). If COPD is not well controlled, treatment might step up to either using both of those or one of those plus an inhaled corticosteroid. If exacerbations remain a problem, an aggressive form of treatment is to prescribe all three drugs, which has become a common practice. They can be given with a single inhaler, which is easier on the patient and reduces the risk of dosing errors. But despite widespread use of triple therapy for COPD, questions remain about just how effective—and safe—it is.

Latest research: To answer these questions, researchers analyzed the findings of 21 controlled trials that compared triple therapy to one- or two-drug therapy in patients with COPD.

First the good news: They confirmed that triple therapy reduces exacerbations, improves breathing and improves quality of life compared with either one- or two-drug therapy…and by 25%.

Now the bad news: Triple therapy also increases the risk for pneumonia because of the corticosteroid, a drug known to increase pneumonia risk in anyone with COPD who takes it. The risk for pneumonia is 50% higher than with the two-drug therapy using LABA and LAMA. Since the risk for pneumonia for anyone with severe COPD is already high due to physical changes that make it harder for the body to fight off infection, a 50% increased risk could be a significant health threat.

Another finding was that triple therapy didn't improve overall survival, so while it's effective, it should be reserved for people with severe COPD who do not respond well to two-drug therapy.

Reducing Your Pneumonia Risk

If your COPD is serious enough to warrant triple drug therapy, take all the steps you can to avoid pneumonia. *These are simple enough and bear repeating…*

• **Get your flu,** pneumonia and pertussis vaccine shots.

• **Wash your hands frequently** with soap and water or use a hand sanitizer.

• **Avoid crowds** during cold and flu season.

• **Don't visit sick loved ones,** and yes, even your grandkids.

• **Get plenty of sleep.**

• **Drink plenty of water.**

If you develop symptoms of pneumonia, let your doctor know right away. Some can be similar to an exacerbation, with cough, difficulty breathing and thick or discolored mucus. But with pneumonia, you may also

Vitamin D Curbs Lung Attacks

Background: Flare-ups of chronic obstructive pulmonary disease (COPD), called lung attacks, cause shortness of breath, coughing and increased mucus production. Nearly all COPD deaths are due to lung attacks.

New finding: COPD patients deficient in vitamin D who took supplements had a 45% decrease in the rate of these attacks.

If you have COPD and suffer lung attacks: Get your blood levels of vitamin D tested. If it's below 10 ng/ml, ask your doctor about taking 2,000 IU of vitamin D daily. (For general health, a recommended level is typically 20 ng/ml to 50 ng/ml.)

Adrian R. Martineau, PhD, MRCP, clinical professor of respiratory infection and immunity, The London School of Medicine, and Dentistry, Queen Mary University of London, UK.

have fever and chills, nausea and vomiting, a rapid heartbeat and/or pain in your chest when you take deep breaths.

Air Pollution Could Ruin Your Vacation

Claire Westmacott, MPH, public health specialist at the International Association for Medical Assistance to Travellers, a Toronto-based nonprofit organization that strives to make travel healthier. IAMAT.org

Will your next vacation take your breath away—in a bad way? Savvy travelers know the dangers of food poisoning and tropical diseases, but there's one health risk that people often fail to consider until they step off a plane and into the acrid environment of a far-away destination—air pollution. Some of the world's most appealing travel destinations have some of its worst air quality. That pollution could make it challenging to breathe during your visit. It certainly wouldn't be pleasant. And it could even put your health or life at risk, especially if you have a preexisting heart or respiratory problem.

Here's how to prevent air-quality issues from ruining your travels…

Before Your Trip

Look up the air pollution levels at your destinations. Two excellent online resources for this are BreatheLife (BreatheLife2030.org)—a campaign led by the United Nations and World Health Organization (WHO)—which provides an easy-to-understand gauge of air quality in many cities…and the outdoor-air-quality section of the WHO website (WHO.int/gho/phe), which provides greater detail including air-quality maps for additional areas.

What to look for: A measure of air quality called the mean concentration of fine particulate matter—abbreviated as PM2.5—that is in excess of WHO guidelines. WHO tracks particles of two different sizes in air, and air is unhealthy when particles of either size exceed a certain level.

Example: The mean concentration of "PM2.5" particulate matter in Mumbai, India, is 64 micrograms per cubic meter of air—more than six times WHO guidelines.

Pay attention to the season when assessing air pollution levels. They can be high at any time of the year, but current evidence suggests that winter and summer months can be the most dangerous. Air pollution can be worse in winter because pollutants get trapped by the colder air and more fossil fuels are burned for heating (especially in places that still burn a lot of coal). In the summer months, high temperatures and humidity can increase the concentration of some pollutants. People with preexisting conditions also can be more sensitive to high temperatures and humidity, especially if they're not acclimatized to the hot weather. The best time to travel may depend on which temperatures you fare better with and the seasonal patterns of pollution at your destination.

Make a precautionary visit to your doctor. This is particularly important when traveling to a destination that has air-quality issues if you have a preexisting heart or respiratory problem such as asthma, COPD, chronic bronchitis or emphysema.

Tell your doctor that you intend to visit an area known for its poor air quality, and ask whether it makes sense for you to bring a short-acting bronchodilator metered-dose inhaler (MDI) even if you don't usually use one…corticosteroid tablets…and/or antibiotics—air pollution has been linked to higher rates of respiratory infections. If your health-care provider recommends any of these, make sure that you understand when and how to use them. (Also, confirm that you have sufficient supplies of any medications you already have been prescribed, and refill these prescriptions if necessary.)

If you have a preexisting respiratory or heart condition and/or you are over age 60, also ask your doctor whether you should have a physical exam that includes a stress and lung-capacity test. These tests could help you and your doctor get a more detailed picture of your heart and lung health, which might suggest that additional precautions are needed—or even that the trip is not safe for you at all.

Ideally, any precautionary medical appointments should occur at least six weeks before your trip departure to ensure that there's time to receive any tests or treatments your doctor recommends.

During Your Trip

Plan indoor afternoons. Air pollution levels tend to peak in the afternoon, so when visiting places with poor air quality, check off your outdoor to-dos in the mornings and evenings…and save indoor activities such as museum visits for the hours between lunch and dinner. Ideally, these indoor activities should be in buildings that have air-conditioning—the air quality inside an ancient, un–air-conditioned castle or cathedral might be no better than that of the surrounding outdoor air.

Indoor locations where many people smoke cigarettes or where there are wood-stoves can be even worse, so avoid these as much as possible.

Safety: Heed any local smog alerts or air-quality warnings that you spot in local news outlets, even if this means spending entire days mainly indoors. The Air Matters app (Air-Matters.com) provides real-time air-quality updates for thousands of locations.

Avoid strenuous outdoor physical activity. Physical exertion makes us breathe more deeply and rapidly, increasing our intake of any pollutants in the air. That means it's a good idea to skip the scenic bike tour during rush hour…and the hike up the mountain during high-smog days.

Don't depend on a mask to protect you from air pollution. You might see people wearing surgical masks outdoors in areas that have air pollution problems. Do not follow their lead—they are not getting the air pollution protection they expect because surgical masks are not designed to filter air. And even with masks that are designed to filter out PM2.5 particles, there is no conclusive evidence to prove that they are effective. If you decide to wear a mask anyway and have a preexisting heart or respiratory problem, ask your doctor whether it is safe for you to wear one or whether the challenges of breathing through a mask will make it even harder for you to get the air you need.

CT Scan for Former Smoker

The US Preventive Services Task Force recommends lung cancer screening with a low-dose CT scan for adults ages 55 to 80 who currently smoke (or who quit only in the last 15 years) and have a history of heavy smoking (the equivalent of at least 20 cigarettes a day for 30 years or more). Studies have shown that undergoing a CT scan reduces lung cancer deaths by 20%, versus a chest X-ray, in those at high risk for the disease. However, you should talk to your doctor about your personal risks and benefits before undergoing a screening CT scan. You will most likely have to bring up the subject—in a recent analysis of 137 doc-tor/patient conversations in which lung cancer screening should have been discussed, only 14 specifically covered the topic, and none of the doctors explained the potential harms of screening. Radiation exposure from a low-dose CT scan is not trivial but should be kept in perspective. The amount is somewhat higher than from a regular mammogram or X-ray of the lumbar spine but is about one-third of that of a regular CT scan.

Michael Steinberg, MD, MPH, director, Rutgers Tobacco Dependence Program, Rutgers Robert Wood Johnson Medical School, New Brunswick, New Jersey.

Long Plane or Car Ride? Beware Pulmonary Embolism

Fred Pescatore, MD, a practitioner of natural and integrative medicine in private practice in New York City. He is author of seven books including The A-List Diet and The Hamptons Diet. DrPescatore.com

Taking a long plane ride? Don't spend a lot of time worrying about crashing—the risk is extremely small. A much bigger risk is developing a life-threatening blood clot, aka deep vein thrombosis (DVT), in your leg during the flight. Most of these clots dissolve harmlessly, but they can instead break off and travel through your bloodstream to the lungs, causing a blockage called a pulmonary embolism, which can block blood flow and be fatal. And signs and symptoms of potential DVT, including swelling of the legs and/or ankles and leg pain, can be very uncomfortable.

The good news is that a simple herbal supplement can go a long way toward preventing swelling and reducing leg pain and, research suggests, DVT. The supplement is Pycnogenol, a registered trademark for an extract from the bark of the French maritime pine.

Preventing DVT

Pycnogenol is a powerful antioxidant that improves circulation and reduces inflammation. In one recent study, 295 people who flew in economy class for more than eight hours were divided into three groups. One group took Pycnogenol, a second wore compression stockings (which help with circulation) and the third control group did nothing special.

Results: Members of the Pycnogenol group had the least leg/ankle swelling of the three groups and the least leg pain. There were two incidents of thrombosis in the control group but none in the Pycnogenol or stocking group.

My recommendation: Pycnogenol had a good showing in this study and makes sense as a blood-clot preventive on long trips—even long car rides. I typically recommend taking 100 milligrams of Pycnogenol twice a day for one week before a long flight, on the day of the flight and for one week afterward. While Pycnogenol generally is considered safe with few side effects, as with any supplement, consult your physician to make sure that it's right for you.

Natural Fix for Colds and More

Jamison Starbuck, ND, is a naturopathic physician in family practice and writer and producer of *Dr. Starbuck's Health Tips for Kids*, a weekly program on Montana Public Radio, MTPR.org, both in Missoula. She is a past president of the American Association of Naturopathic Physicians and a contributing editor to *The Alternative Advisor: The Complete Guide to Natural Therapies and Alternative Treatments.* DrJamison-Starbuck.com

It might be hard to believe that something that's been used as medicine for literally thousands of years could be as effective as an over-the-counter (OTC) drug. But it's true. Essential oils—aromatic oils made from the fragrant parts of various plants—were first used by ancient cultures. But they are now popular among consumers of natural medicine—and for good reason.

Unlike OTC decongestants that can spike blood pressure and OTC antihistamines that can cause drowsiness and other unwanted effects, essential oils battle winter ailments safely and without adverse effects. Your best bet is to use essential oils in diluted topical applications that can be inhaled and improve circulation where applied. This form of aromatherapy works particularly well with respiratory complaints.

Caveat: Because essential oils are very concentrated, when used incorrectly they can irritate or burn the skin and mucous membranes (such as the inside of the mouth and nose) and even the stomach if swallowed. That said, essential oils are high on my list of go-to natural remedies. Some of my favorites for winter (with instructions for safety)…*

For the common cold: Spearmint. Spearmint is less irritating to sensitive, inflamed nasal passages than the more frequently used peppermint or eucalyptus.

What to do: Mix the spearmint essential oil in a carrier oil (such as almond or coconut oil), using a 1:10 ratio. Then put two drops of this mixture above your upper lip—one just below each nostril. This will reduce stuffiness and thin nasal mucus, allowing you to blow your nose effectively and to breathe more easily. Use spearmint oil in this way three times a day.

For sinusitis: Chamomile. Because bacteria are common causes of sinusitis, chamomile's antibacterial properties make it good medicine for this annoying and often painful condition.

What to do: Mix the chamomile essential oil with a carrier oil in a 1:10 ratio (as described above). Then put several drops of this mixture on your skin just below your cheekbones, rubbing it into the skin from beside your nose to the outer corners of your eyes near your temples. Be sure not to get

*To test whether you are sensitive or allergic to essential oils, put one drop of the diluted oil on the inside of your wrist and wait 24 hours. If you see a reaction, do not use the oil elsewhere.

this mixture in your eyes! Put another drop or two above each eyebrow—these are sinus points used for acupressure and the application of topical sinus medication.

Lie down with a hot, moist cloth over your face with your eyes closed (leave a little space for breathing through your nose). Cover with a dry towel for five to 10 minutes. You can do this several times a day. The essential oil vapor will reduce congestion and pain and will help you relax and rest.

For sore throat: Bitter orange. With its soothing citrus scent, bitter orange has antiseptic properties and promotes circulation of blood and lymph.

What to do: Mix bitter orange oil with a carrier oil in a 1:10 ratio (as described above), and then rub several drops into the lymph glands under your jaw and down your neck for relief of sore throat pain. Wrap a moist, hot towel around your neck, and then cover it with a dry towel. Leave in place for 15 minutes. Then gently stroke downward on your jaw and neck—this promotes lymph drainage. Repeat as often as desired throughout the day.

Keep Your Family Safe in Wildfire Areas

Stay indoors as much as possible. Use an air purifier with a HEPA filter if you have one. Leave the air-conditioning turned off unless you can set the air conditioner to recirculate the air inside rather than taking in air from outside. Wear an N95-rated face mask if you must go outdoors—and be sure it fits properly. If anyone in the family has breathing issues, such as asthma, get out of town to an area with better air quality. Anyone with asthma should also have extra rescue inhalers on hand.

Shirleen Loloyan Kohn, MD, pulmonologist, Children's Hospital, Los Angeles.

Liquid Nitrogen Snack Warning (Yes, Really!)

US Food and Drug Administration alert, "FDA Advises Consumers to Avoid Eating, Drinking, or Handling Food Products Prepared with Liquid Nitrogen at the Point of Sale," August 30, 2018.

Have you noticed the newest trendy mall snack? It's bright-colored cereal puffs or cheese puffs that emit a vapor and make you "breathe like a dragon" when you eat them. If you think they look scary, your instincts are right! Those snacks, sold under names such as Dragon's Breath, Heaven's Breath and Nitro Puffs, are so dangerous that the FDA has issued a warning against eating them—or even touching them.

The puffs are doused with liquid nitrogen just before they are handed over to the customer, which is what creates the "dragon's breath" vapor from the mouth and nostrils when they are eaten.

Cereal puffs and cheese puffs might bring to mind Lucky Charms and Cheez Doodles, which aren't exactly health foods—but liquid nitrogen is another matter.

It's true that liquid nitrogen is nontoxic in the sense that it's not poisonous, but it's hardly safe. Liquid nitrogen is a colorless, odorless gas that is really cold—below −320°F...cold enough to instantly freeze skin and flesh. Because it's so cold, liquid nitrogen does evaporate quickly, but it might not have completely evaporated from the snacks before they are eaten. Even if the liquid nitrogen has evaporated, inhaling the vapor is dangerous, as explained below.

The US FDA has received reports of severe injury to skin and internal organs from consuming these snacks. So it has issued a warning to avoid eating, drinking or even touching food products prepared with liquid nitrogen just before they're served. The FDA explains that lingering traces of liquid nitrogen ingested on food can severely damage skin (such as fingers and lips) as well as the tongue, throat and esophagus...and that inhaling the vapor can cause breathing difficulties, including asphyxiation, especially in people with asthma. Liquid nitrogen causes frostbite, destroying both external and internal tissues, including the delicate lining of the lungs and bronchial passages. The FDA asks that injuries from such snacks be reported to MedWatch, its website for reporting safety issues and adverse events.

Note: Other foods, such as alcoholic and nonalcoholic drinks and frozen desserts, are sometimes prepared using liquid nitrogen, but in a way that allows the liquid nitrogen to evaporate completely before they are served. So the desserts and drinks are not dangerously cold when they are consumed.

Next time you're at a mall with a kid who's clamoring to breathe like a dragon, keep walking on past.

Vaping? Your E-Cigarette's Flavor Puts Your Health at Risk

Study titled, "Transcriptomic Response of Primary Human Airway Epithelial Cells to Flavoring Chemicals in Electronic Cigarettes," by researchers in the department of environmental health, Harvard T.H. Chan School of Public Health, Boston, published in *Scientific Reports*.

If you vape e-cigarettes (or know someone who does), you'll want to pass on the flavored varieties. Research is finding that the chemicals used to create these flavors damage lung cells…putting vapers at risk for serious respiratory diseases.

Up to 90% of e-cigarettes are flavored, and the variety of flavors keeps growing. Increasingly, the health impact of the chemicals used to create these flavors is coming under scrutiny. For instance, in 2015, Harvard researchers found the chemical diacetyl in 39 e-cigarette flavors they tested. Diacetyl, a synthetic flavor that mimics butter, has been linked to the irreversible lung disease called "popcorn lung," so-named because it was

first found among workers who inhaled the chemical while working in factories that produced butter-flavored microwave popcorn.

More recently, Harvard University's T.H. Chan School of Public Health looked at another chemical flavoring in e-cigarettes that is used as a safer alternative to diacetyl—2,3-pentanedione. The researchers cultivated cells from healthy human cilia, the fingerlike projections that line the lungs and bronchial passages and help clear them of mucus, debris and unfriendly microbes. They then exposed the cells to diacetyl or to 2,3-pentanedione and analyzed the results.

Results: Both chemicals significantly affected the cilia cells in ways that demonstrated decreased production and function of cilia. Both chemicals also interfered with a gene that breaks down and removes toxins from lungs and interfered with a gene that has been linked to lung cancer. And impaired ciliary function is closely linked to COPD and asthma—suggesting that 2,3-pentanedione is no safer than diacetyl.

Note: These are only two of approximately 25 chemical flavorings used in e-cigarettes considered high-priority respiratory health concerns. And there are thousands of varieties of flavored e-cigarettes.

Of course, the best way to avoid the health risk of flavored e-cigarettes is to not use e-cigarettes at all. But if you do vape—either to help quit regular cigarettes or because you think it's a "healthier" alternative—stick to kinds that don't list flavoring on the label.

Are Your Lungs Really Healthy?

"Healthy" lungs may have damage. A study of lung samples from 34 patients is the first to show that lungs from mild chronic obstructive pulmonary disease (COPD) patients that appear healthy on the surface have already lost more than 40% of their terminal bronchioles (key respiratory passageways). If you are a smoker, former smoker or have a family history of COPD: Ask your doctor for a spirometry test to assess lung capacity. If you are diagnosed with COPD, even if mild, work with your doctor on a treatment plan.

Tillie-Louise Hackett, PhD, associate director, Centre for Heart Lung Innovation, University of British Columbia, Vancouver, Canada.

Weak Hands = Weak Lungs

Study titled "Relationship Between Handgrip Strength and Pulmonary Function in Apparently Healthy Older Women," by researchers at Yonsei University College of Medicine, South Korea, published in *Journal of the American Geriatrics Society.*

Getting older sometimes means getting help with ketchup bottles and pickle jars that used to be easy to open. We might not be happy about it, but it's not surprising. But did you know that the reason you struggle with jar lids can also affect your breathing? Here's why…and what you absolutely should do about it.

Losing muscle strength and mass is a natural process of aging called sarcopenia. How much you lose depends on your health, genetics and lifestyle. Many people think of age-related muscle loss as affecting their arms, legs, torso, etc. But sarcopenia affects all the muscles in the body, including the muscles that control respiration, such as the diaphragm.

Because measuring hand strength is a proven way to infer muscle strength in the rest of the body, researchers at Yonsei University in Korea wondered whether hand strength could predict pulmonary function—how efficiently a person's lungs work. Early detection of impaired lung function can help avert episodic respiratory problems such as bronchitis and pneumonia and help avert cardiovascular disease, chronic obstructive pulmonary disease (COPD), heart failure and early death.

Study: The researchers analyzed data from a health survey of 1,773 healthy women ages 65 to 79. The survey included physical examinations that measured handgrip strength and pulmonary function.

Results: The stronger her hands, the more likely a woman was to have a well-functioning respiratory system—and the weaker her hands, the more likely to have impaired lung function.

Although the study was small and involved only women, and the researchers did comment that research on men is needed, other research has found that grip strength in men is associated with better overall health, including better quality of life and lower risk of dying of from heart disease.

While we can't entirely avoid losing muscle as we age, our lifestyle can minimize the loss. Exercise, both aerobic and resistance, and a healthy diet that includes adequate protein are key. There also are things you can do to keep your lungs in top working order, such as breathing exercises, playing a harmonica or even blowing through a straw.

How to Reduce Household Dust Mites

Best ways to reduce dust mites, which can worsen allergies and asthma: Reduce humidity, which dust mites like—keep home humidity at 30% to 50% by using a dehumidifier or central air-conditioning. Use dust- or allergen-blocking covers on mattresses and pillows. Wash sheets and blankets weekly, in hot water if possible or in cool or warm water with bleach. Vacuum carpets and fabric-covered furniture at least weekly using a vacuum cleaner with a HEPA filter. Clean surfaces with a damp mop or cloth, not dry tools, to avoid stirring up dust. Replace carpets with hard surfaces such as wood or tile if you are especially sensitive to dust mites—and replace curtains with blinds that can be cleaned.

HealthLetter.MayoClinic.com

Pacifier Power!

Parents do their infants a favor if they clean pacifiers by popping them into their own mouths. "Parental pacifier sucking" lowers infant levels of IgE, an antibody linked to allergies and asthma.

American College of Allergy, Asthma and Immunology.

Food Allergies Are Not as Common as People Think

Food allergies are only about half as common as people think they are. 19% of adults asked whether they had food allergies said they did—but only 10.8% actually had reactions to food that constitute typical allergic responses, such as throat tightening and vomiting. The most common allergy found was to shellfish, affecting 2.9% of adults surveyed...followed by milk, affecting 1.9%... and peanuts, affecting 1.8%. Among people who did have food allergies, only 48% said that they had been diagnosed with them by a doctor, and only one-quarter said that they had a prescription for the common allergy treatment adrenaline.

Study by researchers at Northwestern University, Evanston, Illinois, published in *JAMA Network Open*.

Are You Allergic to Cold Weather?

Thomas B. Casale, MD, professor of medicine, department of internal medicine, University of South Florida, Tampa.

If you break out in hives when exposed to winter weather, you may have cold urticaria, which is characterized by an extreme reaction to cold. When temperatures plunge (typically below 39°F), people with this condition can break out in hives (itchy, reddish welts) on areas of exposed skin. Symptoms can occur at a wide range of temperatures, and humidity and wind chill factors are important variables.

Sipping an icy drink or eating ice cream can cause the lips or throat to swell in some people with cold urticaria. In severe cases, it can trigger anaphylaxis, a serious allergic reaction that can lead to shock, trouble breathing or swallowing and even death. For example, swimming in cold water can lead to death from anaphylaxis.

People with cold urticaria have mast cells in the skin that release histamine and other chemicals when exposed to cold. In rare cases, cold urticaria is genetic or associated with a disease such as hepatitis or cancer.

If you have this condition, bundle up during cold weather, leaving as little skin exposed as possible. Also avoid contact with cold objects...cold food and drinks...and swimming in water below 77°F.

Note: Health-care providers should be alerted, as cold IV fluids or surgical procedures can cause an episode.

If these steps don't help, you also can take an over-the-counter (OTC) antihistamine such as *loratadine* (Claritin) when temperatures dip. Or a doctor might prescribe *cimetidine* (Tagamet), an acid reducer that is also used as an antihistamine...the anti-inflammatory drug *omalizumab* (Xolair)...or *epinephrine* (EpiPen), an injection used to treat severe allergic reactions.

Urticaria can be a lifelong affliction, but studies show that symptoms go away after about five years for about half of those with this condition.

Better Travel with a Food Allergy

If you have a food allergy, here are some helpful tips when traveling...

•**Carry a food-allergy card that lists your allergies in the languages spoken at your destinations**—the card should list exactly which foods you cannot eat. Allergy Translation.com offers customizable cards starting at $8.

• **Be extra-cautious when ordering in restaurants**—soups may have shellfish broth …salad dressings may contain nut oils…and other possible allergens may turn up in unexpected places.

• **Pack plenty of your own snacks for your trip**—and a few meal replacements just in case you cannot find anything suitable when you arrive.

• **Consider staying in a hotel or Airbnb rental with a kitchen so that you can make your own meals**—and take your allergy card along when you shop for ingredients.

Roundup of experts on travel recommendations for people with food allergies, reported in *The New York Times*.

You May Depend on Your EpiPen…but Can You Count on It?

Jay M. Portnoy, MD, professor of pediatrics, Missouri-Kansas City School of Medicine.

If certain foods or a bee sting can put you into sudden anaphylactic shock, you probably carry a self-injecting epinephrine device. Most likely that device is an EpiPen. In which case, you really need to read about serious issues with EpiPens that could put your life at risk.

For the 2% of people in the US who have a severe allergic reaction—anaphylaxis—when they are exposed to certain foods or a bee sting or some other allergen, getting epinephrine (adrenaline) immediately is a matter of life and death. Epinephrine is the only drug that can reverse anaphylaxis. Since an anaphylactic reaction can happen too quickly to get to the hospital or even to call 911, people who are known to be at risk for such reactions are advised to carry self-injecting epinephrine devices with them at all times. In the US, an EpiPen is the most common such device. About 3.6 million EpiPens are sold each year, and EpiPen prescriptions have doubled over the past 10 years. *For the most part, EpiPens have indeed saved lives. But there also can be serious problems…*

Malfunctions

From 2013 to 2014, reports of EpiPen malfunctions increased 400%. This led to an FDA inspection of the Pfizer-owned facility where EpiPens are made…the discovery of epinephrine leaks in some devices and failure to fire when triggered in others…and ultimately the recall of several batches of EpiPens. More recently, the FDA sent the distributor, Mylan Pharmaceutical, a warning letter because the company had failed to investigate 228 reported malfunctions, including several incidents in which patients died.

As of November 2017, Mylan has stated that it is confident that EpiPens currently being manufactured are safe and effective. It also pointed out that people can die from anaphylaxis even when medication is delivered properly…that any medical device in the hands of a nonmedical person has a high risk of being used improperly…and that some people can have a severe adverse reaction to epinephrine itself.

Shortages

Shortages of epinephrine auto-injectors have been an increasing problem not just in the US but also in Canada, where EpiPens are available at pharmacies without a prescription. (While US citizens can buy EpiPens in Canada and use them in Canada, border customs officials might not allow them to be brought into the US.) Since 2018 in the US, it has been so difficult to fill a prescription—both for the adult version of EpiPen and for EpiPen Jr, the pediatric version—that the FDA has extended the usual expiration dates on the devices by a few months. Their reasoning is that a weakened injection of epinephrine is better than none. Nor is EpiPen the only epinephrine device in short supply.

Shortages of generic brands marketed by Mylan have been reported, as have shortages of Adrenaclick, an auto-injector made by one of the two EpiPen competitors.

What's causing the current shortage is not known outside of Pfizer and Mylan. It could be a combination of the recall diminishing the supply and an inability of the manufacturer to keep up with increased demand. Food Allergy Research & Education (FARE), a nonprofit advocacy organization, has called on the FDA to declare a national shortage and to demand action from Mylan to explain and address the shortage.

One epinephrine auto-injector is not in short supply—Auvi-Q. The manufacturer, Kaleo, says that it is making sure that commercially insured patients can receive Auvi-Q with no out-of-pocket cost.

Note: Auvi-Q had a voluntary recall in 2015. The new version, which reflects changes made to remedy the problems, is supposed to be reliable. Again, as with EpiPen, there is no way to know for sure.

Affordability

When Mylan bought distribution rights to EpiPen in 2007, it raised the price of a two-pack of injectors from $100 to more than $600, making EpiPens too expensive for many people with poor or no insurance. (*Note*: Current recommendations are to carry two injectors at all times. If you are not able to get to emergency medical care within 15 minutes, it is recommended to inject a second dose of epinephrine.)

Mylan's response to complaints about its pricing was to develop its own generic auto-injectors. But at $300 for a two-pack, they are still not very affordable. Patients who can't or don't want to pay the high prices have taken to carrying prefilled syringes of epinephrine…or carrying auto-injectors that have expired. Prefilled syringes are not a good alternative. They are harder to use—a potentially deadly complication for someone going into anaphylactic shock who is likely to be confused and unable to give himself/herself an intramuscular injection properly.

What You Can Do

To work around the problems of epinephrine auto-injectors' pricing and availability…

• **Ask your doctor for a prescription that doesn't specify a particular brand name.** That way, your pharmacy can dispense to you whatever type is available. Note that other brands do not function mechanically in the same way as EpiPen. If your pharmacist gives you a different brand than you're used to, read the directions very carefully ahead of time…so you'll be able to follow the instructions correctly when you need to use it. Most devices come with a blank "trainer" that can be used for practice. Pharmacists also can show you how to use the device.

• **Plan ahead for refills** because it may take several days for your pharmacy to find an auto-injector for you. EpiPen and Auvi-Q have websites where you can find links for help with availability or financial assistance.

• **In some cases, adult patients have been accepting a pediatric epinephrine auto-injector if an adult one is not available.** The most effective dose of epinephrine needed for an anaphylactic event has not been scientifically established—current doses are more convention than proven by factual data. It is reasonable to carry a pediatric version if that is all that is available. If the dose isn't enough, give a second one.

• **Use the auto-injector if you need it!** You'd think that this advice is unnecessary, but the biggest problem with all auto-injectors is not failure of the device but failure of people to use the device. For example, a recent study found that in more than 2,000 emergency-room visits for an anaphylactic reaction at 34 US hospitals, only about 20% of the patients took or received epinephrine before coming to the ER.

More Cost/Supply Relief?

Relief for at least short supply may be around the corner. The FDA announced in August 2018 its approval of an epinephrine auto-injector made by an Israeli company called Teva. Mylan is suing Teva for patent infringement, but the Teva device is now approved as a generic competitor to EpiPen, although at this writing it is not available in US pharmacies. However, currently priced at $300, the Teva auto-injector is not the cost-saver that was hoped for.

Bye-Bye, Allergies! Surprise Treatment for Lifelong Sensitivities

Andrew Rubman, ND, medical director of Southbury Clinic for Traditional Medicines in Southbury, Connecticut. SouthburyClinic.com

---

The **patient:** "Heather," a woman in her early 60s, who has endured allergic sensitivities as long as she could remember. Her troubling symptoms varied, from skin rashes to intestinal cramping.

Why she came to see me: She initially came to have her diet and allergies evaluated after not having any success with myriad other health care providers over the years. She experienced skin allergies as well as food reactions that came and went without any rhyme or reason. For example, she would react to certain foods at one time and then be tolerant a few weeks later. She developed a skin rash to a wool sweater one season and then the next year tolerated it without a problem. During one of our follow-up visits, I asked her about what other issues she had and she mentioned a persistent cyst on her upper back.

How I evaluated her: The suspicious cyst was located near her shoulder blade adjacent to her spine. It was relatively superficial and the size of a nickel. On palpation, it presented as moderately tender with evidence of some deeper fluid accumulation. At the surface, there was evidence of scar tissue around what appeared to be the opening of a sebaceous gland. (Sebaceous glands are the oil-producing glands that surround hair follicles.)

How we addressed her problem: I explained to Heather that even though I had residential training in minor and orificial surgery, the State of Connecticut did not permit naturopathic physicians to perform surgery. I could, however, use a scalpel to remove superficial scar tissue from the area overlying the cyst. This procedure is called "wound debriding," or removing non-vital tissue, and thus technically not surgery. (*Note:* If it looked either deeply complex, requiring surgical removal, or potentially cancerous, I would have referred Heather to a dermatologist.)

Upon clearing away the overlying scarring blocking the opening to the cyst, I was able to begin to massage out fluid and a small-but-suspicious dark mass the size of a BB. What followed was entirely unexpected. A thin, thorn-like spike approximately $\frac{1}{3}$" in length emerged and I extracted it with tweezers. It was the remainder of a honey bee poison sack and stinger!

Heather remembered being stung in summer camp when she was eight years old, but never did more than take Benadryl at the time. A few years later she experienced a dramatic reaction to allergy desensitization "therapy" provided by a local allergist who pronounced her "strongly allergic" to bees and gave her an EpiPen after seeing her upper arm weep serum where he had administered her "therapeutic" injections.

I was able to express the remaining contents of the cyst and bandaged the wound.

The patient's progress: What surprised both of us is that in the ensuing months, Heather's chronic allergies began to improve, and a nagging muscular stiffness that she had most of her life in her upper back waned as well. Quite amazing that a foreign body, inserted in one's youth, can play havoc over one's entire life.

Vaping Alert for Women

Vaping may increase susceptibility to flu, especially if you're a woman. E-cigarette users' immune response to a dose of FluMist (a vaccine that contains a live attenuated flu virus) was more suppressed than that of cigarette smokers and nonsmokers, suggesting that the immune response to the live virus in the vaccine was less effective for e-cigarette users. Preliminary findings show female response was more affected than male, though researchers still are investigating why.

Meghan Rebuli, PhD, is a postdoctoral research associate at Center for Environmental Medicine, Asthma and Lung Biology, University of North Carolina at Chapel Hill.

Long-Term Risks of Tonsil and Adenoid Removal

Tonsillectomy to treat chronic tonsillitis and adenoidectomy to treat recurrent middle-ear infections both increase the risk for respiratory, allergic and infectious diseases in later life. The risk for diseases of the upper-respiratory tract almost triples when children have had tonsillectomies. For children whose adenoids have been removed, the risk for chronic obstructive pulmonary disease more than doubles—and the risk for upper-respiratory-tract diseases and conjunctivitis nearly doubles.

Sean Byars, PhD, research fellow, school of biosciences, University of Melbourne, Australia, and coleader of an analysis of a database on more than 1,180,000 Danish children, published in *JAMA Otolaryngology Head and Neck Surgery*.

Allergies Can Trigger MS Attacks

Tanuja Chitnis, MD, FAAN, professor of neurology, Harvard Medical School, medical director, Partners Multiple Sclerosis Center, Brigham and Women's Hospital, both in Boston. She is coauthor of a study titled, "Food Allergies Are Associated with Increased Disease Activity in Multiple Sclerosis" by researchers at Brigham and Women's Hospital and Harvard Medical School, published in *Journal of Neurology, Neurosurgery, and Psychiatry*.

There is no cure (yet!) for multiple sclerosis, so it is instead managed with drugs to help mitigate the effects of the disease. Lifestyle adjustments, including a healthy diet, can also help. Now research finds that some healthy foods might be a problem for certain people who have MS.

It's already known that certain environmental factors can trigger MS and/or make it worse. But until now, the association between one environmental factor—allergies—and MS has not been clear.

So researchers at Brigham and Women's Hospital and Harvard Medical School had 1,349 adult MS patients fill out questionnaires about their current history of three kinds of allergies—environmental (dust, mold or hay fever), food (eggs, dairy, wheat, soy, fish, shellfish, fruits, nuts or other food) and/or drugs. The patients also had gadolinium-enhanced MRIs of their brains. These scans are taken to show lesions, which confirm that inflammatory cells have crossed into the central nervous system, as happens during an MS attack.

Results: Compared with patients who had no known allergies, patients with food allergies had 27% more MS attacks. The brain scans of these patients also were more than twice as likely to have MS lesions in their brains as patients without food allergies. No association was shown for environmental or drug allergies and either MS attacks or brain lesions.

Note: The study authors point out that they did not distinguish between true food allergy and food sensitivity.

Researchers believe that inflammation may be one reason for the association between food allergy and MS activity and lesions. Since environmental and drug allergies did not have the same effect, the researchers believe that there may be a unique mechanism associated with food allergies and MS relapses. The researchers also suggest that having a food allergy may alter the gut microbiome and produce changes in brain chemicals that affect the central nervous system. This study did not investigate whether active avoidance of the allergen reduced risk. They hope to pursue this important question in future research.

MS is a progressive autoimmune disease of the central nervous system that destroys myelin, the protective covering of nerve fibers, and eventually destroys the nerves themselves. Symptoms include numbness or weakness on one side of the body, vision problems, tingling, pain, tremor, unsteady gait, slurred speech, fatigue, dizziness and bowel and bladder problems.

Typically, the disease is characterized by periods of relapse, when symptoms worsen and disease severity increases…followed by periods of remission, when symptoms typically clear at least partially. Besides taking drugs that can speed recovery from attacks and slow progression of the disease, certain supplements and lifestyle changes—such as avoiding stress, smoking, heat, infection and fatigue—can also help lessen its severity.

More research is needed to better understand the results of this latest study. But in the meantime, if you or a loved one has MS and a known food allergy (or sensitivity), in light of this research it makes sense to be even more scrupulous about avoiding your allergen. And if you have MS but aren't sure whether you have a food allergy or sensitivity, it's a good idea to discuss with your doctor whether you should be tested. Most adults with food allergies have had them since childhood—but food allergies can also start in adulthood.

Chapter 15

STROKE ALERTS

Stroke Risk for Women Is Different

Stroke is not an equal-opportunity health issue. Even accounting for women's average longer life spans, more women than men in the US die of stroke—it's the fourth-leading cause of death for women but only the fifth for men. And women with diabetes and abnormal heart rhythms are more likely to have strokes than men with these conditions. While doctors have long known these facts, their cause has not been clear. Now new research sheds light on what could be driving women's increased stroke risk.

Recent finding: Researchers at Brigham and Women's Hospital in Boston reviewed the scientific literature on ischemic stroke (when blood flow through an artery in the brain is blocked) looking for clues as to why women are more prone to stroke than men. They evaluated the data according to factors specific to women such as sex hormones, pregnancy and menopause.

Results: As expected, the researchers found that the most common causes of stroke for both men and women were conditions such as smoking, high blood pressure, diabetes and abnormal heart rhythms. However,

they also found specific hormone-based risk factors unique to women that could be contributing to their higher stroke rates. Some of these factors are already known to raise stroke risk—early menopause (before age 45)…use of oral contraceptive pills that contained synthetic estrogen…being pregnant… and taking oral synthetic estrogen hormone therapy for menopausal symptoms. However, researchers also found two unsuspected factors associated with stroke—having begun to have monthly periods early (before age 10)…and having a low level of DHEA-S, a naturally occurring hormone that is a building block of testosterone and estrogen and that decreases with age and stress.

Bottom line: The researchers point out that more studies are needed to find out exactly how these hormonal characteristics might increase stroke risk and the best way to address the risk. However, while not much can be done about some risk factors, such as when periods begin or menopause starts, knowing more about unique risks they face reinforces for women—now maybe more than ever—why it's good to take charge of

Kathryn M. Rexrode, MD, associate professor of medicine, Brigham and Women's Hospital, Boston, and senior author of a study titled, "Stroke Risk Factors Unique to Women," published in *Stroke.*

what is within their control. According to the American Heart Association and the American Stroke Association, 80% of strokes are preventable, and recommendations for everyone (women and men) to reduce their stroke risk include maintaining healthy blood pressure, blood sugar, weight and cholesterol, eating a healthy diet that includes at least five daily servings of fruits and vegetables, getting adequate exercise, limiting alcohol and not smoking.

Diet Drinks Linked to Stroke and Heart Disease

Study titled, "Artificially Sweetened Beverages and Stroke, Coronary Heart Disease, and All-Cause Mortality in the Women's Health Initiative," led by researchers at Albert Einstein College of Medicine in New York City and published in *Stroke*.

Enjoying a cool, refreshing diet drink is a daily habit for many people who are trying to improve their health by dropping unwanted pounds. For postmenopausal women, however, consuming artificially sweetened sodas and juices may not be a harmless way to cut calories, according to a startling new study published in *Stroke*.

Here's how the research unfolded—and the risks that were discovered…

Study details: As part of the Women's Health Initiative, a long-term study investigating strategies to prevent heart disease, breast and colorectal cancer and osteoporosis in postmenopausal women, health data was tracked for nearly 12 years on 81,714 participants who reported how often they drank diet drinks, such as low-calorie, artificially sweetened colas, sodas and fruit drinks.

Compared with study participants who consumed diet drinks less than once a week or not at all, those who drank two or more of these drinks daily were 31% more likely to have an ischemic stroke (caused by a blood clot). *In addition, the frequent consumers of diet drinks were…*

• **29% more likely to develop heart disease (fatal or nonfatal heart attack).**

• **16% more likely to die from any cause.**

The news was even worse for obese women—they were more than twice as likely to have a stroke if they downed two or more diet beverages a day. African-American women without previous heart disease or diabetes were nearly four times more likely to have a stroke. The results were adjusted for known stroke risk factors such as age, high blood pressure and smoking.

Caveats: Even though this study found a link between intake of diet drinks and stroke and heart disease, it was observational and does not prove that the heavy consumption of these drinks causes cardiovascular disease. The study also did not specify which artificial sweeteners or specific drinks the women had consumed, nor was there any attempt to extrapolate these results to men or younger women.

The American Heart Association (AHA) recently published an advisory stating that there is inadequate scientific research to conclude that low-calorie sweetened beverages do—or do not—affect risk factors for heart disease and stroke in young children, teens or adults. The association recognized that diet drinks may help replace high-calorie, sugary beverages but added that water (plain, carbonated and unsweetened flavored) is the best option for a no-calorie drink.

How to Stop a Stroke Before It Happens

Bruce A. Perler, MD, MBA, a practicing vascular surgeon at Johns Hopkins Medicine and the Julius H. Jacobson II, MD, Endowed Chair in Vascular Surgery at Johns Hopkins University School of Medicine, both in Baltimore.

Feeling perfectly healthy? Chances are, your doctor still orders certain tests—called "screening tests"—that check for conditions such as colon cancer or osteoporosis that might be lurking and could be treated.

So why not a screening test for stroke risk? We know that people living in the US have nearly 800,000 strokes each year and that 80% to 90% of those strokes are caused by blood clots. Many of these strokes originate from clogged carotid arteries—large arteries in the neck that feed blood to your brain. Like the arteries that feed your heart, these can be narrowed by plaque buildup as you age.

This may surprise you: There is a test that can detect such blockages. It's a simple ultrasound of your neck that costs about $70 to $300 (depending on where you live) and sometimes is covered by insurance.

However, no major medical group advises checking the carotid arteries of all adults—due to concerns that many questionable results will turn out to be wrong, leading to needless worry, costly follow-up testing and risky surgeries.

But some medical groups, such as the Society for Vascular Surgery, the American Heart Association and the American Stroke Association, think it makes sense to test certain people who are at increased risk for a stroke from a clogged carotid artery.

The danger: Without testing, too many people, while clinically asymptomatic, will unknowingly suffer one or more symptomless "silent strokes"—small, repeated insults to the brain caused by inadequate blood flow, which over time can lead to decline in cognitive function. Unsuspecting people with blockages also may ignore signs of transient ischemic attacks, or TIAs (also known as "ministrokes")—brief attacks that produce passing stroke symptoms that may last only for a few minutes, such as weakness of an arm or leg, brief loss of vision or difficulties speaking. Ministrokes can be the precursor to a bigger and permanently damaging stroke. Still other people will get no warning before a stroke that leaves them disabled or dead, further adding rationale for the screening test.

Should You Get Scanned?

While guidelines from medical groups vary, many doctors—including myself—say that you should consider a potentially lifesaving scan of your carotid arteries if one or more of the following apply to you…

• **A "bruit" in your neck is detected by your doctor.** This abnormal sound, detected by a stethoscope during a routine physical exam, can indicate a narrowed artery—especially when it's accompanied by other stroke risk factors, such as high blood pressure.

Note: Your doctor should listen for a bruit on both sides of your neck. In some cases, patients actually can hear a "whooshing" sound in their ears.

• **You are over age 65 and have multiple stroke risk factors,** such as smoking, elevated cholesterol, high blood pressure and/or diagnosed coronary artery disease.

• **You have been diagnosed with peripheral artery disease (PAD).** This narrowing of the leg arteries can cause leg pain, particularly when walking. If the arteries feeding your limbs are clogged with plaque, the arteries in your neck may be, too.

• **You have worrisome results from an ankle-brachial index test.** With this test, your doctor compares your blood pressure readings at your ankle and upper arm. The test can indicate PAD, so it's recommended for people with suspicious symptoms in their legs, including pain, numbness or weakness, but also is sometimes used as a broader screening tool for artery health.

• **You have had symptoms of a ministroke.** This might include weakness or numbness on one side of your body or slurred speech. Even if the symptoms lasted for just a minute or two, they are serious. People who have a ministroke are at high risk for a bigger stroke, most often in the first few days, but also in the months and years ahead.

If you have possible ministroke symptoms in the future: Treat them as a medical emergency, and call 911 right away.

Important: If you decide, in consultation with your doctor, to get a carotid ultrasound, make sure that you get the gold-standard test, called a carotid duplex ultrasound, from a laboratory accredited by the Intersocietal Accreditation Commission (IAC). The test, which requires no preparation, can take up to 30 to 60 minutes. You will be asked to wear loose-fitting clothing that allows the technician to access your neck. If there is significant plaque in a carotid artery, the lab report should say how extensive the blockage is and describe the characteristics of the plaque in a way that will help your doctor assess your risks.

What's Next?

If your carotid scan shows no significant blockage, continue taking steps to lower your stroke risk—control blood pressure and cholesterol, maintain a healthy body weight and don't smoke.

What if your carotid testing indicates trouble? *Here are the rules of thumb…*

• **If less than 50% to 60% of your artery is blocked and you have no symptoms,** you will likely be advised to continue or add medications that reduce your stroke risk, such as a statin for high cholesterol, aspirin to reduce clotting and medication to lower your blood pressure. If you smoke, you will have a powerful new reason to quit.

• **If your blockage is 60% or more but you have no symptoms,** surgery (called a carotid endarterectomy) to remove the plaque may be needed, depending on the severity of the narrowing and the character of the plaque…or if there has been increased narrowing over time. If surgery is not indicated, drugs and lifestyle changes are recommended, and scanning should be repeated every six to 12 months to watch for progression.

• **If you have a blockage of 50% to 99% and symptoms,** the choices are clearer. Unless you have a condition, such as severe, noncorrectable coronary artery disease, heart failure or severe chronic obstructive pulmonary disease (COPD), that makes such procedures too risky, endarterectomy or a stent to open your clogged artery likely will be offered. Stenting is considered more appropriate for symptomatic patients who are too high risk for endarterectomy.

Caution: These procedures can reduce your long-term stroke risk, but they both carry risks of causing an immediate stroke or death by dislodging plaque and sending it to your brain.

My advice: If you are considering one of these procedures, look for a highly experienced surgeon and hospital—and ask for their complication rates. With a top-notch team, stroke or death rates following endarterectomy or stenting should be no more than 2% to 3% for asymptomatic patients… and no more than 5% to 6% for symptomatic patients.

Your Eyes Could Give Important Clues About Stroke

Richard Leigh, MD, assistant clinical investigator, Neuro Vascular Brain Imaging Unit, Intramural Stroke Branch, National Institute of Neurological Disorders and Stroke of the National Institutes of Health. He is lead author of a study titled, "Blood-Ocular Barrier Disruption in Acute Stroke Patients," published in the journal *Neurology*.

Your body has amazing ways of protecting itself. For example, one of the most important natural protective mechanisms is the blood-brain barrier, a semipermeable layer of cells that prevents blood from leaking out of blood vessels and into the brain.

A similar mechanism (known as the blood-ocular barrier) protects the structures of our eyes. But when a person has a stroke, all bets are off as to the effectiveness of this eye-protecting barrier.

A recent study came about after what seemed to be a serendipitous finding—MRI scans of the brain, taken right after a person suffered a stroke, showed that material used for contrast in those scans (gadolinium) was leaking into the eyes. Gadolinium is clear and harmless, so its presence in the eyes does not affect vision. But researchers hope that this new information will lead to more studies and, possibly, to an eye exam that can provide helpful information about what is going on inside the brain of stroke patients.

Study details: Researchers carefully analyzed the brain MRIs that were taken of 167 people who were admitted to the hospital after having an ischemic stroke (caused by a blood clot). MRIs with gadolinium, the tracer that allows structures to be seen more easily, were taken immediately upon arrival to the hospital and then again two hours and/or 24 hours later. The researchers then made observations about the "leakage" of gadolinium into the eyes during this time frame and tried to identify associations with other important characteristics of the stroke.

Results: Based on the MRIs, three-quarters of stroke patients were found to have evidence of gadolinium in their eyes during the 24 hours after the contrast agent had been administered. There was minimal difference in the occurrence of leakage into the eyes between patients who received the clot-busting treatment tissue plasminogen activator (tPA) after their strokes and in those who didn't receive the drug (79% versus 71%). In most cases, the gadolinium was found in both eyes.

Eighteen percent of people with scans at two hours had severe gadolinium leakage, and they were more likely to have had more damaging strokes. It is possible that this finding provides insight about the stroke that would not be seen on a routine CT or MRI of the brain. In patients with scans taken 24 hours after introduction of the gadolinium, those with a history of high blood pressure were twice as likely to have leakage into the eyes. Leakage was also more common in older patients.

Note: In an unrelated action, the FDA recently issued a warning that gadolinium can linger in the brain, skin and bones for years. Some patients have complained of pain, burning sensations and weakness after injection of the contrast agent. Currently, however, there is no scientific evidence for negative effects from gadolinium when used in patients with adequate kidney function. The FDA advises the use of formulations of gadolinium with macrocyclic agents, which do not deposit in the body.

What's Your Stroke Risk If You Have AFib?

Enrique D. Garcia-Sayan, MD, assistant professor of cardiovascular medicine at the McGovern Medical School at University of Texas and director of echocardiography and associate chief of cardiology at LBJ General Hospital, both in Houston. Study titled, "Reassessment of Risk for Stroke During Follow-up of Patients with Atrial Fibrillation" by researchers from National Yang-Ming University in Taipei, Taiwan, and University of Liverpool, UK, published in *Annals of Internal Medicine*.

The main danger of living with atrial fibrillation, or AFib, is that it increases your risk for stroke. With AFib, an irregular (often too-fast) heartbeat causes blood to pool in the left atrial appendage (an upper chamber of the heart), where it can form into a clot that can travel to the brain and cause a stroke.

At the same time, AFib is the number one preventable cause of stroke. Taking a blood-thinning medication called an oral anticoagulant can prevent clots from forming. But there is a downside…anticoagulants can increase your risk for significant bleeding by about 2% to 4% per year. The challenge is to figure out for whom the benefit of taking these drugs outweighs the risk.

To do this, doctors use a scoring system called CHA2DS2-VASc (you can simply say "chad-vasc") that assigns points for various stroke risk factors. *Give yourself one point for each of these characteristics that applies to you…*

- **Congestive heart failure**
- **Hypertension**
- **Diabetes**
- **A history of vascular disease**
- **Being a woman**
- **Being between the ages of 65 and 74**

And two points for the following…

- **Having a history of stroke or transient ischemic attack (TIA, often called a mini-stroke)**
- **Being age 75 or over**

People who score zero have no increased yearly stroke risk due to AFib. The yearly risk for a score of one is just under 1%, and the risk increases as your score goes up.

The American Heart Association and other organizations recommend considering aspirin (a medication that prevents blood platelets from clotting) or an anticoagulant (a blood thinner) for anyone with a score of one. Anyone with a score of two or higher is a definite candidate for an oral anticoagulant. *But there are two steps to take to make sure that your CHA2DS2-VASc is as useful as possible…*

- **Recheck your score every year.** Scores change over time, especially as people age. In fact, a study of about 14,600 people newly diagnosed with AFib found that patients initially considered low risk according to CHA2DS2-VASc and not prescribed an anticoagulant had about a 40% risk of moving into a high-risk range within three years. Within a single year after diagnosis, 16% of the patients in the study had added at least one point to their score.

- **Have your doctor individualize your score.** There are some gray areas in the scoring system, notably for people with a score of one. For example, if you scored one point only because you're a woman—and you have no other risk factors, taking an anticoagulant might convey more risk than benefit. On the other hand, if you have a score of one and are just one year shy of age 65 or 75, the benefit may outweigh the risk. Similarly, the risk of bleeding is not the same in every patient, and this can be estimated by your doctor by using a different assessment called the HAS-BLED score. These variations are perfect examples of why treatment should be personalized.

If you have AFib, the best decision for you will come from a discussion of drug risks and benefits with your doctor and some shared decision-making.

Important if you take fish oil/omega-3 supplements: Fish oil is not an anticoagulant and should not be used as a substitute for one if you have AFib. That being said, there is much controversy about the perceived increased risk of bleeding in patients taking fish oil for other health reasons. Though high doses of omega-3 fatty acids including fish oil may increase bleeding time, clinically significant bleeding has not been clearly demonstrated in studies of people who were on anticoagulants and took these supplements, nor has evidence been found of increased risk of bleeding or serious adverse events with the addition of fish oil. So, once again, the recommendation is for individualized decision-making and discussion with your physician about whether the benefits of continuing fish oil supplements when starting an anticoagulant outweigh the still-unproved risk of bleeding.

It should be noted, however, that nonsteroidal anti-inflammatory drugs (NSAIDs), such as ibuprofen and naproxen, should be stopped or minimized while on anticoagulants, as they can increase not only the risk of bleeding but also of stroke. Also, if you were taking aspirin prior to starting a blood thinner, talk to your doctor about whether you should continue to do so because, for many patients, the increased bleeding risk does outweigh the benefits—but don't stop taking aspirin until you have this discussion.

Overtreating Thyroid Disease May Raise Stroke Risk

Among 170,000 people tested for blood levels of the hormone free thyroxine (FT4)—low levels indicate an underactive thyroid—those with the highest levels, but within what is still considered the normal range, had a 40% greater risk of developing atrial fibrillation (AFib) than those with the lowest levels. AFib, a common heart-rhythm disorder, increases risk for stroke.

Jeffrey L. Anderson, MD, distinguished clinical and research physician, Intermountain Medical Center Heart Institute, Murray, Utah.

Atrial Fibrillation Gone? You're Still at Risk for Stroke

Tom Marshall, PhD, professor of public health and primary care in the College of Medical and Dental Sciences at University of Birmingham, UK.

Your doctor has given you good news. Your atrial fibrillation (AFib)—an irregular heartbeat that greatly increases stroke risk—has gone away. Your heart rhythm has returned to normal.

But you're not out of the woods, according to new research. You're still at increased risk for stroke—and you might need a drug to counter that risk. In a study in *The BMJ*, researchers examined the records of about 50,000 patients in the UK, 11,000 of whom had a history of AFib but whose physicians had determined it was resolved. Some had undergone treatment to eliminate AFib, while others had experienced a spontaneous return to normal heart rhythms.

Key finding: These patients were not only still at higher risk for stroke than people who had never had AFib, their risk was similar to that of people with ongoing AFib.

How could that be? For one thing, AFib can come and go. The heart may resume its normal rhythm for a time, prompting some to consider the condition "resolved," even "cured." Plus, treatment effects can diminish over time.

Example: One out of four patients treated successfully with catheter ablation, which uses radiofrequency waves, has his/her AFib return within a year.

Finally, while some patients with AFib have symptoms (heart palpitations, extreme fatigue, lightheadedness, confusion, shortness of breath), others have none. So the first "symptom" that their AFib has returned may unfortunately be a stroke.

Most patients whose AFib has been resolved spontaneously or through treatment, study authors concluded, should not stop taking stroke-preventing anti-coagulant medication such as *warfarin* (Coumadin) or *rivaroxaban* (Xarelto). Even if you've been successfully treated for AFib, talk to your doctor about these medications.

This Vitamin Really Protects Against Stroke

Study titled, "Most Vitamin, Mineral Supplements Not Shown to Lower Heart Disease Risk: Naturally Derived Nutrients from Plant-Based Foods Recommended to Cut Heart Disease Risk," led by researchers at University of Toronto, published in *Journal of the American College of Cardiology*.

You already know that vitamins are good for you and that it's important to get them from food, not only from pills. But a new study has found that supplements of a certain B vitamin are protective against stroke. So should you take supplements of this vitamin? *Here's how to know…*

The study: University of Toronto researchers reviewed 179 studies published between 2012 and 2017 that looked at heart-health benefits of vitamin and mineral supplements and concluded that nearly all of them were not effective for preventing or treating cardiovascular disease. Included were the most popular supplements—vitamin C, calcium, vitamin D and multivitamins.

However, researchers found a notable exception: vitamin B-9, more commonly known as folic acid (the synthetic form) or folate (the natural form). Taking a folic acid supplement or a B-complex supplement that included folic acid was found to reduce the risk for stroke by a very significant amount—20%.

This finding builds on earlier research suggesting cardiovascular benefits of folic acid supplements. For instance, a 2015 study that involved 20,000 people from the China Stroke Primary Prevention Trial (CSPPT) found that folic acid supplements reduced the risk for cardiovascular disease and stroke. And another CSPPT study published earlier this year found that patients with high blood pressure and a low blood platelet count who took the blood pressure drug *enalapril* (Vasotec) and folic acid were 73% less likely to have a first stroke than those who took only the drug.

While these associations do not prove cause and effect, all of this would seem to be evidence that it's a very good idea to make sure you're getting enough folic acid.

Folic acid is in many foods. Spinach, asparagus and brussels sprouts are especially rich sources, but you can also get it from green leafy vegetables, fruits, nuts, beans, peas, dairy products, meat, eggs, seafood and grains. Also, most bread, cereal, pasta and rice are enriched with folic acid.

Even with the 20% reduction in stroke risk, researchers from the latest study did not suggest that there's enough evidence to recommend taking folic acid supplements for stroke prevention. But if you have any particular stroke risk factors, such as diabetes, high blood pressure or being obese or overweight, you might want to ask your doctor about the study and discuss whether taking folic acid supplements (or folate supplements) would be a good idea for you.

Can Yoga Give You a Stroke?

Loren Fishman, MD, physical medicine and rehabilitation specialist, assistant clinical professor, Columbia Medical School, New York City, and yoga teacher.

S ome yoga poses twist your neck so much, you may have heard that it could cause a stroke. How much danger of stroke is there really?

Twisting poses have not been known to cause strokes, and your risk for stroke from yoga is low...as long as you avoid certain poses and take a few reasonable precautions.

The *possibility* of stroke from yoga first rose to public attention in 2012, when a Pulitzer Prize–winning *New York Times* reporter, William Broad, published a book called *The Science of Yoga*. He reported that yoga poses that flex the neck extremely could cause tears in neck arteries...which could cause blood clots to form...and the clots could flow into the brain and cause a stroke.

A 2009 survey of more than 1,000 yoga teachers from 34 countries published in *International Journal of Yoga Therapy* did confirm that the neck was the most common site for injury, including severe injury...followed by the shoulder, back, knees and wrists. And it's true that a few cases of stroke attributed to yoga poses that extremely flex the neck have been reported—but not many. Between 1969 and 2012 there were three published case reports.

That said, if you have risk factors for stroke, such as high blood pressure—or if you simply have neck problems—it's best to avoid certain yoga poses. Poses that can potentially put the neck arteries at risk are those that extremely bend or stretch the neck or put pressure on the neck, such as Shoulder Stand and Plow. Even if you aren't at higher risk for stroke and don't have neck problems, it's a good idea to avoid these poses when you are new to yoga and have not yet mastered proper technique and balance. (In case you wondered, no stroke danger has been found from Headstand and poses that exert pressure on the head.)

With the Shoulder Stand, the whole weight of your body is on your shoulders and the back of your neck, which is forced into an extreme flex position. So, too, with Plow, which extends the stretch of the Shoulder Stand to lower your legs so that your toes touch the ground behind your head. In fact, even seasoned teachers almost always put blankets under the shoulders to make the neck angle less acute.

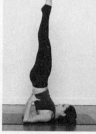
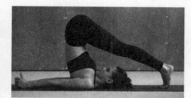

Shoulder Stand   Plow Pose

A far more common yoga injury is worsening of glaucoma. Intraocular pressure is already high with glaucoma, and any position that inverts the body—for instance, a Headstand, Shoulder Stand, Standing Forward Bend or Downward-Facing Dog—can increase eye pressure further and injure the optic nerve. Research has found that some inversion poses can cause intraocular pressure to *double in just 15 seconds*. This is fine for most people, but dangerous for anyone with glaucoma.

Be sure to let your yoga instructor know if you have glaucoma—or any other any physical or medical issues, including high blood pressure, osteoporosis, disc problems and spinal stenosis. If you have multiple sclerosis (MS), take a pass on Bikram yoga. Room temperature can reach 105°F, which can trigger an MS flare.

Most yoga injuries are sprains and strains, which can be avoided, or risk can at least be minimized, by making sure you have a good teacher and by not going beyond your fitness level and ability.

Learn more about common injuries caused by yoga poses and how to avoid them, as well as which yoga poses are safest for more than 90 medical conditions on the Yoga Injury Prevention website YIP.guru. (*Note*: You'll need to sign up. The first week is free, after which access to the site is $4.33/month.)

Bottom line: For most people, the advantages of yoga far outweigh the risks of injury. You're in much greater danger crossing the street!

Stroke Risk Lingers Long After Heart Attack

Study titled, "Duration of Heightened Stroke Risk After Myocardial Infarction," led by researchers in the department of neurology at Weill Cornell Medical College, New York City, presented at the annual meeting of the 2018 American Neurological Association.

I t's long been known that your risk for a stroke is increased during the month after a heart attack. But after that, it was thought, your stroke risk returns to normal. However, one month is too soon to relax your stroke watch, according to the latest research.

Because a heart attack (myocardial infarction) interrupts normal blood circulation, it's easy for a blood clot to be released into the bloodstream, which then can travel to the brain and cause an ischemic stroke. Studies have found that this risk is highest in the first month after a heart attack. However, those studies were done on small numbers of patients.

To get a more detailed picture of post–heart attack stroke risk, researchers at Weill Cornell Medical College looked at data from 1.7 million people on Medicare over a period of about 4.6 years, including more than 46,000 patients over age 65 who were hospitalized after a heart attack.

Results: As expected, risk for stroke was almost three times higher than normal risk in the first month after a heart attack. However, stroke risk was doubled during the second month...and was still elevated during the third month (about 60% higher). Risk did not return to normal until after the third month.

The researchers surmise that increased stroke risk is partly the result of decreased heart function post–heart attack, during which time the heart is not beating efficiently, and blood tends to pool and form clots. For this reason, heart attack patients typically are prescribed a blood thinner, such as aspirin, after a heart attack. These new findings suggest that patients may need to take a more powerful anticoagulant...and possibly for longer. The researchers suggest that more research is needed to develop guidelines.

Meanwhile, if you or a loved one has recently had a heart attack, alert your doctor that your stroke risk may be higher than previously thought—and discuss strategies to reduce risk.

And stay alert for the "F.A.S.T." warning signs of stroke: Face drooping...Arm weakness...Speech difficulty...and Time to call 911.

Chapter 16

VERY PERSONAL

Ladies, Let's Talk about Orgasms

Has your doctor ever asked you how often you use your vibrator? Or if you even have a vibrator?

If the answer is "Certainly not!" you're not alone. Almost no doctors ask women about vibrators—or orgasms—at all. Most women won't bring up or even think about this topic on their own. Yet for many women whose sex lives decline after menopause, as often is the case, the use of a vibrator is a safe and effective way to restore the joyful (and healthful) sex that they miss. It's good for relationships, too.

Gynecologist Lauren Streicher, MD, often recommends vibrators as a health device. She is on a mission to get women to talk about sexuality, including the inability to have an orgasm, with their doctors. *We talked with her about what that could accomplish…*

Why should women talk about sexual problems, including a lack of orgasms, with their doctors?

Because sexual pleasure is important for most women's physical and emotional health and, if a woman has a partner, for her romantic relationship. Vibrators can help—and doctors should feel comfortable recommending them. More than half of American women ages 18 to 60 have used them at some point in their lives, but that means nearly half never have.

That is a missed opportunity because vibrators can help many women, both before and after menopause, with desire, arousal, lubrication and, yes, orgasm.

Is not being able to have an orgasm really a health condition?

It is if it's negatively affecting a woman's life. Many women enjoy sex without orgasms, and in fact, most women don't have orgasms during intercourse and they still consider it a pleasurable experience.

But when a woman—or a man, for that matter—has an orgasm, it not only feels good, it also can be profoundly relaxing for him/her. Often, it decreases stress and helps a woman sleep better.

Plus, levels of the hormone prolactin go up after orgasm—and that's true for both men

Lauren Streicher, MD, clinical professor of obstetrics and gynecology at Northwestern University Feinberg School of Medicine and medical director of Northwestern Medicine Center for Sexual Health and Menopause, both in Chicago. She is author of *Sex Rx: Hormones, Health, and Your Best Sex Ever.* DrStreicher.com and women—which increases bonding with your partner. Men also really like their partners to be orgasmic and to enjoy themselves, and it can strengthen a relationship.

Many women, particularly as they get older, are distressed that they can no longer achieve orgasms. Some are not able to have an orgasm at all, while others find that their orgasms are not as strong as they once were and/or take a very long time to happen. Most women I see with these issues used to have orgasms just fine, and then something changed.

The medical term for this is "female orgasmic dysfunction." Often, it's related to menopause. That said, if a woman doesn't have orgasms but it doesn't bother her, she does not have a dysfunction.

How does menopause affect sexual pleasure and orgasms?

There are several ways. One is a decline in libido that is related to the decline in estrogen that starts around perimenopause and continues for the many years that follow. That estrogen drop also reduces genital blood flow—and the ability to have an orgasm is tied to good blood flow.

It's similar to erectile dysfunction in men. Also, medical conditions such as cardiovascular disease, diabetes or pelvic surgery can reduce blood flow. For a woman, good blood flow to the clitoris allows the tissue to become engorged, aroused and stimulated and keeps nerve endings healthy and responsive.

How exactly does a vibrator address all that?

Most women need direct clitoral stimulation to have an orgasm. For younger women, manual or oral stimulation, or even just the contact during intercourse, can be sufficient. But as women age, they may need something to increase the intensity of the sensation. Even women who are not able to have an orgasm with other kinds of stimulation very often can have them with vibrators.

The clitoris actually has receptors that specifically respond to vibration. That vibrating stimulation also increases blood flow, which in turn increases lubrication. If it is a dildo-type vibrator, regular use also can help maintain elasticity of vaginal tissues.

If it doesn't seem like a comfortable topic, how can a woman bring up to her partner the idea of using a vibrator?

She might say something like, "I love when we have sex, but I think it would be fun to try something different, and I hear that using a vibrator can make sex more pleasurable." She might mention that she read a health article—such as this one—reporting that vibrators can help women her age and that many women use them.

Aren't many men put off by the idea of their partners using vibrators because it implies that the men aren't "enough"?

That's sometimes true, but not as often as you might think. In one national survey, published in *Journal of Sex & Marital Therapy*, 70% of men said that vibrators are not intimidating. In fact, a man can take the lead on this and say to his female partner, "I've heard it's much more pleasurable for many women with a vibrator, and I'd love for you to have that kind of pleasure, so I bought you one." How any particular couple handles this topic is very individual—in some, the woman takes the lead, in some the man, and some couples like to shop for vibrators together.

Of course, vibrators also can enhance same-sex relationships. Nor does anyone's sexuality have to stop when the person's not having sex with a partner. By discovering more about your own body and how to sexually satisfy yourself, you'll facilitate your ability to achieve orgasm in an intimate relationship, too.

Can older women who have never had orgasms start having them?

Absolutely. A typical woman who has never had an orgasm—and who is likely to be quite reticent about all these matters that we've been discussing—just needs "permission" from a health professional to use a vibrator…and in some cases, a little help finding her clitoris. And then, she usually is just fine.

Do you hereby give all our readers permission?

I do!

More from Lauren Streicher, MD

The Doctor's Guide to Sexual Aids

One type of vibrator that I recommend is a small, external bullet-style clitoral vibrator that you can hold on the right spot—either on your own or while you're having intercourse with your partner. There also are couples' vibrators that are U-shaped. They slide in the vagina so that the man can put his penis in at the same time as the woman is getting direct clitoral stimulation.

Many women also benefit greatly from lubricants after menopause. For intercourse, I recommend silicone-based lubricants—they're very slippery and won't damage vaginal tissue. Water-based lubricants are good, too, and are the best choice if you are using a vibrator or other sex toy, because silicone lubricants do not mix with silicone toys.

If you are using a water-based lubricant, however, be sure to choose one that has low osmolality—a measure of dissolved particles. Many popular lubricants have high osmolality, but that can dry out tissue (the opposite of what you are trying to accomplish!) and increase the chance of irritation and infection.

Recommended: Water-based low-osmolality lubes include Pulse H2Oh!, Good Clean Love, Sylk, System JO and Slippery Stuff. When using a vibrator, use a water-based lube only—silicone-based lubes can damage the silicone used in many vibrators.

Steer clear of lubes with chemicals in them for flavor or warming—these can damage delicate vaginal tissue. But warming your lube is a really nice option. Pulse is a lubricant-warming dispenser sold with low-osmolality water- or silicone-based lubricant pods.

Many women are nervous about shopping for vibrators.

Tip: Look for women-friendly erotic shops near where you live. There's also a big selection of products available online, of course. That can be overwhelming, but if you shop for my recommendations above, it should be less daunting. I don't have any financial connections to any of these companies.

The Secret to a Better Sex Life for Women with Sleep Apnea

The study titled, "Association of Continuous Positive Airway Pressure Treatment with Sexual Quality of Life in Patients with Sleep Apnea," led by researchers at University of Washington, Seattle, and published in *JAMA Otolaryngology-Head & Neck Surgery.*

If someone asked you to give some sage advice on ways to boost a couple's sex life, a clunky CPAP mask probably wouldn't even make your list. But a surprising new study shows that this device might be just what's needed—at least for women with sleep apnea.

That's good news for females who have this sleep-disturbing breathing disorder, but why didn't men get the same boost?

The researchers had set out to investigate how CPAP (known clinically as continuous positive airway pressure) affects sexual quality of life for both male and female sleep apnea sufferers. The disorder is known to reduce libido in men and women and contribute to erectile dysfunction, but most of the previous research has focused on men—perhaps because fewer women have the condition.

It was a good bet that the use of CPAP, which delivers continuous air to keep the airway open and prevent snoring, gasping and waking up, would improve the sex lives of sleep apnea patients who used the device. After all, a good night's sleep works wonders in knocking out the troubling symptoms of sleep apnea, including daytime sleepiness, depression and irritability.

But not all the findings lined up the way the researchers had expected.

Study details: A total of 182 men and women who were newly prescribed CPAP to treat obstructive sleep apnea took part in the research, and information about the participants' quality of life, including their sex lives, was collected before and after the nearly three-year study.

Researchers then analyzed the difference in sexual quality of life scores between the 72 CPAP "users" who wore the mask for more than four hours per night and the 110 "nonusers" who wore the mask for fewer than 30 minutes per night. The CPAP users came out on top—averaging 0.6 points (12%) higher (on a scale of zero to 5) than the scores for the nonusers.

Here's the surprising kicker: With further analysis, the researchers discovered that the higher sex scores applied only to the women in the study—not the men. This finding contradicted many of the earlier studies, which tended to focus on men with sleep apnea and a sexual dysfunction such as erectile dysfunction.

Compared with the current research, the men who were previously studied "might have been starting from a relatively worse-off place, which may have resulted in higher self-reported improvement," explained Sebastian Jara, MD, the study's lead author and a resident physician in otolaryngology-head and neck surgery with UW Medicine/Seattle.

Even so, the health benefits of CPAP, which include reduced risk for heart disease, stroke and diabetes, are so well-recognized that men with sleep apnea should still be motivated to use CPAP—even if this study didn't show that their sex lives would improve.

A larger future study may indicate that both sexes enjoy better sleep—and a better sex life—with CPAP.

Bottom line: If your doctor prescribes CPAP to treat obstructive sleep apnea, it's definitely worth using. The mask may not be

a turn-on, but a well-rested partner with a renewed sex drive certainly can be!

Natural Pain Relief for Ovarian Cysts

Laurie Steelsmith, ND, LAc, naturopathic physician, acupuncturist and medical director of Steelsmith Natural Health Center in Honolulu, Hawaii. She is coauthor of Natural Choices for Women's Health *and writes the blog "Natural Healing Secrets for Women." DrSteelsmith.com*

O varian cysts are fairly common among women of childbearing age, but most are small and harmless. If symptoms, such as pelvic pain or bloating, occur, they tend to be subtle...but not always, depending on the type of cysts that you have.

Cysts generally fall into one of two categories—both of which are related to a woman's monthly menstrual cycle. A follicular cyst occurs when a woman's egg is not released from the follicle and continues to grow...and a corpus luteum cyst develops when a follicle releases an egg, as normally occurs during ovulation, but the follicle accumulates fluid that turns into a cyst. Both of these types of cysts typically disappear on their own within a few months. Other, less common types of ovarian cysts, such as the multiple small cysts (often called a "string of pearls") that are symptomatic of polycystic ovarian syndrome (PCOS), may require a different form of treatment than the "watchful waiting" approach often used for follicular and corpus luteum cysts.

Regardless of the type of cyst you have, you'll want relief if you're experiencing pelvic pain, painful intercourse or uncomfortable bloating. Fortunately, there are natural therapies available to both ease discomfort and promote hormonal balance—this, in turn, will also help reduce bloating associated with ovarian cysts. Your hormones play an important role in the smooth transition of follicle development, the release of a healthy egg and the production of progesterone. Most cysts are caused by an imbalance in the orchestration of a woman's hormones. If there is too much estrogen, cysts can form...if a woman doesn't ovulate (which results in low progesterone), a cyst can form...and if she has too much testosterone, as is the case in PCOS, she can form small cysts.

Large cysts will most likely need to be treated surgically (these typically fall in the greater than 5-centimeter category). Smaller cysts can often be helped with natural therapies. Because the majority of cysts disappear on their own, I often recommend to my patients that they get through any associated discomfort by using castor oil packs each night for up to two weeks, which can ease pain by increasing circulation and moving lymph through the pelvis. Whenever there is stagnation of blood, body fluids or lymph—or what we call qi in Traditional Chinese Medicine (TCM)—there can be pain. The castor oil pack increases circulation and blood flow through the area, decreasing stagnation.

To make a castor oil pack: Rub a teaspoon of castor oil onto your lower abdomen, then place a piece of clean flannel or cotton on the area. Cover this with a heating pad or hot-water bottle. The heat itself—with a heating pad or hot bath (preferably with Epsom salts)—may alleviate pelvic pain.

Important: If you experience sudden, sharp pain in your lower belly with vaginal bleeding—especially if it's accompanied by fever or vomiting—get to an emergency room or call your doctor. This could signal a ruptured cyst that requires prompt treatment including ultrasound to monitor internal bleeding and, in rare cases, surgery to remove the cyst.

To improve your overall ovarian health, which will also help ease your symptoms, I urge you to discuss the classic herbal tonic known as Turska's formula, which can effectively treat ovarian cysts, with your naturopathic physician. (To find a naturopathic physician near you, check the website of the American Association of Naturopathic Physicians.)

A number of other herbal remedies can also be taken to promote hormonal balance, increase circulation to your reproductive organs, and—importantly—reduce ovarian pain. These include maca...milk thistle...black cohosh...and, my favorite herbal supplement for hormonal balance, chaste tree berry (also known as Vitex). Chaste tree berry has a long history of supporting fertility by promoting healthy ovulation.

Diet can also make a big difference. Organic vegetables, wild-caught salmon, flaxseed and quality fats (such as avocado) support hormonal equilibrium and may reduce your symptoms, while magnesium-rich almonds may help ease pain. Chamomile tea may diminish the dull ache that can accompany ovarian cysts.

And even though you may be tempted to stay in bed due to your discomfort, exercise can provide enormous relief. Yoga, in particular, may offer the very release from tension that you might need. Last but not least, strive to stay relaxed. In TCM, ovarian issues are due to liver imbalances and qi stagnation driven by stress.

Think You Can't Get an STD at Your Age? Think Again!

Edward Hook, III, MD, professor in the division of infectious diseases at the University of Alabama at Birmingham School of Medicine, codirector of the UAB Center for Social Medicine and STDs and director of the STD Control Program for the Jefferson County (Alabama) Department of Health.

You might think that sexually transmitted diseases, or STDs, are health issues that mostly teens and young adults have to worry about. But anyone of any age who's not in a totally (and we mean totally) monogamous relationship where both partners have been tested for STDs is at risk.

Right now, there's a dramatic surge in cases of chlamydia, gonorrhea and syphilis in the US, with all three hitting record numbers in 2016 and again in 2017. The number of people over age 45 getting these diseases more than doubled between 2012 and 2016, according to the latest record-keeping from the CDC. Better news is that HIV is on the decline—but it's still a concern along with HPV, the human papillomavirus, which causes cervical cancer in women (and can cause other cancers in women and men), and trichomoniasis, a sexually transmitted parasite that can increase your risk of getting an STD including HIV.

What in the world is going on? Put simply, Americans have become lax about practicing safe sex because of advances in the treatment of HIV—the fear of getting AIDs from HIV is not as strong as it used to be. We have, as a country, gone backwards in protecting ourselves. But here's what hasn't changed: STDs can still be dangerous or even deadly…you can never fully rid yourself of some of them once you have them…and most STDs don't produce early symptoms, so you can't "spot" warning signs in a potential partner any more than you can in yourself, leaving you open to infections.

If you're at a time in your life when you don't want to be in a serious relationship yet want to enjoy an active sex life, here's how to keep yourself from becoming another STD statistic…

•**Keep practicing safer sex.** Use a condom every time, especially if you don't know for sure that your partner has been screened and is negative for all STDs. This also keeps your partner safe should you have an infection you're unaware of. Condoms alone don't do it, though—that's why the term is "safer"—it's not possible to protect yourself 100%.

Condom use is even lower among people engaging in oral sex than in purely genital contact. Since more and more STDs appear to be transmitted through oral contact, infections could be prevented with use of condoms and oral barriers or dams (placed over the vulva during oral sex).

•**Get regular sexual-health checkups.** This includes a physical exam and screening tests. Advancing age might not make it feel any less awkward to talk to your doctor—primary, ob-gyn or urologist—about your private life, but he/she needs to know if you have new partners because this helps determine whether and when you should have STD tests.

This talk about your sex life need not be complex. Just two facts will tell your doctor whether additional history is needed: How many sexual partners you have had in the past six months…and whether you think that any of your partners currently has or might have had other partners in the past six months.

•**STD screening isn't painful or complex.** Women are tested for chlamydia, gonorrhea, trichomoniasis and HPV with a vaginal swab or a urine sample. Men are tested for gonorrhea and chlamydia with a urine sample… trichomoniasis is harder to detect in men, but a urine sample or swab can be used if there's a discharge. Both men and women are tested for syphilis and HIV with a blood sample.

If you and your partner decide to be exclusive—and avoid condoms and/or engage in oral sex in the process—you should both have a sexual-health checkup first. Remember that monogamy doesn't confer protection from an STD that came from a former partner.

Putting an End to Painful Sex

Laurie Steelsmith, ND, LAc, naturopathic physician and acupuncturist. She is coauthor of three books—the *Natural Choices for Women's Health, Great Sex, Naturally* and *Growing Younger Every Day*. DrSteel smith.com

The Patient: Sara, a 43-year-old attorney and mother of one.

Why she came to see me: Following an unexpected divorce after the birth of her daughter, Sara deliberately chose to be single and celibate for three years—she wanted to focus on her career and child, and to take the necessary time to grieve her marriage. But when an attorney named Seth joined her firm, they struck up a flirtation that led to four months of courtship.

When Sara walked into my office, they'd been intimate but had had sexual intercourse only once. "It was dreadful," Sara said. "I love him, and I see a future with him, but the sex itself was excruciating." Pelvic pain during intercourse was accompanied by burning, stinging, achiness, throbbing, and a feeling of being "raw." A self-described "problem solver," Sara was determined to seek out natural help not only for her relationship with Seth but also, and most importantly, with herself.

How I evaluated her: Sara and I began with a candid discussion about sex and her overall health. Prior to her pregnancy, she and her ex-husband had relished a robust sex life. After their daughter's birth, however, she found herself turning away from him. Stretch marks, a "sagging belly," residual weight gain, and new-mom fatigue made her feel far from desirable. Moreover, she'd had a grueling labor—so much so that the mere idea of intercourse filled her with anxiety. When she and her husband did have sex again before their separation, it was agonizing. While certainly not the reason for their unanticipated but amicable split, Sara had become fearful of sex ever since, even admitting it may have been one of the reasons she shunned the idea of dating.

Outside of the bedroom, Sara was in terrific health: She practiced yoga daily, went on long hikes, swam, and played in the park with her daughter. Sara rarely drank, and followed a nutrient-rich, flexitarian diet. In addition, her menstrual cycle had returned to normal two years earlier.

To rule out any underlying health problems, I ordered a full gynecological exam and a urine test. In particular, I wanted to test for a UTI (bladder infection), ovarian disorders and cysts, a yeast infection, sexually transmitted diseases, and cervical dysplasia (abnormal cells that grow on the cervix and can become cancerous). When these tests came back normal, I also ordered a 24-hour urine collection test to evaluate for oxalates.

What my evaluation revealed: To our relief, most of Sara's examinations came out clean, but my inability to see a blatant reason for her pain was indicative of a pervasive problem. Pelvic pain—which can be experienced in the vulva, vagina, or anywhere else in the pelvis—can be difficult to diagnose or treat. Solving pelvic pain can not only transform one's sex life, it can also unburden one's libido and encourage well-being.

Given the symptoms Sara described, as well as a vaginal exam that revealed slightly inflamed, swollen tissues (though no latent signs of tearing from childbirth) and the high levels of oxalates in her urine, I suspected she had vulvodynia—a rather elusive pain syndrome, characterized by irritation, tenderness, burning, and painful intercourse, that may affect as many as six million women worldwide. While the cause of vulvodynia remains inconclusive, researchers list possibilities that range from frequent antibiotic use to trauma—like the arduous delivery Sara experienced.

How we addressed her problem: To take Sara from pelvic pain to pelvic pleasure involved a multi-pronged approach…

•**Removing possible irritants.** I encouraged her to switch her chemically-laden detergent to an all-natural, perfume-free brand, and to use soft, unscented toilet paper to minimize the risk of irritating her vulvar and vaginal tissues. Likewise, I advised her to start using chlorine- and perfume-free tampons and pads. Since she both swam and worked out regularly, I asked her to remove wet or damp clothing (such as her swimsuit and yoga pants) immediately after use, and to start wearing all-cotton underwear. Further, I suggested refraining from using bubble bath, which can intensify symptoms.

•**Low-oxalate diet.** The late Clive Solomon, PhD—a researcher specializing in vulvar pain—discovered that many women who suffer from vulvodynia (VVD) secrete, like Sara, high amounts of oxalates in their urine. (Whether oxalates are a cause of VVD or simply aggravate vulvar tissue that is already irritated is not known.) Oxalates are commonly found in many foods we ordinarily deem "good" for us: leafy greens, soybeans, wheat germ, leeks, green peppers, beets, sweet potatoes, berries, and peanuts, to name a few. If one's vulvar tissues are unhealthy, oxalates can generate irritation, histamine release, and pain.

●**The right supplements.** I recommended that Sara take 200 mg of calcium citrate three times a day, as calcium citrate can reduce the effects of oxalates in the body, making it more difficult for them to irritate one's tissues. Her supplement protocol also included taking 250 mg of N-acetyl glucosamine (NAG) twice a day to strengthen the connective tissues of her vulva. I also urged her to begin taking a probiotic to encourage more "friendly" gut bacteria. Intestinal problems can exacerbate—even create—oxalate sensitivity.

●**Physical therapy.** I advised Sara to work once week with a therapist who specializes in women's pelvic pain. In addition to muscle and soft-tissue release techniques, the therapist also did biofeedback with Sara to help her strengthen and release the muscles of her lower pelvis.

●**Vaginal steam baths.** Traditionally used in Korea and parts of South Africa, vaginal steam baths can loosen and relax one's pubococcygeus (PC) muscle, promote increased circulation (always a boon for better sex), and may allow for easier penetration during intercourse for those with pelvic pain.

●**All-natural lubricant.** To encourage delightful, pain-free sex, I proposed trying a product such as Aloe Cadabra, to both replicate the effects of Sara's natural lubrication and to hydrate her vulvar and vaginal tissues.

●**More foreplay.** Abstinence can change a woman's sexual response time (in short, extra arousal may be needed).

●**Talking openly about sex—and more.** I gently encouraged her to communicate with

Seth to nurture their relationship as a whole. For as helpful as my suggestions might have been, there is no greater aphrodisiac and pain reliever than a loving, solid, and honest partnership.

The patient's progress: Taking her sexual health into her own hands proved to be hugely beneficial to Sara. Within two weeks of starting our treatment plan, she returned glowing from head to toe. Changing her diet had not only mitigated her pelvic pain but it also led to smoother skin and smoother digestion. She found vaginal steam baths particularly calming and nourishing, allowing her much-needed time to focus on her body's needs and wants (her favorite bath-enhancement was rose essential oil—a fitting choice, given that rose can bolster feelings of safety and self-esteem). As for sex—and her relationship with Seth? "It is so much better," she said, "most likely because I've never felt so empowered."

The Right Medication to Improve Sex after Heart Failure

The right medication improves sex for heart failure patients. It also increases energy for household chores and walking/jogging. The drug Entresto—a combination of *sacubitril* and *valsartan*—was more effective than the standard drug treatment (*enalapril*) and has been shown to help patients live longer.

Caution: It sometimes can reduce blood pressure too much.

Scott D. Solomon, MD, is professor of medicine at Harvard Medical School, Boston, and senior author of a study of 7,618 heart failure patients, published in *JAMA Cardiology*.

Drug-Free Help for PCOS

Laurie Steelsmith, ND, LAc, naturopathic physician and acupuncturist. She is coauthor of three books—the *Natural Choices for Women's Health, Great Sex, Naturally* and *Growing Younger Every Day.* DrSteelsmith.com

The patient: "Simona," a 35-year-old dancer and business executive.

Why she came to see me: Simona came to my clinic because of infrequent periods that were suddenly causing her concern. Throughout adulthood, her periods had arrived every other month; in the last two years, however, her periods had dwindled down to three or four annually. While her primary care physician had urged her to take birth control pills to help regulate her cycle, she was keen on taking a different approach—one that would not only feel more in tune with her health-centric, organic lifestyle, but would also address the reason beneath her irregularity. She and her fiancé were also planning on trying for a child in the next year or two, and the Pill simply didn't fit into their "long-term plans."

How I evaluated her: An in-depth discussion revealed that irregular periods were not the only source of Simona's distress. She was also experiencing mood changes, headaches, an increase in facial hair that sent her to her esthetician more frequently, and sporadic acne. She further complained of extremely tender breasts 10 days to two weeks before her period started…bloating…day-time fatigue and nighttime insomnia…increased anger and "the blues"…and dark patches of skin. When her period did arrive, it was the heaviest it had ever been. Having spent much of her life on the slender side, she was also shocked to find that she'd recently gained 12 pounds—a "mystery" to her given that neither her diet nor her commitment to dancing had changed.

Five years earlier, she and her ex-husband had stopped using birth control because they were open to the possibility of getting pregnant but nothing happened. At the time, she hadn't thought that there was anything particularly wrong and chalked it up to lifelong irregular cycles, problems in her relationship and the feeling that it "just wasn't meant to be." After the stress of her divorce coupled by an increase in her workload, she noticed that her periods "made an appearance" less and less. She "managed to ignore this"—that is, until her recent inexplicable weight gain, even less frequent periods and changes in appearance compelled her to take action. That, and the man she'd recently gotten engaged to dreamed of having children with her—a dream she "passionately shared."

Simona followed a low-fat, vegetarian diet that included a lot of rice, pasta, potatoes, beans, salads, protein bars and shakes. She also claimed to have constant sugar cravings, which she would often try to satisfy with fruit, "healthy" cookies and cereal.

Following our discussion, I gave her a full pelvic exam, including a PAP smear and a pregnancy test for which she tested negative. I also ordered a blood test to evaluate her estrogen, progesterone, testosterone and DHEA levels as well as her fasting insulin, fasting glucose and hemoglobin A1c (HbA1c). Finally, I ordered a thyroid panel and a transvaginal ultrasound.

What my evaluation revealed: I called Simona immediately after receiving the results from her ultrasound as the images exposed multiple small cysts on her ovaries. Dubbed a "string of pearls," these cysts are often indicative of a hormone disorder. Further, while her thyroid test was normal, she had low levels of estrogen and progesterone as well as elevated androgens—namely, high testosterone and DHEA levels. She was also showing sign of insulin resistance, or metabolic syndrome, as revealed in her fasting insulin, glucose and HbA1c.

The combination of Simona's symptoms and results led me to diagnose her with Polycystic Ovarian Syndrome. Commonly known as PCOS, the hormonal condition, which affects 1 in 10 women of childbearing age, is characterized by a surplus of androgens (what we consider "male hormones") and often results in infertility, metabolic problems and weight gain. In addition to irregular periods, acne, hirsutism (excessive body hair), headaches and mood issues, PCOS can cause precisely these type of cysts—fluid-filled sacs that are prevalent among women in their reproductive years.

How I addressed her problem: As with all of my patients, I outlined a strategy to manage Simona's PCOS from a natural, holistic perspective.

PCOS—which is often referred to as "the silent disorder"—may not only exhibit complications in the present but can also lead to issues down the line, including high blood sugar, mood disorders, heart disease and type-2 diabetes. This is because insulin resistance underlies nearly all cases of PCOS. By supporting Simona's ability to increase insulin sensitivity, she would have enhanced hormone balance, improved ovulation—and, thus, a better chance at getting pregnant when she and her fiancé were ready.

We began with a look at her diet. While her daily salads were admirable, there was room for improvement. Given that women with PCOS often have higher rates of inflammation and oxidative stress, I urged Simona to shift away from the high-carbohydrate foods (rice, pasta, potatoes, protein bars, shakes) that had served as cornerstones of her diet to an eating regime that would support insulin sensitivity. To that end, I encouraged her to religiously fill her plate with anti-inflammatory, blood sugar-stabilizing foods such as organic vegetables, wild-caught fish, organic lean chicken, nuts and seeds, and "quality" fats like avocados and olive oil. I also instructed her to rid herself of sugar, high-glycemic fruit, preservatives and excessive caffeine—all of which can impact hormone levels.

We turned to other aspects of her lifestyle next. On average, she slept five to six hours a night—an amount that's far below what's prescribed (and ideal). I urged her to start prioritizing sleep as much as she prioritized dancing as sleep deprivation can result in elevated cortisol, which can disturb hormone equilibrium. To address her level of stress in general, Simona agreed to start delegating work tasks when she could and to take on only as many classes per week as she could realistically handle.

I also prescribed botanical medicines. First, I urged her to get a daily of dose of spearmint tea. As the National Institutes of Health reveals, spearmint tea can have anti-androgen effects, which help foster hormone harmony. It also aids with acne.

Second, I put her on an herbal formula called Ovablend. Created by Vitanica, Ovablend was formulated by the esteemed naturopathic physician Dr. Tori Hudson to support women with PCOS. The formula contains nutrients to support healthy insulin response, blood sugar control and herbs to balance hormones. It's used along with Soy Choice, a product containing non-GMO soy isoflavones to facilitate better hormone regulation.

Next, I recommended a supplement called Sensitol. This form of inositol (classified as one of the B vitamins) can help "pop open" insulin receptors, which could further encourage hormone balance.

I also prescribed two months of weekly acupuncture sessions. In Traditional Chinese Medicine, PCOS is considered a damp condition with stagnant energy in the lower pelvis, and I have seen acupuncture profoundly influence women's ovulation and fertility. (Research substantiates this by showing that acupuncture can be an effective treatment in regulating menstrual cycles.)

Finally, I explained that if she didn't respond to this approach, we would need to consider taking a prescription medication called Metformin. Primarily used in the treatment of type-2 diabetes, it can also significantly impact healthy ovulation and fertility in women with PCOS.

The patient's progress: Simona responded beautifully to her treatment protocol—so much so we were able to shelve the idea of medication (while also remaining watchful of her progress). She returned to her "normal" body weight, her acne diminished and, within a few months, she started having cycles every 40 days. A follow-up ultrasound also revealed that her cysts had disappeared. Furthermore, her hormone test demonstrated that while her androgens were still elevated, they were much less so—a solid indication that she was well on her way to greater hormone balance. As such, the litany of symptoms she first reported—from mood changes to heavy periods—had also subsided. While not "cured" of her condition, she claimed that the lifestyle changes she'd implemented were buoying her hope for the future—and allowing her to handle PCOS with the very grace she practiced on the dance floor.

Five Surprising Causes of Postmenopausal Bleeding That Aren't Cancer

Frederick "Ricky" Friedman Jr, MD, associate professor, Icahn School of Medicine at Mount Sinai, director, division of obstetrics and division of generalists, department of obstetrics, gynecology and reproductive science, Mount Sinai Health System, New York City.

If you've reached menopause, you probably thought that your days of any bleeding down there were over—but then you saw blood. You might have even panicked because you know that can be a sign of cancer.

But take a deep breath, says Frederick Friedman, Jr, MD, director of obstetrics at the Mount Sinai Health System in New York City. While there is a link between bleeding and cancer in the uterine lining (endometrial cancer), in 90% of postmenopausal women when bleeding occurs, it's something else.

Note: Even if it is just spotting, any postmenopausal bleeding should prompt a visit to your doctor to figure out what is going on. If you can see your doctor while you are actively bleeding, it is easier to identify the cause.

That being said, here are some of the surprising reasons a postmenopausal woman can have bleeding…

You Have an STD

You might not realize that you're at risk for a sexually transmitted disease during this chapter of your life, but if you're not in a long-standing, monogamous relationship, you are. There's been a dramatic rise in STDs among older Americans in recent years. A lot of this can be traced to increased sexual activity because of drugs, such as Viagra, that make men more able to have sex, but that's not the only reason for the increase—there's a female connection, too. After menopause, vaginal tissue grows thin due to the lack of the female sex hormone estrogen, making it more prone to tearing, which can leave you more vulnerable to an STD. Gonorrhea, chlamydia, herpes and syphilis can all cause bleeding, especially early on. Other symptoms that may suggest your bleeding is an STD include discolored cervical mucus and pain during urination. Your doctor will ask for a urine sample or swab your cervical discharge and send it off to the lab for a diagnosis.

It's Really a Bladder Infection

You may think the bleeding is coming from your vagina, cervix or uterus, but it may be trickling down from your bladder. That's because bladder infections or the bladder condition interstitial cystitis can sometimes cause bleeding. Other clues include needing to go to the bathroom often and urgently and/or pelvic pain. A urine sample will identify a bladder infection. Additional testing may be needed for suspected interstitial cystitis including a biopsy of tissue from the bladder wall.

Yes, It Can Be a Polyp

Polyps inside the uterus or cervical canal are fairly common, but the amount of blood they cause can be scary, especially after menopause. As your uterine lining thins due to the drop in estrogen, these polyps also grow thin, and your body may shed the surface of the polyp—causing the bleeding. It's usually light spotting or staining, but at times it can be surprisingly heavy. Your doctor will run a series of tests including a sonogram to locate the polyp and likely remove it to make sure it's not cancerous.

Hormones Gone Haywire

While vaginal or endometrial thinning can lead to postmenopausal bleeding due to atrophy or too little estrogen, being on hormone replacement therapy can do so for the opposite reason: The lining of the uterus—the endometrium—thickens, and then bleeds. In the perimenopause, many women are still making some estrogen, which causes the lining to thicken due to cell growth. However, they might not be ovulating. Since progesterone is generally made by the ovary only after ovulation, the "unopposed estrogen" causes a very thickened lining of growing cells. This is called endometrial hyperplasia, and this condition often occurs when a woman has too much estrogen and not enough progesterone to balance it out (hormone replacement therapy that includes both estrogen and progesterone can help avoid this). The uterine lining may shed in this circumstance for several reasons. If the lining is too thick, the buildup may outgrow its blood supply and be shed. Similarly, as the hyperplasia develops, the attachment of cells to each other weakens. It's important to find out whether hormone replacement is causing your bleeding because endometrial hyperplasia has been linked to the development of endometrial cancer.

It's Really a Hemorrhoid

If you see blood on toilet paper or in your toilet bowl, it could actually be rectal bleeding from hemorrhoids. Other possible causes of rectal bleeding include a fissure or cut, a bacterial infection or inflammatory bowel disease. If the source of your bleeding turns out to be rectal, your doctor will likely suggest a stool test and, if it could be more than a hemorrhoid, possibly an imaging test such as a colonoscopy to find the cause.

Every one of the above causes of postmenopausal bleeding is far more common than uterine cancer, so again, if you've seen blood, don't panic...but do see your doctor right away.

Do Probiotics Really Improve Vaginal Health?

Mary Jane Minkin, MD, clinical professor of obstetrics, gynecology and reproductive services at Yale School of Medicine, New Haven, Connecticut.

Research has shown that an oral probiotic supplement can help ease certain digestive conditions, such as irritable bowel syndrome—and it can help anyone maintain a healthy balance in the gut for proper digestion. But these supplements promote vaginal health, too, by helping to prevent bacterial infections, known as bacterial vaginosis (BV).

Here's why: Though most women don't realize it, the bacteria that we have in our vaginas are the same bacteria that we have in our guts. A healthy balance of the so-called "good" and "bad" bacteria in the vagina contributes to a normal vaginal pH (level of acidity). Many factors, including the use of oral steroid drugs and the hormonal changes of menopause, can disrupt the vaginal pH level, putting a woman at higher risk for BV. Antibiotics, in particular, can affect the vaginal pH since these drugs kill not only bad bacteria but also good bacteria, such as lactobacilli, that protect vaginal health.

Taking a probiotic supplement will boost protective lactobacilli levels. But one of the problems with taking a probiotic is that there are many different strains of lactobacilli, and some seem to be more helpful than others.

Research has found that various types of lactobacilli benefit vaginal health, including lactobacillus reuteri, salvarius and/or plantarum. Several studies have shown that the lactobacilli found in the oral feminine probiotic supplement RepHresh Pro-B, including lactobacillus rhamnosus, also promote a healthy balance of vaginal bacteria and yeast.

Important: Probiotics are generally safe for everyone to take, but it's best to check with your doctor before using any new supplement—especially if you take medication or have a chronic health condition.

Note: Yogurt does not contain the species of lactobacillus that helps keep the vagina healthy. However, some strains of yogurt may be good for the gut—and yogurt is generally a good source of dietary calcium.

The Detox Cure for Irritable Bowel Syndrome

Laurie Steelsmith, ND, LAc, naturopathic physician and acupuncturist and author of the blog "Natural Healing Secrets for Women" at BottomLineInc.com. She is coauthor of three books—*Natural Choices for Women's Health, Great Sex, Naturally* and *Growing Younger Every Day.* DrSteelsmith.com

---

Why she came to see me: It was immediately clear that Carolyn was troubled when she arrived at my office. Hunched over, with a slight grimace on her face, she told me about the bout of intestinal distress she'd recently experienced, a spell that had been going on for the last two months and that was marked primarily by persistent bloating, gas and constipation—in short, nearly the entire gamut of digestive problems. While her primary care physician had given her a "probable diagnosis" of irritable bowel syndrome, she intuited that something else was amiss, and wanted to address the issue naturally before turning to more medication.

How I evaluated her: Over the course of a thorough discussion, I learned that Carolyn had endured complications with her gut health since her late teens. That was the era in which her pediatrician first prescribed Carolyn antibiotics to treat her acne. "The medicine didn't clear it up; instead, it caused some major side effects in my digestion," she said. Nevertheless, she heeded different doctors' orders throughout her twenties (and part of her thirties) and continued to try antibiotics and other medications to remedy the acne

that persisted into adulthood. For nearly six years, however, both her acne and her stomach troubles had diminished. Now that she was up for tenure at a private university—which naturally arrived with a great deal of stress—her stomach woes had returned with a vengeance.

"I've become so uncomfortable that I don't want to put on a bathing suit, let alone participate with my paddling team," she said. What's more, the stress caused by both her career and her digestive health was compelling her to turn to sweets...and often. "It's ridiculous, I know," she admitted, noting that she'd gained weight and wasn't exercising as much as she used to. She also mentioned that she'd been feeling simultaneously apathetic and anxious, which only exacerbated her urge to hunker down with cookies, candy and Netflix. It wasn't until a recent, severe stomach ache forced her to miss an important faculty meeting that she realized she needed to get help—and fast.

In addition to reviewing her symptoms and their patterns, I conducted a full physical exam, which included a blood test to determine if she had anemia (a relatively unknown side effect of IBS). Furthermore, I ordered a lactose intolerance test, a stool culture to assess for intestinal flora imbalances and parasites, and a blood test, through ELISA/ACT Biotechnologies, to see if she had any food allergies.

The test I ordered looks at "delayed food reactivities," which means that a patient can eat a food on Sunday but have an immunological reaction on Monday, Tuesday or Wednesday—or, to phrase it differently, anywhere from 24 to 72 hours after the food was consumed. As I discussed with Carolyn, the fact that food can take time to present adverse reactions is one of the reasons it can be so difficult to determine which foods a person is sensitive to (tests such as these are akin to elimination/challenge diets, as well as blood tests that address immediate reactions to a food). Further, as I also explained, most cases of IBS are associated with delayed food reactions—and removing these foods can have profound health benefits.

What my evaluation revealed: Overall, Carolyn was mostly healthy—she was neither anemic nor lactose intolerant, and she didn't have parasites. At the same time, her tests did demonstrate that she had an intestinal flora imbalance—namely, yeast overgrowth and food reactivities.

Based on her symptoms and medical history, it was abundantly clear that the medications she'd taken over the years had done a number on her digestive health. What's more, the specific foods she was reactive to were foods that she consumed regularly, primarily gluten products like crackers, pasta and those aforementioned cookies. There were other compounds she was reactive to as well, including paprika and a food additive called guar gum, which we discovered she inadvertently consumed twice a day in her morning and afternoon protein shakes. This, too, was presumably contributing to her symptoms.

How I addressed her problem: As I explained to Carolyn, digestion consists of several processes to make what you eat a part of every cell in your body. When the digestive system becomes compromised—whether due to medications, a diet that includes low-nutrient, high-sugar, high-calorie foods, an allergy, or an infection—it can wreak havoc on your whole health, including your spirit and motivation.

A large part of this comes down to the small intestine. Your small intestine has a difficult and complex job sorting through everything you eat and separating what should be absorbed from what should be eliminated. If your small intestine, like Carolyn's, is chronically irritated, it will allow more toxins and other undesirable chemicals to pass into your bloodstream. This can lead to food allergies, poor liver detoxification, fatigue, skin rashes and acne as well as a host of additional complications—not to mention recurrent, even debilitating, intestinal upset.

Her large intestine had also been compromised over the years, mainly by an excessive amount of yeast, which was most likely due to years of taking antibiotics. This was a huge contributing factor to her gas, bloating and constipation as well.

To this end, I put Carolyn on a one-month intestinal detox—a strategy that would help restore the friendly bacteria in her gut, decrease her discomfiting symptoms and return her to health.

This detox entailed a low-carbohydrate diet that consisted of less than 50 grams of carbohydrates per day. I have dubbed this a modified ketogenic diet—a plan that follows the traditional keto diet's requisite of eliminating carbs (albeit with a bit more wiggle room) and deriving the lion's share of one's calories from healthy fats such as olive oil and avocadoes. (My amended plan also includes adequate protein and lots of low-carb, fiber-rich vegetables like broccoli and spinach, which would, in this case, help ease Carolyn's constipation.) I also urged Carolyn to avoid all of the items to which she showed a food reactivity, particularly gluten products.

Furthermore, I gave her a product called Candaclear, a terrific supply of antifungal herbs and supplements that can help eradicate yeast, partly through its inclusion of probiotics. (This product is marketed to consumers as Clear Four; "Candaclear" is part of the manufacturer's professional line.)

I additionally encouraged Carolyn to take 300 mg of magnesium citrate per day (magnesium operates as a gentle laxative) and to drink three cups of pau d'arco tea daily. This South American tea, whose roots trace back to 1873, is famed for its antifungal properties, such as lapachol and beta-lapachone.

Finally, I asked Carolyn to give up those sweets she loved, as well as fruit and alcohol.

The patient's progress: While skeptical about her willpower over sweets—"it's the only thing that comforts me sometimes," she said—Carolyn's pending promotion, unpleasant symptoms and desire to be at her best served as excellent inspiration. Her sugar cravings "radically decreased" within a few days' time, which is often the case when one's digestion gets back on track and the absorption of key nutrients improves.

A week after the start of her intestinal detox, she found that her clothes fit better, her bloating had significantly diminished and her constipation had given way to a bowel movement every day. The closer she adhered to the diet I gave her, and the more exercise and sound sleep she got, the better she felt—less fatigued and more energetic, with greater clarity, focus and stamina to face life's challenges.

"I feel lighter, freer, and yet stronger," she claimed—so much so she'd rejoined her paddling team. She saw the month-long intestinal cleanse as less of a 30-day commitment than a lifelong guide to optimal health, which was, in the end, quite similar to the tenure position she was ultimately offered.

Quick and Easy First-Aid for Stomach Troubles

Andrew L. Rubman, ND, founder and medical director, Southbury Clinic for Traditional Medicines, Southbury, Connecticut. He writes the "Nature Doc's Patient Diary" blog at BottomLineInc.com/blogs.

Even if you eat a healthy diet and get plenty of exercise, digestive problems still happen. If they happen a lot, you should check with your doctor to rule out underlying serious health issues. But for once-in-a-while indigestion, constipation and/or diarrhea, there are easy, natural remedies that will soon have your gut feeling better.

For Occasional Indigestion

If you ate too much…or too fast…or if something you ate "didn't agree with you," you can try…

•**Baking soda.** Sodium bicarbonate, commonly known as baking soda, neutralizes the acidity in your stomach. Mix about one-half teaspoon of baking soda with four ounces of water, and slowly sip the mixture.

Relief should come quickly (and maybe a belch or two).

Important: Wait for at least two hours after eating to drink this remedy—you do not want to partially neutralize the acid that is needed to digest food and absorb nutrients.

For Occasional Constipation or Diarrhea

Both of these conditions can be the result of a poor diet…the wrong mix of organisms in the gut microbiome…and/or certain medications. Not drinking enough water also can cause constipation. *What can help…*

•**Probiotics.** There are many different kinds of beneficial probiotic bacteria that we need to have in our guts for good digestive health. Some of the most well-studied strains with evidence of gut benefit are Lactobacillus casei, Lactobacillus acidophilus and Lactobacillus rhamnosus GG—all particularly good for treating diarrhea but also helpful for treating constipation. Lactobacillus supplements are available over-the-counter in grocery and drugstores.

Align is a good product with a patented strain of another probiotic (Bifidobacterium infantis) that works well with Lactobacillus and that has shown gut benefits in industry-sponsored studies.

Follow the label directions for the correct dose. You should get relief within 12 to 18 hours, although complete healing can take three to five days.

Bonus: Probiotic products containing Lactobacillus have been found to significantly reduce flatulence.

•**Glucomannan.** This water-soluble fiber supplement is made from the root of the konjac plant. It is an effective "bulk-forming" laxative, so it helps with constipation but not diarrhea. As a bonus, glucomannan also helps relieve nausea.

This type of laxative swells in the intestine, softening the stool and making it easier to pass. When using to relieve constipation, take one 575-mg capsule of glucomannan with at least a full eight ounces of water up to three times a day, away from meals.

How to Keep Your Digestion Working Great

While the remedies above are good to have on hand, it's best if you don't have to use them often. *Here are some strategies to keep your digestion functioning smoothly…*

•**Chew thoroughly.** You'll eat more slowly, enjoy your food more—and give your stomach a break. Chewing sufficiently allows enzymes in saliva to start digestion in your mouth, as they're meant to do—and breaking the food into smaller particles lets your intestines better absorb nutrients.

•**Drink water, but not with your meal.** Drinking water or other liquids at mealtime dilutes the hydrochloric acid your stomach needs to digest food, slowing digestion and inhibiting absorption of nutrients.

It's OK to slowly sip just enough liquid at a meal to help you wash down mouthfuls of food if you want—but keep it to no more than four ounces. It's best to not drink close to meals—aim for a half hour before to an hour after. On the other hand, do be sure to drink enough liquids during the rest of the day.

•**Omega-3 fatty acids.** These essential fats not only help fight inflammation, they also promote a healthy gut microbiome. Unless you regularly consume wild-caught cold-water fish, you probably do not get enough from diet alone. One good brand of omega-3 supplements is Nordic Naturals. Whatever brand you use, aim for a daily dose of at least 650 mg of eicosapentaenoic acid and 450 mg of docosahexaenoic acid.

Important: Digestive ailments that are more than just occasional or that are accompanied by other symptoms, such as fever, pain or blood in your bowel movements or vomit, should be checked out by a healthcare provider.

Help for Severe Constipation

Biofeedback therapy relieves serious constipation. Called dyssynergic defecation, it affects one-third of constipated patients and is the result of nerves and muscles in the pelvic floor not working properly. Research has shown that instrument-guided biofeedback therapy is effective. It usually is done in a medical office, but it may be available at home in the future.

Satish S.C. Rao, MD, PhD, is professor in the department of gastroenterology at Augusta University, Georgia, and lead author of a study published in *The Lancet*.

Treat Your Skin from the "Inside Out"

Alan M. Dattner, MD, a board-certified dermatologist and pioneer in integrating nutrition, holistic medicine and dermatology. He is author of *Radiant Skin from the Inside Out: The Holistic Dermatologist's Guide to Healing Your Skin Naturally*, as well as several professional articles and book chapters relating to holistic dermatology. HolisticDermatology.com

If you have a skin problem and go to a conventional dermatologist, you're likely to get a diagnosis and a prescription for medication that in actuality may only help keep your symptoms in check.

A different approach: In the world of holistic dermatology—where treatment is all about finding the root cause of a problem rather than just controlling the symptoms—the skin serves as a window to what's happening deep inside the body.

A Leaky Gut

In healthy people, the inside of the small intestine has a cellular barrier that prevents incompletely digested food molecules and toxins from crossing through to the bloodstream. In a condition known as "leaky gut," the cellular bonds holding the intestinal lining together are broken, allowing these materials to slip through, activating the immune system to cause inflammation (see box page 332).

Leaky gut is often caused by an overgrowth of yeast (frequently from a high-sugar diet)…or from specific food components like gluten, a protein found in wheat, barley and rye. In fact, 40% of gluten-sensitive patients analyzed in a study published in 2017 in *World Journal of Gastroenterology* cited eczema or a rash as symptoms.

If you find that you're sensitive to gluten, a gluten-free diet can give a leaky gut time to begin healing. A diet that's low in sugars and simple carbohydrates can reduce the inflammation caused in the gut by yeast and also improve leaky gut. In addition, you should eliminate high-yeast foods such as bread (even gluten-free bread can contain yeast)…cheese…wine…and beer.

Also: Probiotic supplements and probiotic-rich foods like sauerkraut (eaten daily) can replace yeast in the gut with more diverse, healthy bacteria. In addition to the steps described above, try the following holistic strategies to fight…*

Eczema

The rough, red, inflamed patches of eczema can cause itching so intense that it's nearly impossible not to scratch. *What to do…*

• **Stop the scratching.** Ice cubes in a wet towel applied to eczema patches for five or 10 minutes provide a satisfying sensation that calms the instinct to itch.

Helpful: The anti-itch supplement Nettle Quercetin from Eclectic Institute.

• **Cure infections.** Cracks, crusting and open scratch marks are vulnerable to infection. For protection, take an antimicrobial herb such as olive leaf. Check with a doctor who has experience prescribing herbal medicine for advice on dosage—it varies depending on the patient. Redness, swelling, tenderness, pus and honey-colored crusting are all signs that an infection should be treat-

*To find a holistic practitioner near you, consult the American Holistic Health Association, AHHA.org.

ed by a doctor. At this point, the organism should be cultured to determine an appropriate antibiotic to use.

• **Ease inflammation.** Try a chamomile or chickweed anti-inflammatory ointment.

• **Try digestive enzymes.** These supplements can improve leaky gut by reducing the size of food molecules to simple building blocks like amino acids that do not trigger a reaction.

What helps: A digestive enzyme that contains dipeptidyl peptidase-4 (DPP-4).

Rosacea

Rosacea is an inflammatory skin condition marked by facial redness, blood vessel enlargement and tiny pimples known as pustules.

• **Avoid problematic foods.** Certain foods dilate facial capillaries. Common triggers: Spicy foods…hot liquids such as coffee…and alcohol.

• **Watch out for extreme weather conditions.** Protect the skin from wind, cold and sun whenever possible—all can contribute to redness.

• **Get more vitamin C and the bioflavonoids that accompany it in fruits and vegetables.** Bioflavonoids reduce capillary fragility, which often manifests as broken blood vessels or easy bruising. Eat vitamin C–rich foods such as kale, spinach and broccoli (citrus fruit can aggravate rosacea)…or take a vitamin C supplement (500 mg twice daily).

• **Control your emotions.** Anger, anxiety and embarrassment can cause blood to rush to the face, intensifying rosacea.

What helps: Deep breathing and meditation.

Dandruff

This white and red scaling of the scalp, forehead, eyebrows or chest is caused by an inflammatory immune reaction to a specific type of yeast (called Malassezia) that normally lives on the skin.

Even though antidandruff shampoos containing *ketoconazole* (Nizoral), *selenium sulfide* (Selsun Blue) or *pyrithione zinc* (Head

The Inflammation Factor...

Even though chronic inflammation is widely known to fuel health problems ranging from heart disease and diabetes to cancer and rheumatoid arthritis, it also plays a crucial role in skin conditions.

Here's what happens: When the immune system becomes triggered—due to a variety of causes (see main article)—it can attack cells, tissues or organs, as well as the skin, showing up as inflammation. That's why if you have a skin problem such as eczema, rosacea or seborrheic dermatitis (better known as dandruff), it's likely signaling a problem elsewhere in the body.

& Shoulders) are designed to kill Malassezia yeast, they won't fix dandruff at its root cause.

• **Reduce yeast.** With dandruff, it's crucial to cut sugar, use probiotics and take an anti-yeast supplement such as caprylic acid.

• **Get the right oils.** Omega-3 fatty acids calm inflammation. Try eating two servings of cold-water fish, such as wild salmon, a week. Use cold-pressed, organic olive oil or safflower oil, and avoid oils heated to a high temperature.

Helpful: Supplementation with vitamin E as well as vitamin C, B-complex, zinc and magnesium will help the body keep inflammation-fighting oils in their more usable forms.

Does Your Fingernail Have a Big Dent?

Debra Jaliman, MD, a dermatologist in private practice in New York City and assistant clinical professor of dermatology at Icahn School of Medicine at Mount Sinai, also in New York City. She is the author of *Skin Rules*. DrJaliman.com

An indentation on the fingernail and a bump at the edge of the cuticle mean that the matrix (the tissue beneath the fingernail) is affected. The matrix, which contains blood vessels and nerves, constantly produces new cells. These new cells force old cells to clump together to create your fingernail. By the time the nail emerges from beneath the skin, the cells are dead. Otherwise, it would be very painful to cut your nails!

To find out what's causing an odd bump, you should consult a dermatologist. The bump at the edge of the cuticle could be a wart, cyst or other benign condition...or it could be malignant (melanoma, squamous cell carcinoma or basal cell carcinoma). The only way to know for sure is to have a sample (a biopsy) of the bump taken and analyzed. If the bump is malignant, your dermatologist can recommend treatment, such as complete removal of the tumor, and refer you to a cancer specialist. If the bump is due to a cyst, it will need to be surgically removed. A wart can be removed by freezing it with liquid nitrogen, but the treatment will need to be repeated.

There could be a variety of explanations for the indentations in your fingernails. Skin conditions such as psoriasis or a fungal infection can sometimes cause small dents or pits in fingernails. A deficiency of vitamin B-12 or iron can often result in nail ridges or dents. A large indentation can also be due to "spoon nails," so-called because the nail becomes concave and shaped like a little spoon. Spoon nails can be caused by iron-deficiency anemia, heart disease or an underactive thyroid.

A deep, horizontal ridge across the nail, sometimes called Beau's lines, can also resemble a dent. This condition can be caused by a reaction to a drug, such as chemotherapy, or even a zinc deficiency that interrupted nail growth and then the growth resumed once you stopped the drug or corrected the nutritional deficiency. In some cases, Beau's lines can signal a chronic underlying health condition, such as diabetes or peripheral vascular disease.

A dermatologist can examine your nail ridges to determine whether you may have an underlying health condition and refer you to an appropriate specialist, if needed, for treatment.

INDEX